Register Now for Online Access to Your Book!

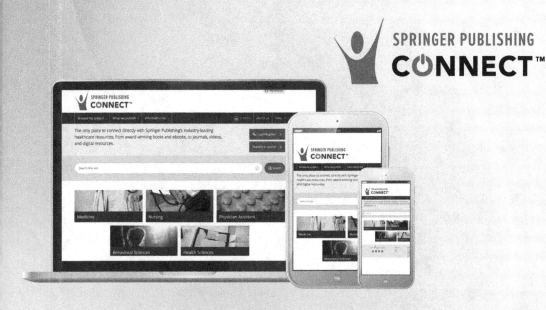

SPRINGER PUBLISHING CONNECT™

Your print purchase of *Case Study Approach to Psychotherapy for Advanced Practice Psychiatric Nurses* **includes online access to the contents of your book**—increasing accessibility, portability, and searchability!

Access today at:
http://connect.springerpub.com/content/book/978-0-8261-9504-3
or scan the QR code at the right with your smartphone
and enter the access code below.

73YBKRHV

Scan here for quick access.

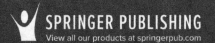

SPRINGER PUBLISHING
View all our products at springerpub.com

Case Study Approach to Psychotherapy for Advanced Practice Psychiatric Nurses

Candice Knight, PhD, EdD, APN, PMHCNS-BC, PMHNP-BC, is an associate professor and director of the Psychiatric-Mental Health Nurse Practitioner Program at New York University College of Nursing in New York City, New York. Dr. Knight received her doctorate in clinical psychology from Fielding University, a doctorate in social and philosophical foundations of education from Rutgers University, a master's degree in clinical psychology from Fielding University, a master's degree in psychiatric nursing from Hunter College, and a post-master's in psychiatric nursing in the psychiatric nurse practitioner program from Rutgers University. She is a licensed clinical psychologist, a psychiatric nurse clinical specialist, and a psychiatric mental health nurse practitioner. Dr. Knight is a well-known regional and national speaker on many diverse topics related to psychotherapy. Her research, writing, and teaching interests are how to become an exceptional psychotherapist, how to create moments of healing in psychotherapy, and how to teach psychotherapy to aspiring psychotherapists.

Dr. Knight has been in private practice in Flemington, New Jersey, since 1982, and is co-owner of Park Place Practice, a large private practice that works with clients across the life span. She conducts psychiatric and psychological evaluations, prescribes psychiatric medication, and provides psychotherapy for children, adolescents, adults, and older adults. Dr. Knight is a certified Gestalt therapist who practices psychotherapy from a humanistic–existential framework. Whether providing psychotherapy or prescribing medications, she believes in the primacy of the therapeutic relationship and understanding her clients from an in-depth, phenomenological perspective. Dr. Knight has also received advanced training in person-centered psychotherapy, existential psychotherapy, emotion-focused therapy (EFT), redecision therapy, expressive arts therapy (music, art, and movement), structural family therapy, group therapy, play therapy, Eye Movement Desensitization and Reprocessing (EMDR) therapy, cognitive-behavioral therapy (CBT), Dialectical Behavior Therapy (DBT), and interpersonal therapy (IPT). She integrates aspects of these approaches into her work as a humanistic–existential psychotherapist, and especially enjoys integrating music and the creative arts into her psychotherapy approach and to create moments of healing. Dr. Knight also has special interests in somatic symptom disorders, anxiety disorders, obsessive-compulsive disorders, trauma and stressor-related disorders, and enjoys working with clients across the life span.

Kathleen Wheeler, PhD, PMHNP-BC, APRN, FAAN, is an advanced practice psychiatric nurse and a professor and coordinator of the Psychiatric Mental Health Nurse Practitioner (PMHNP) program at Fairfield University Egan School of Nursing and Health Studies in Fairfield, Connecticut. She developed this program in 1994 and it was one of the first PMHNP programs in the United States. Dr. Wheeler has been a leader in projects that are highly significant for psychiatric nursing. These include cochair of the National Panel that developed the first PMHNP Competencies and the first chair of the National Organization of Nurse Practitioner Faculties' (NONPF) PMHNP special interest group. Both editions of her book, *Psychotherapy for the Advanced Practice Psychiatric Nurse: A How-To Guide for Evidence-Based Practice*, have been awarded AJN Book of the Year Awards. This book has been widely adopted by graduate PMHNP programs in the United States. Her leadership extends beyond psychiatric nursing as past president and advisory director of the Eye Movement Desensitization and Reprocessing International Association (EMDRIA) and in the development of an Integrative Trauma Psychotherapy Certificate Program for licensed mental health professionals at her university. Her awards include induction as a Fellow in the American Academy of Nursing (FAAN); the American Psychiatric Nurses Association (APNA) Media Award; the APNA Excellence in Practice Award; the APNA Excellence in Education Award; the EMDRIA Award for Outstanding Contributions and Service; and Distinguished Alumni of Cornell University-New York Hospital School of Nursing. Dr. Wheeler is a psychoanalyst and an EMDR trainer and consultant with expertise in treating trauma. Recently, she chaired the Expert Panel that developed Trauma and Resilience Competencies for Nursing Education, which are now copyrighted and available online. The Delphi survey supporting this work is published in the *Journal of the American Psychiatric Nurses Association*. She is on the Editorial Board of that journal as well as on the Editorial Board of the *EMDR Journal of Practice and Research*.

Case Study Approach to Psychotherapy for Advanced Practice Psychiatric Nurses

Candice Knight, PhD, EdD, APN, PMHCNS-BC, PMHNP-BC

Kathleen Wheeler, PhD, PMHNP-BC, APRN, FAAN

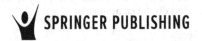 SPRINGER PUBLISHING

Springer Publishing Company, LLC
11 West 42nd Street, New York, NY 10036
www.springerpub.com
connect.springerpub.com/

Acquisitions Editor: Adrianne Brigido
Compositor: diacriTech

ISBN: 978-0-8261-9503-6
ebook ISBN: 978-0-8261-9504-3
DOI: 10.1891/9780826195043

20 21 23 24 25 / 5 4 3 2 1

The author and the publisher of this Work have made every effort to use sources believed to be reliable to provide information that is accurate and compatible with the standards generally accepted at the time of publication. Because medical science is continually advancing, our knowledge base continues to expand. Therefore, as new information becomes available, changes in procedures become necessary. We recommend that the reader always consult current research and specific institutional policies before performing any clinical procedure or delivering any medication. The author and publisher shall not be liable for any special, consequential, or exemplary damages resulting, in whole or in part, from the readers' use of, or reliance on, the information contained in this book. The publisher has no responsibility for the persistence or accuracy of URLs for external or third-party Internet websites referred to in this publication and does not guarantee that any content on such websites is, or will remain, accurate or appropriate.

Library of Congress Control Number: 2020907794

Contact us to receive discount rates on bulk purchases.
We can also customize our books to meet your needs.
For more information please contact: sales@springerpub.com

Publisher's Note: **New and used products purchased from third-party sellers are not guaranteed for quality, authenticity, or access to any included digital components.**

Printed in the United States of America.

We dedicate this book to our current and future advanced practice psychiatric nursing students with the hope it will ignite the flame of excitement in them to enthusiastically learn and embrace the art and science of psychotherapy, the heart of our profession.

—Candice Knight
—Kathleen Wheeler

Contents

Dedication   *vii*
Contributors   *xi*
Foreword Mary D. Moller PhD (h), DNP, ARNP, PMHCNS-BC, CPRP, FAAN   *xiii*
Preface   *xv*
Acknowledgments   *xvii*

1. Psychodynamic Psychotherapy: Healing Attachment Wounds   *1*
   Kathleen Wheeler

2. Gestalt Therapy: A Client With a Conversion Disorder   *17*
   Candice Knight

3. Person-Centered Therapy: A Client With Postpartum Depression   *41*
   Laura Kelly

4. Existential Psychotherapy: An Older Adult Client at a Crossroad   *55*
   Candice Knight

5. Humanistic and Psychoanalytic Play Therapy: A Child With Attention
   Deficit/Hyperactivity Disorder and Oppositional Defiant Disorder   *73*
   Amelia Muir

6. Group Therapy: Stages of Group Development   *95*
   Richard Pessagno

7. Family Therapy: A Family Over Time   *113*
   Candice Knight

8. Cognitive Behavioral Therapy: A Grieving Client   *139*
   Sharon M. Freeman Clevenger

9. Manualized Cognitive Behavioral Therapy: An Adolescent With Anxiety
   and Depression   *161*
   Pamela Lusk

10. Dialectical Behavior Therapy: A Client With Complex Trauma   *183*
   Danielle Conklin

11. Interpersonal Psychotherapy: A Client With Complicated Bereavement   *205*
   Candice Knight

12. Motivational Interviewing: A Client With Depression   *223*
   Susie Adams

13. Harm Reduction Psychotherapy: A Client With a Substance Use Disorder   *241*
   Michelle Knapp and Adam Kozikowski

14. Eye Movement Desensitization and Reprocessing Therapy: Healing
   Trauma   *259*
   Kathleen Wheeler

15. The Trauma Resiliency Model®: A Client With Chronic Trauma   *273*
   Linda Grabbe

Index   *291*

Contributors

Susie Adams, PhD, APRN, PMHNP-BC, PMHCNS-BC, FAANP, FAAN Professor of Nursing and Faculty Scholar for Community Engaged Behavioral Health, Vanderbilt University School of Nursing, Nashville, Tennessee

Danielle Conklin, DNP, NP-P, PMHNP-BC Clinical Assistant Professor, New York University College of Nursing, Psychiatric-Mental Health Nurse Practitioner Program, New York, New York; Faculty, National Institute for the Psychotherapies, Integrative Trauma Treatment Program, New York, New York; Candidate, New York University, Postdoctoral Program in Psychotherapy and Psychoanalysis, New York, New York; Private Practice, New York, New York

Sharon M. Freeman Clevenger, MA, MSN, CARN-AP, PMHCNS-BC CEO Indiana Center for Cognitive Behavior Therapy, P.C.; Cognitive Psychotherapy and Integrative Medicine Psychiatric Practitioner Doctor of Science in Integrative Healthcare Candidate, Huntington University of Health Sciences; Adjunct Professor, Purdue University, Fort Wayne, Indiana

Linda Grabbe, PhD, FNP-BC, PMHNP-BC Clinical Assistant Professor, Nell Hodgson Woodruff School of Nursing, Emory University; Psychiatric/Mental Health Nurse Practitioner, Community Advanced Practice Nurses, Inc., Atlanta, Georgia

Laura Kelly, PhD, APN, PMHCNS-BC, PMHNP-BC Clinical Associate Professor and Director, Psychiatric-Mental Health Nurse Practitioner Program, Columbia University New York, New York; Private Practice, Eatontown, New Jersey

Michelle Knapp, DNP, NP-P, PMHNP-BC, FIAAN Clinical Assistant Professor and Director, Substance Use Sequence, New York University College of Nursing, New York, New York; Private Practice, New York, New York

Candice Knight, PhD, EdD, APN, PMHCNS-BC, PMHNP-BC Associate Professor and Director, Psychiatric-Mental Health Nurse Practitioner Program, New York University College of Nursing, New York, New York; Licensed Psychologist and Psychiatric Nurse Practitioner, Park Place Practice, Flemington, New Jersey

Adam Kozikowski, MS, NP-P, PMHNP-BC Clinical Adjunct Professor, New York University College of Nursing, New York, New York

Pamela Lusk, DNP, RN, PMHNP-BC, FAANP Clinical Associate Professor, Ohio State University College of Nursing, Columbus, Ohio

Amelia Muir, MS, NP-P, PMHNP-BC   Psychiatric Nurse Practitioner Private Practice, Brooklyn, New York

Richard Pessagno, DNP, PMHNP-BC, CGP, FAANP   Psychiatric-Mental Health Nurse Practitioner, Private Practice, Wilmington, Delaware; Adjunct Faculty PHMHNP Program, Catherine McAuley School of Nursing, Maryville University, St. Louis, Missouri

Kathleen Wheeler, PhD, PMHNP-BC, APRN, FAAN   Professor and Director of PMHNP Program, Fairfield University, Egan School of Nursing, Fairfield, Connecticut

Foreword

The *Case Study Approach to Psychotherapy for Advanced Practice Psychiatric Nurses* by Candice Knight and Kathleen Wheeler is a long-awaited companion to the foremost nursing psychotherapy book, *Psychotherapy for the Advanced Practice Psychiatric Nurse*. Written for both the novice and experienced advanced practice psychiatric nurse (APPN), this book comes at a critical juncture in time in the evolution of our role. Even though all APPNs are required to have academic and clinical content in two psychotherapeutic modalities, this requirement does not necessarily translate to experience in two schools of psychotherapy. The marketplace often does not include psychotherapy in the provider job description, thus not allowing or encouraging the APPN to practice at the full scope of the role for which we have been educated.

With many educational programs today providing only survey courses and in-class role-play experiences, graduates often report feeling intimidated at the thought of conducting formal psychotherapy. This book fills an important gap as it provides a practical, yet invaluably rich guide to a more thorough understanding of the major psychotherapies. The unique chapter format delivers a straightforward description of the psychotherapy school, followed by a synopsis of the leaders and developers of the school/approach to therapy and a summary of the philosophy and key concepts. The reader then steps into and experiences excerpts from real psychotherapy sessions presented in a longitudinal manner that progresses from the initial session to termination. The sessions are drawn from the files of the chapter authors, replete with the development of goals, interventions, and techniques, what worked, and what didn't work. A novice APPN will soon appreciate the value of psychotherapy through a new and practical lens while experienced APPNs will have a refresher course at their fingertips!

Edited by two of the most revered psychotherapy exemplars in our profession, Drs. Candice Knight and Kathleen Wheeler have collaborated to create a unique resource for our personal libraries that heretofore has not existed. They have not only written a majority of the chapters, but have also selected their exemplar students, proteges, and discipline-specific authorities to share specific psychotherapy expertise. They have given our profession a guidebook through the confusion that often envelops an APPN when confronted with the realization that medication is not the only answer for the distress our patients are experiencing. When we as providers know that psychotherapy is the answer but we do not know how to start, the *Case Study Approach to Psychotherapy for Advanced Practice Psychiatric Nurses* can help us overcome our own discomfort and give us an informed and practical point from which to begin.

My own patients have benefitted from the personal enrichment I have experienced from my interactions and consultations with both authors over the past 25 years. For years, many of us have asked them to share cases that illustrate how they navigate the various psychotherapy processes. They have given our discipline, our patients, and their family members a precious gift that will enrich our professional lives for years to come. On behalf of the advanced practice psychiatric nursing community, we owe a sincere debt of gratitude to my friends and colleagues, Candice and Kate. You listened to our requests, you collaborated, and you have delivered what our profession has desperately needed. Please accept the sincere sentiment with which the words *thank you* are most genuinely written to both of you and your collaborators.

Mary D. Moller, PhD (h), DNP, ARNP, PMHCNS-BC, CPRP, FAAN
Associate Professor
Coordinator, PMHNP DNP Program
School of Nursing
Pacific Lutheran University
Tacoma, Washington

Preface

Psychotherapy is regarded as an essential competency for the advanced practice psychiatric nurse (APPN). Teaching students how to conduct psychotherapy is a complex and multifaceted endeavor that cannot be reduced to a technical mechanistic enterprise, but necessitates a well-thought out, comprehensive approach. It requires that the APPN student acquire knowledge of the major theoretical orientations including psychodynamic, humanistic–existential, and cognitive-behavioral approaches, as well as group therapy, family therapy, trauma-based therapies, and short-term, evidence-based approaches, and to have the ability to apply the knowledge in clinical practice. In addition, it requires that the APPN be involved in their own self-growth experiences, to pursue personal psychotherapy, and to engage in clinical case supervision.

Most experienced faculty use a variety of methodologies to teach psychotherapy to APPN students in order to aid them in acquiring the requisite knowledge. This usually includes lecture and discussion, viewing psychotherapy films by the masters, classroom demonstrations, and small group experiential training sessions. Many existing APPN faculty are not well versed in different types of psychotherapeutic approaches and have difficulty providing classroom demonstrations and expert clinical case supervision. They may not have had the opportunity to participate in training institutes nor have undertaken the years of personal psychotherapy and case supervision that is required for a seasoned teacher of psychotherapy. In addition, due to the recent and demanding role of prescribing, much classroom time, formally devoted to teaching psychotherapy, has been lessened in our graduate programs. Concomitantly, APPN students often have a paucity of psychotherapy experiences at their practicum sites because of a focus on psychopharmacology and prescribing. In this context, a case study approach to psychotherapy is a methodology that can be effectively used to teach psychotherapy and bridge the gap between the theory and practice of psychotherapy. The *Case Study Approach to Psychotherapy for Advanced Practice Psychiatric Nurses* is intended to fill this void.

The *Case Study Approach to Psychotherapy for Advanced Practice Psychiatric Nurses* was developed as a companion book to the groundbreaking APPN psychotherapy book, *Psychotherapy for the Advanced Practice Psychiatric Nurse* by Kathleen Wheeler (Wheeler, 2021). It is hoped that the *Case Study Approach for Psychotheraphy*, written for both the novice and experienced APPN, will supplement this psychotherapy textbook and add additional materials and activities to learn the art and science of conducting psychotherapy. We suggest that each chapter in *Psychotherapy for the Advanced Practice Psychiatric Nurse* be augmented by reading the corresponding chapter in this book in order to obtain a rich and robust learning experience. The session dialogues may be read as homework assignments or enacted in the classroom for a lively experience and discussion.

The case studies in this book have a range of diverse theoretical approaches and varied client problems and psychiatric diagnoses. The book is organized into 15 chapters, with each chapter presenting a case study using a different theoretical approach. Each chapter follows a similar format, allowing for comparison among the psychotherapy approaches. The format begins with the author's personal experience, providing the reader with the understanding of how various theoretical orientations were chosen by the authors. This is followed by a background on the founders and leaders and the philosophy and key concepts of the approach. Next illuminated is how the approach describes mental health and psychopathology, therapeutic goals, assessment perspectives, and therapeutic interventions.

The chapter then presents the case study, starting with a background of the client, followed by a selection of verbatim transcript segments from the beginning, middle, and final phase of therapy. The transcripts highlight the key interventions used in the therapy, allowing readers to see concrete examples of how the therapy works. The therapeutic process is illustrated by client–therapist dialogues, which are frequently augmented by process commentaries explaining the rationale for the interventions. A final commentary on the case is presented to enhance the reader's clinical reasoning skills. The chapter ends with questions for reflection to help the reader apply the material to his or her personal life and offer guidelines for continuing to work with the theoretical orientation. References are included with each chapter.

Candice Knight
Kathleen Wheeler

REFERENCE

Wheeler, K. (Ed.). (2021). *Psychotherapy for the advanced practice psychiatric nurse* (3rd ed.). New York, NY: Springer Publishing Company.

Acknowledgments

I am most appreciative to the expert advanced practice psychiatric nurses (APPN) who contributed chapters to this book. The chapters illustrate many diverse approaches to conducting psychotherapy and provide the reader with the opportunity to observe psychotherapy over time through segments of verbatim session transcripts. The transcripts bring the psychotherapeutic process to life and allow a rare and privileged glimpse of the dialogue that occurs within sessions.

I am also grateful to the clients who contributed their personal narratives and life stories to this book. Although pseudonyms and significant changes were made to protect the clients' identities, the essence of their sessions was preserved. The clients were eager and willing to share their work in the service of training future APPNs in the art and science of psychotherapy as well as to add to the knowledge of experienced APPNs.

I also want to acknowledge all of my therapists, supervisors, and trainers who inspired me to become a skilled psychotherapist. Special thanks is extended to Hermene Terry, Gene Kerfoot, Will Kouw, Bud Feder, Laura Perls, Sal Manuchin, Violet Oaklander, Les Greenberg, Albert Ellis, and Natalie Rogers.

I am also deeply grateful to Timothy Brown, my husband, colleague, and collaborator, for his many editing contributions to the book. As a licensed clinical social worker, psychotherapist, and lifelong **logophile**, his review of the chapters contributed in important ways to the clarity of this book.

—*Candice Knight*

I am very grateful to the expert clinicians who contributed chapters to this book. I remain in awe of my colleagues who have achieved expertise in specific psychotherapy approaches. Their knowledge and compassion inspire us to learn more so we too can help others heal and be all we can be. I echo Candice's thanks to our patients who teach us how to be better therapists.

There are so many supervisors and colleagues who I have learned from over the years. Special thanks to my friends and colleagues, Karen Alter-Reid and Cheryl Kenn, who reviewed the Eye Movement Desensitization and Reprocessing (EMDR) chapter included in this book. And thank you to Robert Broad, my husband, a psychologist and a training analyst, who encouraged and supported me for the past 40+ years so I could follow my passion.

—*Kathleen Wheeler*

Psychodynamic Psychotherapy: Healing Attachment Wounds

Kathleen Wheeler

■ PERSONAL EXPERIENCE WITH PSYCHODYNAMIC PSYCHOTHERAPY

Soon after completing my master's and doctoral degree in advanced practice psychiatric nursing at New York University in the mid-1980s, I wanted to start my own private practice. However, I knew that in order to gain the clinical skills and confidence for this enterprise, I needed first to get more training in psychotherapy. I decided to apply to a 4-year psychoanalytic program at The Training Institute for Mental Health in New York City. Notably, I was the first nurse to apply and be accepted by this institute. Following this rigorous program, which required 4 years of coursework, my own personal analysis three to four times per week, a 10-hour caseload of patients at the Institute weekly, and supervision three times a week, I felt ready to see patients on my own.

■ FOUNDER OF PSYCHODYNAMIC PSYCHOTHERAPY

Psychodynamic psychotherapy is derived from psychoanalytic psychotherapy, which was developed by Sigmund Freud at the end of the 19th century. Sigmund Freud's classic model of psychoanalytic psychotherapy is based on drive theory; that is, that all behavior is determined by unconscious forces or instincts, either sexual or aggressive. Freud's structural model of the id, ego, and superego explains the idea of psychic conflict. That is, symptoms are thought to develop through a conflict between an instinctual wish (id) and the person's defense against the wish (ego). The superego is part of the unconscious that is formed through internalization of moral standards of parents and society and acts to censor and restrain the ego. Freud delineated the psychosexual stages of development based on the idea that libidinal energy shifts between various erogenous zones in each stage. The concept of *psychic determinism* is embedded within this model and refers to the idea that nothing happens by chance; everything on a person's mind and all behavior, pathological and nonpathological, has a cause, and is determined by multiple factors.

Freud's seminal ideas have contributed to the evolution of many different psychodynamic schools of thought. Each psychodynamic model evolved from previous approaches while establishing a new perspective that placed different emphases on human development and motivation for behavior. Each psychodynamic school of thought that followed—that is, ego psychology, interpersonal analysis, object relations, Lacanian psychoanalysis, intersubjectivity, and relational and attachment-based psychotherapy—developed its own theoretical constructs and techniques. The evolution of Freudian thought parallels paradigm shifts in science in the 20th century from Freudian drive theory to relational, intersubjective, and attachment models, with each contributing theory about what constitutes motivation for human behavior.

▪ DEFINITION OF MENTAL HEALTH AND PSYCHOPATHOLOGY

Underpinnings of psychodynamic therapy are rooted in developmental theory, with the basic premise that what has happened in the past determines what the person is doing today. It is posited that through understanding these factors and the unconscious, the individual is empowered and then free to make more conscious decisions and consequently live a more satisfying and useful life. Thus, the mentally healthy person is able to regulate their anxiety, be in relationships, make conscious decisions, and live a satisfying, useful life. The mentally healthy person is succinctly stated in Freud's well-known phrase "the ability to love and to work."

Historically, psychodynamic schools emphasize the centrality of conflict among powerful desires, wishes, and fears. Psychopathology arises when there is a conflict among desires, wishes, and fears. This may arise from any developmental level and symptoms develop as a result from problems occurring during any phase of development. Freud posited that if a person has not successfully negotiated the previous stage, specific problematic character traits or psychopathology is thought to continue throughout life. More recent psychodynamic theorists stress the importance of relationship in the development of mental health and illness.

▪ THERAPEUTIC GOALS IN PSYCHODYNAMIC PSYCHOTHERAPY

Psychodynamic psychotherapy can be seen as a continuum from supportive psychotherapy to expressive psychotherapy to psychoanalytic psychotherapies. The goals and focus of each type of psychodynamic psychotherapy differ. The goals for the supportive end of the continuum are aimed toward stabilization through restoring functioning, reducing anxiety, strengthening defenses, and facilitating more effective problem-solving, whereas the psychoanalytic end is aimed toward processing through interpreting unconscious conflict and gaining insight (Gabbard, 2017).

Most clinicians believe that the decision to use supportive psychodynamic psychotherapy should be based on the person's ego strength and weaknesses, present coping skills, highest level of functioning previously achieved, recent losses, and other life stresses and circumstances. McWilliams (2011) states that the overall goal for expressive psychodynamic psychotherapy is the development of an integrated, complex, and positively valued self. This means that the person is able to tolerate ambivalent feelings and self-regulate emotions. The goal for psychoanalytic psychotherapy is resolution of the transference neurosis and effecting deep personality or trait change. The transference neurosis is an intense repetition of childhood conflicts, where the patient re-experiences feelings that originally developed in relation to the parent but now are felt toward the therapist because of the frequency and intensity of the sessions. The degree to which the therapy is supportive versus psychoanalytic is based on the focus of transference issues and the frequency of sessions (Gabbard, 2017).

In moving toward the psychoanalytic end of the continuum, as the transference deepens, the focus on interpretations increases, as does the number of sessions per week. Through transference, unconscious conflicts are illuminated and then worked through. Those who embark on psychoanalytic psychotherapy need the time and resources to invest in several sessions per week and treatment may require several years. These individuals are often in training to be psychoanalysts and need to be in their own analysis as part of their training program.

■ PERSPECTIVE ON ASSESSMENT IN PSYCHODYNAMIC PSYCHOTHERAPY

Assessment of ego functioning, relationships, and attachment style are all important in formulating a treatment plan for psychodynamic psychotherapy. See Chapters 3 and 5 in Wheeler (2022) for specific assessment tools to measure these constructs. Ego functioning refers to components of executive functioning such as self-awareness, problem-solving, memory, adaptability, affect regulation, and interpersonal functioning. Like the solid foundation of a well-built house, ego strength supports the individual in the pursuit of life goals, dreams, and ambitions, especially during times of trouble. It ensures coping abilities, provides an individual with a sense of identity, can be recognized during initial assessment and throughout therapy, and increases as patients grow in maturity (Bjorklund, 2000). To the degree each ego function can be identified and assessed in the clinical situation, ego strength can be acknowledged, rated, reinforced, supported, built upon, or "loaned" to some degree to lower-functioning patients by their relatively higher-functioning therapists in the process of identifying with the therapist's own ego strength (Bjorklund, 2000).

Developmental theories and the level of defenses are also considered in order to determine what type of psychodynamic therapy should be offered. In assessing ego strength, it is important to identify the primary defenses the person uses to ward off anxiety. McWilliams (2011) lists the types of defenses most commonly associated with those in the psychotic level of personality organization and identifies these defenses as originating early in development. These include denial, projection, splitting, primitive idealization and devaluation, withdrawal, omnipotent control, and dissociation. These defenses protect the person who is terrified of annihilation, who lacks a basic security in the world, and who is vulnerable to psychotic disorganization. Those on this end of the developmental continuum struggle with identity issues and confusion about who they are. Even if not overtly psychotic, the person is thought to be functioning at the symbiotic level of development, with little self–other differentiation. A therapeutic focus based on the assessment provides a realistic expectation for treatment. This flows from conceptualizing presenting issues developmentally and understanding intrapsychic conflict. See Figure 1.1 for components of a psychodynamic case formulation.

■ THERAPEUTIC INTERVENTIONS IN PSYCHODYNAMIC PSYCHOTHERAPY

The job of the psychodynamic therapist is to help the person understand both how fears and inhibitions in early life have led him or her to react to healthy feelings as if they were a threat and how the resulting anxiety plays an active role in generating his or her difficulties in the present. The person inadvertently and consistently brings about

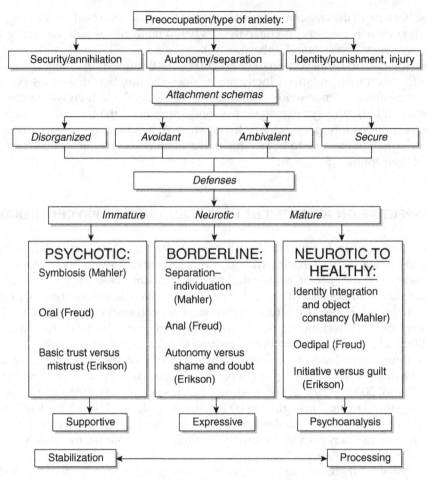

FIGURE 1.1 Case formulation and psychodynamic therapy algorithm.

Source: Reproduced from Wheeler, K. (2021). *Psychotherapy for the advanced practice psychiatric nurse: A how-to guide for evidence-based practice* (3rd ed.). New York, NY: Springer Publishing Company.

consequences that are not consciously intended. For example, the person who is fearful of feelings of anger may act overly nice, unassertive, and maintain a passive stance toward others. This allows others to ignore his or her needs and, consequently, he or she begins to feel frustrated and devalued, which leads to more anger and more anxiety, and the pattern is repeated. Another example is a person who fears hostility from others because it triggers their experience with an early unsafe caretaking environment. Thus, the person interprets every interaction as potentially hostile, then preemptively enacts self-protective hostility toward others, which evokes hostility from them, which leads to more anxiety (Wachtel, 2011).

The psychodynamic therapist uses interpretations to expose the person to previously avoided experiences while offering empathy in a safe, therapeutic environment. Interpretations are important in order to assist the person in deepening their understanding of their motivations, feelings, and how they needed to obscure the threatening aspects of their caretaker. Therapeutic interpretations are not just aimed toward intellectual understanding, but also emphasize the facilitation of emotional experiencing at a gradual pace. Re-experiencing painful affect allows adaptive processing so that dissociated or disconnected memory networks can be integrated with other, more adaptive neural networks (Cozolino, 2017). The emphasis is on the past and past relationships; focus on the expression of emotion; identification of patterns in actions, thoughts, feelings, experiences, and relationships; exploration of and working with resistances that impede treatment; exploration of intrapsychic issues through asking about dreams; and a focus on the transference and the working alliance. The therapist needs to remain cognizant that the patient may in reality have been in an unsafe environment.

■ CASE STUDY

Background

Michelle is a single 28-year-old woman from France and a full-time student majoring in creative writing and journalism who works part-time as a waitress in New York City. Her parents and two older siblings live in France. She sought treatment after returning to New York from a visit home because she felt "confused, depressed, and was losing control." She lived with her boyfriend for the past 2 years and things were not working out as he "wanted his freedom" and was going out with other women. Michelle's anxiety reached panic proportions when she was alone in her apartment and she began to fear being attacked and possibly raped. These feelings left her breathless with heart palpitations. It was these episodes that brought Michelle into treatment.

Michelle reported that her father is an angry, impulsive, verbally abusive, and critical man who would scream and explode over trivial incidents. She was never sure how to please him. However, she idealized him as he was there in a way for her that her mother never was there for her. Her mother's unavailability and absence were a constant theme in her memories of her childhood. She believes that her mother did not like her and recounted many childhood memories of waiting for her mother who did not come home or pick her up when she was supposed to from school. Even when Michelle's mother was there physically, she says that her mother was never there emotionally. Michelle describes the frequent headaches and illnesses of her mother, which kept her in bed for days with Michelle playing a caretaking role for her mother. Her mother would often cry unconsolably in Michelle's arms when her mother felt her lovers were abandoning her. Michelle found letters when she was 8 years old from her mother to her lover and remembered crying for days; however, upon confronting her siblings about the letters, she learned that everyone already knew about her lover and that her mother had had other affairs before this. Her father agreed with Michelle that her mother was never there for her. Michelle remembers no happy memories of childhood but remembers always crying and wanting attention.

Throughout her childhood Michelle suffered from constipation and intestinal pain. After many diagnostic tests, she had an appendectomy but then was told nothing was wrong with her appendix and it was all in her head. During early adolescence, Michelle said she was very promiscuous and had many one night stands, often with her older sister's friends. She drank a lot of alcohol and smoked marijuana, coming home many nights drunk and/or stoned. At the age of 17, Michelle was so distraught that she stood on a window ledge threatening to commit suicide. It was after this that she sought therapy for the first time but had to quit after a few months because her father said he would not pay for it. Between the ages of 17 and 18, she was bulimic, eating the pies her mother made and then throwing up. At age 19, she came to New York City to work as an au pair for an American family. Shortly after this, she was mugged and raped by a man who told her he was a policeman.

Psychodynamic Formulation

Michelle's history of maternal deprivation left her hungry for love and affection and with deep feelings of worthlessness. Although her father was there for her at times, he was an angry, domineering man who demanded perfection. Michelle's superego is harsh as she is hard on herself and has internalized and identified with her demanding, critical father. Michelle was scapegoated in her family by her older siblings who told her she was stupid and fat and made fun of her for crying all the time. Her sister and brother would discipline Michelle; for example, slapping her hands when she bit her nails. Being a victim has been a constant theme throughout her life. Her masochism is multidetermined. Preoedipal issues are apparent in her neediness, demandingness, and fragility. She describes herself as attention-seeking, social, and provocative in relationships. She states that she is desperate for love and so needy that she goes along with anything, and then begins to feel used. She then becomes demanding, angry, and provocative, which may be an attempt to turn the tables, gain control, and get even with those who have hurt her. Michelle described her relationship with her boyfriend as a fantasy, in which she demanded affection and was so emotionally needy that she turned him off. He told her: "You need someone to take care of you." It was toward the end of this 2-year relationship when Michelle sought treatment.

Major defenses for Michelle include denial and projection. Her need to control others and paranoia that she might be hurt may in part be due to her rage toward her mother and father, which is projected onto others. Her idealization of her father and her belief that her mother would be there for her despite her constant unavailability demonstrate her use of denial. Michelle's repression is apparent in her inability to remember many details of her childhood. Her search for love is about suffering and pain. Being given attention from the loved one even if the attention is negative becomes all consuming.

Developmentally, Michelle experienced her childhood in a depriving, turbulent milieu and her parents' stormy marriage served to heighten and exacerbate Michelle's infantile conflicts. Her early needs may not have been met adequately by either parent. Her oral hunger is apparent in her demanding, dependent, love-seeking behavior, while her negativism and difficulty maintaining her own autonomy reflects unresolved anal developmental issues. Michelle's unavailable, absent mother contributed to her sense of defectiveness, inadequacy, and shame. Persistent intense anxiety permeates most aspects of her life. In her mother's absence, psychically as well as physically, Michelle turned to her father, who forced her to go along with his wishes; thus, her struggle for autonomy was thwarted. In the context of her mother's absence, she took her mother's place and filled in socially and emotionally her mother's role with her father. Thus, she was the oedipal victor winning her father's love and attention.

A secure attachment to her mother was threatened because she could not count on her mother to be there for her. All children need to feel safe in order to survive. This type of attachment pattern can be conceptualized as ambivalent/anxious. Ambivalent/anxious attachment results in the person feeling insecure; difficulty with separation; difficulty being soothed upon reunion; too much anxiety due to the caregiver's unreliability; high emotionality that interferes with functioning; and confusion about the integrity of relationships in the present. This left Michelle with deep feelings of defectiveness and the false-negative belief that there was something wrong with her. This was a safer position for her than recognizing that her life was in danger. It would cause even greater anxiety for a child to let in the reality that perhaps they are not cared about as they should be, and due to the child's normal cognitive immaturity (Piaget, preoperational, magical thinking), the child concludes that the emotional or physical abuse occurs because they caused it to happen. Thus, it is the child's fault if there is chaos and neglect, which then preserves the image of the parents as loving and benevolent. This is a safer conclusion for the child, so they feel they have some control over the situation. As a result, Michelle had pervasive feelings of guilt and low self-esteem without consciously understanding to what these feelings were connected.

It is important to note that Michelle's early years were nurturing enough in that some self-object differentiation was attained. She has received scholastic honors this year in college and has been able to work and live productively in a foreign country, which attests to her ego functioning.

Treatment and Goals

Michelle came to her sessions one to three times a week over the next 2 years for psychodynamic psychotherapy. Psychodynamic techniques employed were analysis of resistance and transference, dream interpretation, free association, clarification, observation, reflection, and analysis of defenses. Goals of treatment included (a) to develop a working alliance; (b) to understand and interpret transferences when necessary; (c) to enlarge the sphere of Michelle's observing ego; (d) to assist Michelle in modifying her overly harsh superego; (e) to assist in the development of healthier defenses; (f) to help Michelle in the working through of her rage toward her mother and father; (g) to aid Michelle in the process of gaining insight and acceptance of her mother's absence; (h) to assist in the transfer of the soothing function of the therapist; (i) to promote autonomy of Michelle's ego from drives; and (j) to attain at greater level of self-object differentiation.

Michelle's pervasive sadness and anxiety were in the foreground the first year of treatment with major themes of intense neediness and her ensuing struggle to obtain love and safety. She was conflicted about seeking help in psychotherapy. On one hand, seeking and asking for help was difficult for Michelle as she had been encouraged to be independent from an early age and ridiculed when she requested assistance from her parents. On the other hand, Michelle felt that others should know what she wanted without her telling them. The latter is rooted in the early mother–child interaction and wish for symbiotic oneness with the all-giving mother. As the treatment process unfolded, a transference evolved with Michelle needing me to mirror and validate her experiences for her. She felt I should know what she wanted. On a more latent level, being close to another person meant she would be abandoned, and she felt she could not rely on anyone to be there for her. Michelle fought the ensuing regression triggered by therapy in an effort to avoid the inevitable hurt and disappointment which she felt would result from counting on me.

In exploring deeper into Michelle's feelings of anxiety, she realized how bitter and angry she felt toward her mother for not being there for her as she had needed. This was demonstrated in a provocative, angry stance toward others. She recounted that she cried from age 8 until 19 and was often inconsolable. Sessions early in treatment focused on the many instances in her childhood when her mother had not been there for her. Tearful and angry, Michelle mourned the loss of her mother. As she understood and felt her anger, her anxiety lessened and she had no further panic attacks.

After 6 months of treatment, I told Michelle about my upcoming vacation in August. She replied that she needed a break anyhow and wanted space. She felt angry about coming for her sessions and thought it was a waste of time. She sadly remembered as a little girl wanting desperately for someone to listen to her. Michelle would invite herself over to her friend's home to stay overnight, but her friend would want to be alone. Michelle would feel so hurt and would beg her friend to allow her to stay anyway, which she did and then Michelle would feel even worse as her friend would ignore her. Michelle felt that her boyfriend needed his space and that something was missing. He was not there for her in the way she needed him to be. I asked Michelle whether she felt

I too needed my space and would not be there for her as I was going on vacation. She denied caring whether I was there or not and left slamming the office door.

The next session Michelle felt confused, moody, and sad. She was angry at work and felt that she could not count on anyone. She had entertained a houseguest from France and felt taken advantage of by him . . . he was not there for her and not supportive. As her litany of grievances mounted, I gently asked if she could be talking about how she felt here too? That I would not be there for her and that she felt she could not count on me? Tearfully, Michelle said she thought it was too important to her to come here and that it had become a part of her life. This was Michelle's first acknowledgment of transferential feelings and I felt it was an important step in her therapy. Michelle spent the next several sessions talking about her mother and her feelings that she had not been wanted. Michelle knew her mother had an abortion after she was born, and also felt that she had been a "mistake." She believed that her mother did not really love her. Unlike her brother and sister, who both had a baby book created for them, there was no baby book about Michelle, which reinforced her belief that her mother did not love her. As a child she had entertained thoughts of being the child of her mother's lover and not her father's child. Consequently, it was difficult for her to believe that anyone could care for her and be there for her.

Upon my return from vacation, Michelle said she felt stronger and more separate from her parents. She had always felt caught in the middle, with her mother stating that Michelle was always on her father's side, and her father buying her love with money and the attention she so desperately craved. Michelle said she felt less needy and enjoyed her alone time now in a way she had never felt before. Her recently experienced good feeling brought a new anxiety to the fore, that of being afraid to feel good and the need to be prepared for the worst. The week of feeling stronger was quickly followed by a period of anger and anxiety. Michelle feared being hurt, that someone would break into her apartment and strangle her. In exploring this with her, she recounted that, around the age of 7, she was molested by a neighbor boy in her building who came into her bathroom while she was taking a bath and touched her genitals.

Her recent setback now was the first of many clinical regressions occurring during her treatment. Any sign of clinical improvement resulted in her dramatically losing therapeutic ground. Michelle's libidinal tie to her family was through pain and suffering. She only experienced caretaking when she was in a crisis that demanded attention. Her unhappy ideal self was the only time she was ensured concern and attention from her parents. In addition, her unconscious idealization of unhappiness may represent the struggle against identification with a devalued maternal figure. Michelle stated: "My mother had no power at home. My father denied her feelings."

Michelle had also been experiencing difficulties in her sexual relationship with her boyfriend. She felt he only wanted her physically "for my face and my body." When they would have sex, she would begin to feel as if she could not breathe and that she was being suffocated and might die. She stated that she would push him away in an angry violent fashion and felt repulsed by his advances. In exploring this feeling with her, Michelle stated that she had this experience when she had an abortion at the age of 22. I wondered whether this related to her difficulty in establishing firm boundaries for herself. Michelle reported this dream: "A friend of my sister's left her baby in the room, a bar. The baby was pale and sitting there. I try to take the baby in my arms but all these naked bodies are on the floor. I had to crawl over a naked man. The friend asked me to leave the baby alone. I'm upset. She doesn't want to take care of the baby. There was a naked man's body under me that I couldn't avoid. I was so ashamed. I touched the sexual part of the man." Michelle's associations to the dream were that: "Maybe the baby was me . . . I want to be taken care of." She had no thoughts about the image of naked bodies and wanted to move away from this material. Perhaps this dream symbolized her growing awareness of her desire to be cared for and how she desperately sought love and affection through her promiscuity.

Although Michelle's dependent, love-seeking orientation allowed her to form a strong transference with me, she continued to complain throughout therapy that it was not helping and that she was thinking too much about herself. My role as a psychodynamic psychotherapist was to listen and interpret Michelle's resistance in an effort to help deepen her understanding of her underlying dynamics, because what happens in the transference with the therapist also happens in other relationships as well. Michelle's complaints would start as she entered the office stating that she did not want to be there. She felt that she wanted to stop and needed a break from treatment and that she was being forced to come to her sessions. This struggle can be seen as a defense against passive submissive wishes, that is, fear of fusion with an early depressed mother. This is a form of a negative therapeutic reaction, that is, negativism is a way of being close while denying the wish. Michelle reported a dream seeming to highlight this negativism: "I was with family and friends. I was in the wrong place. They were saying no. I was saying yes." Michelle continued to feel negative about treatment for the next year. Although she had the option to leave, she continued to come and complain. I began to feel depressed before her sessions and wondered what I could do to help her. It seemed that nothing I said was enough. I also found myself extending her sessions by 5 to 10 minutes in an effort to make up for her dissatisfaction with me. As patient and understanding as I felt, it did not seem to matter. Michelle seemed entrenched in devaluing treatment and wanted out. I began to feel badly for her that she had me as her therapist and felt as she did, that she had gotten short-changed. My own feelings of inadequacy proved a fertile ground for her criticisms. Supervision with a senior psychodynamic psychotherapist helped me to stay the course and respond therapeutically, nonjudgmentally, and compassionately in sessions.

In extratransferential relationships, too, Michelle stated that she was making an issue out of everything, saying the opposite of what everyone was saying and felt aggressive at work, arguing with coworkers and provoking others. She had been angry at her boyfriend and went to a party where she felt he was not paying enough attention to her, so she took off her slacks and walked around in her underpants, shocking everyone there. The following dialogue reflects Michelle's dependency and how our therapeutic relationship was reflective of her relationship with her mother in the past.

Michelle: When I feel helpless, I provoke others and this protects me. By keeping people on edge, I hurt them and it's my way to survive.

APPN: I wonder, do you think that could be going on here too? That you feel helpless and need to also keep me at a distance?

Michelle: (*Smiles*) Maybe . . . I do feel too dependent here. Therapy was giving me strength over the summer, but somehow, I felt relieved to not be here. But now, I don't need to come.

APPN: When in the past have you felt that way?

Michelle: I remember I would scream and cry whenever my mother came into my room. I felt robbed by her. Her presence made me feel that she was taking something away from me.

APPN: It seems that both here with me and as an adolescent with your mother, you felt similarly, that you want to push us away. Perhaps it feels scary to feel so dependent. . . .

Michelle: Yes, I can give up everything to have someone take care of me.

Another theme that emerged at this time was that of Michelle feeling she was doing something wrong and that I was judging her. For example, Michelle thought that her desire to quit treatment was seen by me as dumb. In exploring this with her, she remembered her father as quite critical and demanding. She recalled being taken by her father to her horseback riding lessons and then being so anxious that she would fall. He would scream that she was wasting his time and money. Michelle felt it was important for her to be able to say no to me now, that is, that she was not going to come just because I wanted her to. I agreed that it did seem important for her to be able to say no to her boyfriend and now to me. It seemed though that she was feeling about therapy as her father had about her horseback riding lessons, that it was just a waste of time and money. In exploring this with her, she expressed fears of becoming too dependent on me and felt it would be hard to leave therapy. "Since my needs aren't met in a relationship, I get frustrated." I thought that perhaps Michelle had internalized her father's harsh, critical messages.

As Christmas vacation approached, Michelle began to feel increasingly anxious, especially at night when home alone. She would be taking a bath and begin to worry that someone was going to attack her and strangle her. She also had been feeling claustrophobic and fearful in the subway. Upon questioning Michelle about the origin of these feelings, she stated that as a child she felt the same when she was shut in her room by her dad after he said goodnight. Michelle would cry and at times feel panic stricken, upon which her father would scream at her: "Take control of yourself!" Michelle's recurring paranoia seemed to coincide with her impending separation from treatment over the holidays and earlier from her separation from her father. Michelle's rage at the abandoning loved one precipitated a decompensation of ego defenses with projection of her hostile impulses. In part her paranoia stemmed from Michelle's unmet dependency needs, resulting in projected rage.

Indeed, in the next several sessions Michelle stated that she was feeling angry at me but knew that she should not be mad at me. She stated that somehow, she felt I should know what she wanted. She felt bitter and angry about coming to therapy. She had a sense of struggle, of pain, loneliness, and fragility. She felt everyone was against her. She stated: "I'm never doing the right thing." She recalled sadly feeling that her mother's lover had taken her place, with Michelle then taking her mother's place with her father. Michelle would fill in for her mother by vacationing with her father. She recalled how scared she would feel driving with her father as he would drink and drive recklessly. Once they were in an accident and she was injured and nearly killed. Michelle said that no one else would go with her father and her siblings could not understand why she went along. Thus, as a result of her mother's unavailability, Michelle was literally in life-threatening situations. It seemed that the impending separation from treatment revived abandonment feelings from her past which were closely aligned with fearful feelings based on real dangerous past situations experienced in the context of her mother's abandonment.

Another important dimension of Michelle's fear related to her feeling that something was wrong with her and that she had done something wrong. The cognitive egocentricity of childhood contributed to Michelle's pervasive guilt and her low self-esteem. Therapeutic interventions focused on questions exploring specifically how Michelle felt she had caused her mother's neglect and abandonment. I pointed out to Michelle that she had deserved better and that her mother's problems prevented her mother from being there for Michelle and that she did nothing wrong to cause her mother's neglect.

Transcript of Therapeutic Interventions

The following is a verbatim transcript from a session transcribed toward the end of Michelle's treatment. This session illustrates several psychic shifts that took place for Michelle and are elucidated in the discussion immediately following the session.

Michelle:	I seem to end up in these situations. I was doing my captions at work and do you remember that lady I told you about who I thought had some problems and who I thought I should keep away from? She's the one who was recently divorced from the boss.
APPN:	Yes.
Michelle:	Well, anyhow I was working with Barbara doing the captions and she came up and said I wasn't doing it right. She should realize that I'm new and that I don't know everything and am still learning. But no, she starts screaming at me that I've fucked it up and makes this whole big scene in front of everyone. I was so humiliated. She could have told me quietly and alone but no, she starts screaming in front of everyone and I'm so embarrassed.
APPN:	That is a very humiliating situation. What did you say?
Michelle:	At first, I didn't say anything. I was too stunned. Then I decided I had to say something to her, that it was important for me to talk to her. So, I asked her if I could see her alone and then told her that she could not speak to me again like that and that if she wanted to correct my work to do so without screaming and in private. She started crying and telling me all about her problems and that she was under a lot of stress and how sorry she was. I couldn't believe it. All of the sudden she's crying in my arms and confiding in me.
APPN:	And once again you end up caretaking.
Michelle:	Yes. Just like with my mom. She used to cry in my arms and tell me how bad things were and I never knew what to say or do. She would tell me how bad things were for her with my father. Then, that afternoon, this photographer guy from France, who's a friend of my boss, came to the office. I was joking around with him. You know goofing around and the people at work were saying why don't you go with him shopping. He said he was going to go buy a pair of jeans that afternoon. They said to him: "Why don't you take Michelle with you? She can help you pick out some jeans." I think he really wanted me to go. He said: "Yeah, come Michelle, let's go." I felt confused at first but then thought why should I go with this guy to help him out? I don't really know him and I get paid by the hour so if I leave, I'll lose out on my money. You know, what's in it for me? So, I said: "No, I'm not going."
APPN:	It sounds like with both the woman who humiliated you at work and this man, you decided what was in your best interests and let them know and you were able to say no, I'm not going to do something that isn't good for me.
Michelle:	Yes, I felt it was good that I did that . . . (pause) I don't know. Things have been up and down lately.
APPN:	What do you mean?
Michelle:	Friday night I was so lonely and hurt. I went home and cried.
APPN:	What was going on?
Michelle:	I don't know. Nothing really had happened to make me so sad.

APPN:	You were here for your session that evening. How did you feel when you left?
Michelle:	It was a good session. I didn't feel bad when I left.
APPN:	Do you remember what you said as you were leaving?
Michelle:	No.
APPN:	That the session had gone by so quickly and you could stay here forever.
Michelle:	Yes, I remember being so surprised that the time was up. Then I went home and cried. I had a dream that night that I was in a huge apartment where the light was warm and it was comfortable. Someone came and told me that my mother was dead.
APPN:	Anything else about the dream?
Michelle:	No, it's funny though that I've been thinking a lot about my mother lately and I feel like for the first time I really understand that my mom wasn't there and before I knew it, but I didn't know it. Do you know what I mean?
APPN:	I'm not sure. Tell me.
Michelle:	Well, I know you have told me that so many times that she wasn't there for me, but I feel that I never really realized it before now. And, all I can say is that I see it now.
APPN:	So maybe the dream is not about your mom physically dying but about your new awareness and acceptance of her absence in your life.
Michelle:	Yes, I guess so.
APPN:	Also, the setting in the dream sounds very nice. You are in a huge, warm, light apartment. Do you think that could be about some of the feelings you have been having here lately?
Michelle:	Yes, I thought of that. Maybe. I feel I am changing and looking at things differently. I'm beginning to remember things from my childhood that I didn't remember before.
APPN:	Oh? Tell me.
Michelle:	About who I was and how I was laughing and having fun. I had friends who liked me and we would laugh together.
APPN:	Tell me more about what you are remembering.
Michelle:	I was thinking of my friend, Pierre, and how much fun we used to have. I was such a tomboy. He and I learned to ride our bikes together. We kept falling off and laughing and making fun of each other. We taught ourselves to ride.
APPN:	What a spunky little girl to teach yourself to ride a bike! You know, you have told me before about learning to ride your bike but never about the fun you had doing it, only about how disappointed you were about your mom not coming down to see you ride. It is as if the disappointment and sadness about your mom not being there for you poisoned all your experiences as a child so you could not remember until now anything positive that happened.

Michelle: Yes, I only felt the pain. Funny, but it's as if something is alive, what's missing is found.

Commentary

This session illustrates several intrapsychic shifts. In contrast to Michelle's previous resistance, which was manifested by her feeling forced to come to session, the overall tone of the session is quite positive with Michelle wanting to come and eager to tell me what had happened. This represents a highly significant change from her previous negative stance. I feel that our relationship revived abandonment experiences for Michelle and served as a focal point in treatment with the resulting intensification of the transference leading to subsequent therapeutic growth. The negative maternal transference of the abandoning mother served to heighten Michelle's resistance. The resistance was worked through and disproved by the reliability of the psychotherapeutic frame, that is, the consistency, structure, and reliability of the sessions, and my return after my vacations and holidays. My emotional availability, despite her negativity, disproved her transference. I was not like her inconsistent, unavailable mother. Here was a reliable, consistent, caring person whom she could count on. Michelle also experienced the choice of having phone sessions when she could not come to my office for sessions, so my availability could then be on her terms. I was not like her father who forced her to do things and be there for him. Insight derived from interpretive work, linking her distorted views of me with their origin in her childhood, promoted further ego growth. Clearer representations of herself from others emerged, leading to a kinder, more accepting view of herself. There was thus a modification of her harsh superego.

The incident at work that Michelle talks about in the session demonstrates an increase in ego strength in that Michelle has less need for approval and can withstand criticisms better and say no to the woman at work and the man, who represented aspects of both her mother and father. Her need for nurturing and dependency was so great when she entered treatment that she went along with anything in order to be loved. She illustrates in this session that she can deal with others better as they are in the here and now. Contributing to her increased ego strength is the enlargement of the sphere of her observing ego. She is able to reflect on her past dysfunctional patterns of behavior and see choices that are available. Her awareness of the genetic roots associated with her interaction with the woman and the man at work represents a relatively recent insight for Michelle.

It is also interesting in the session that Michelle demonstrates a mini therapeutic regression. She relates that she had felt good after the last session, but then went home and cried. Although nothing in reality had happened to make her feel bad, intrapsychically she retreated with each move toward autonomy, which was associated with positive transferential feelings. Michelle quickly loses therapeutic ground and regresses to her former ,more familiar self, that of feeling pain. Michelle's positive feeling about therapy is a new experience, which she has difficulty sustaining.

Michelle's dream represents an important shift for Michelle in that she is acknowledging her mother's absence in a new way, which in the past she defensively needed to deny. Michelle's guilt over having caused her mother's abandonment is abating through her understanding of her mother's own problems and Michelle's relinquishment of her denial of her mother's deficits. Her statement "I knew it but I didn't know it" demonstrates her denial and the shift in her defensive structure.

In the session, I focused on the apartment in the dream as a metaphor for Michelle's feelings about therapy. In retrospect, this may also represent her feelings about herself and the internal changes that have taken place. It is light and the apartment is huge, indicating that with the light she can see clearly. Thus, the denial is lifted and, with that, a larger intrapsychic space is created with more room for growth. The apartment is also warm, which may relate to Michelle's increase in positive feelings about herself. Michelle's awareness of her parents' limitations has allowed her to feel more positively about herself. Previously, she felt that she was such a bad person and that it was not her parents who were at fault.

Michelle's remembering positive things from her childhood indicates a lifting of repression has taken place. With the relinquishing of denial, she can now let in more positive feelings and memories about herself. This may be what Michelle has found, a new affective coloring of her self representation. Her previous defensive structure consisted of the use of more primitive defenses, projection, and denial while now she can sublimate her aggressive and sexual drives through her work as witnessed by a heightened interest in the creative aspect of her photography work. Michelle's expression and understanding of her anger at her parents has enabled her to own her anger and she does not need to project it onto others; thus, her paranoia has decreased. As illustrated by the verbatim session, she uses denial less and has moved toward resolution and acceptance of her mother's absence. When she entered treatment, she idealized her father and only had hostile feelings for her mother. Through the therapeutic process she became in touch with the sadism she experienced at the hands of her father.

When Michelle came to therapy, she was drowning in her own experiences. She was not able to look at her dysfunctional patterns of behavior and see how she contributed to her own unhappiness. She is now able to reflect on her experiences. She has made many gains in this area and is aware of how she transfers maternal and paternal feelings onto others. She has enlarged the sphere of her observing ego which has contributed to structuralization of her ego.

Although Michelle is still subject to clinical regressions after therapeutic gains, she is able to sustain happiness for longer periods of time. She actively pursues her own happiness and now does not wait for others to take care of her. Further ego strength is demonstrated by her ability to look after herself. She set appropriate career goals and has moved into an apartment with a roommate she likes and gets along with. Through internalization of the soothing function of the therapeutic relationship, Michelle now has the capacity to be alone and to enjoy her time alone. Previously, she became highly anxious when in her apartment alone and would frantically call her friends. When sick or feeling vulnerable, she did not know how to go about nurturing herself. She tries now to take better care of herself. Over the course of the past 2 years, she has cut back on her drinking and smoking and is now taking yoga classes that she finds helpful in relieving stress.

Michelle can now postpone gratification and regulate her emotions. Recently she waited 10 days for her boyfriend to call her. In the past, she would call her boyfriend constantly demanding attention, much as she would call her mother when she was at work. Also, Michelle's reactive approach to her environment has been modified, resulting in greater autonomy of her ego from drives. Further strengthening of her ego is illustrated by her increase in self-esteem and lessening of her need for approval. Michelle's neediness previously prevented her from using good judgment. She is now better able to say no to men and set appropriate boundaries in relationships with others. Her sexualized aggression and obsession with men was modified as she understood the needs served by her behavior. Through her work in psychodynamic psychotherapy, she has deepened her understanding of herself, thus enlarging the sphere of her observing ego. Our work together has resulted in a kinder, more compassionate relationship with not only others but toward herself.

DISCUSSION QUESTIONS

1. Can you identify any aspects in your current relationships with others that may have arisen because of significant past relationships with your parents or siblings when you were growing up?
2. Are there any problems in your life that you think psychodynamic psychotherapy could help you deal with better?
3. Discuss aspects of a case formulation for psychodynamic psychotherapy using the table included in this chapter.

REFERENCES

Bjorklund, P. (2000). Assessing ego strength: Spinning straw into gold. *Perspectives in Psychiatric Care, 36*(1), 14–23. doi:10.1111/j.1744-6163.2000.tb00685.x

Cozolino, L. (2017). *The neuroscience of psychotherapy: Healing the social brain* (3rd ed.). New York, NY: W. W. Norton.

Gabbard, G. O. (2017). *Long-term psychodynamic psychotherapy: A basic text* (3rd ed.). Washington, DC: American Psychiatric Publishing.

McWilliams, N. (2011). *Psychoanalytic diagnosis* (2nd ed.). New York, NY: Guilford Press.

Wachtel, P. (2011). *Therapeutic communication: Knowing what to say when* (2nd ed.). New York, NY: Guilford Press.

Wheeler, K. (2022). *Psychotherapy for the advanced practice psychiatric nurse: A how-to guide for evidence-based practice*. New York, NY: Springer Publishing Company. Psychodynamic Psychotherapy: Healing Attachment Wounds

Gestalt Therapy: A Client With a Conversion Disorder

Candice Knight

■ PERSONAL EXPERIENCE WITH GESTALT THERAPY

Almost 40 years ago, I was introduced to Gestalt therapy serendipitously while teaching an undergraduate psychiatric nursing course. I had given my students a group assignment to select a type of psychotherapy, develop a comprehensive understanding of the approach, and then present it to the class. In addition, I encouraged them to visit a psychotherapist who practiced in the modality. One group chose Gestalt therapy and contacted Laura Perls, who agreed to meet with them for an afternoon in New York City at her apartment, which doubled as her office. The students had no inkling that they had contacted the world-renowned psychotherapist who, along with her husband Fritz Perls, was the founder of Gestalt therapy. Brimming with excitement, I seized the opportunity and decided to accompany my students. When we arrived at Laura Perls' Central Park West apartment, the door was open, beckoning us to look inside. We beheld a majestic floor-to-ceiling painting of Fritz Perls. Our ears were serenaded by Laura Perls playing Beethoven on her grand piano. And, the fragrant aroma of blueberry muffins, freshly baked for the occasion, pleasantly wafted from a nearby table. She greeted us with warmth and elegance, and, soon after introductions, the students somewhat timorously informed her that they had composed a list of questions for her to answer. Laura pronounced grandly and with a flourish, "I don't talk about Gestalt therapy. I do Gestalt therapy. You cannot learn Gestalt therapy by talking—only by doing. Who would like to volunteer to do a piece of work?" She concluded this declaration by imperiously fixing her gaze on no one and everyone. Not one of my students had ever crossed the threshold of a psychotherapist's office, and they were thoroughly frightened by the prospect of volunteering. As their professor, I experienced a momentary dilemma vis à vis what behavior was appropriate, but heeded the voice from my internal dialogue that urged, "Don't squander this opportunity to work with a master therapist!" Accordingly, I threw caution to the wind and volunteered. Laura and I worked on one of my repetitive dreams. The experience was profound and healing. And so, it came to pass, on November 18, 1983, that I discovered my theoretical orientation—Gestalt therapy.

Months later, I enrolled in a 3-year Gestalt therapy training program and commenced my own personal individual Gestalt therapy. Over the subsequent years, I trained with some of the master therapists in Gestalt therapy including Irv and Miriam Polster, Joseph Zinker, Violet Oaklander, Mariah Fenton Gladis, Bud Feder, Jack Aylward, and

Phil Lichtenberg. In 1988, I founded the Gestalt Center of New Jersey, a Gestalt training institute in Flemington, New Jersey. I have been involved in national and international Gestalt therapy organizations and continue to remain an active member of the Gestalt therapy community. Over the years, I have received training in many other types of therapies including Existential therapy, Person-centered therapy, Redecision therapy, Expressive arts therapy, Emotion-focused therapy, Family therapy, Psychoanalysis, Eye Movement Desensitization and Reprocessing (EMDR), and Cognitive-behavioral therapy; nevertheless, Gestalt therapy still remains my theoretical orientation and psychotherapeutic home. I find it to be theoretically rich, relationally engaging, and a powerful healing approach in working with clients of all ages and with most types of psychological issues and/or psychiatric disorders.

■ FOUNDERS AND LEADERS OF GESTALT THERAPY

Fritz and Laura Perls, the founders of Gestalt therapy, were both psychoanalysts and the directors of the South African Institute for Psychoanalysis when they integrated concepts from classical psychoanalysis with concepts from interpersonal and Reichian analysis, holism, organismic theory, gestalt psychology, phenomenology, and existentialism. Their first book, *Ego, Hunger and Aggression: A Revision of Freud's Theory and Method* (1942/1992), was intended to add to the field of psychoanalysis, but instead it became a modality in and of itself, based on its radical departure from psychoanalysis. Fritz and Laura Perls subsequently immigrated to the United States and officially launched Gestalt therapy in 1951, with the publication of the book *Gestalt Therapy: Excitement and Growth in the Human Personality* (Perls, Hefferline, & Goodman, 1951/1994). In 1952, they established the New York Institute for Gestalt Therapy where they provided training in Gestalt therapy for psychotherapists.

As Gestalt therapy evolved over the next seven decades, it further expanded its concepts and methodologies (Perls, 1969/1992, 1973; Polster & Polster, 1973; Wheeler, 1991; Yontef, 1993; Zinker, 1977/1998, 1994) as well as its application to different populations such as children (Oaklander, 1978), families (Resnikoff, 1995), groups (Feder & Ronall, 1980), older adults (Fodor, 2015), and organizational systems (Nevis, 1987). It also applied the theory and techniques to disorders such as addictions (Matzko, 1997), anxiety (Herera, Mstibovskyi, Roubal, & Brownell, 2018), attention deficit hyperactivity disorder (ADHD) (Root, 1996), body image (Clance, Thompson, Simerly, & Weiss, 1994), gender identity (Kolmanskog, 2014), personality disorders (E. Greenberg, 2019), posttraumatic stress disorder (Serok, 1985), psychoses (Gagnon, 1981), and schizophrenia (E. Greenberg, 2015). Gestalt therapy also has an extensive research base (Brownell, 2008; Gestalt Review, 1997; Harman, 1984; Roubal, Brownell, Francesetti, Melnick, & Zeleskov-Djoric, 2016) and is considered an evidence-based psychotherapy. There are a number of national and international Gestalt therapy journals. Gestalt therapy has a worldwide presence with over 100 training institutes throughout the Americas, Europe, Asia, and Australia, and it continues to grow and thrive (O'Leary, 2013).

■ PHILOSOPHY AND KEY CONCEPTS OF GESTALT THERAPY

Gestalt therapy embraces a humanistic–existential worldview and thus believes that people are endowed with an inherent tendency to develop their potential and are free to choose how to live their lives. It has a commitment to holism, the phenomenological perspective, and the existential themes of authenticity, freedom, and personal responsibility. Gestalt therapy emphasizes the notion of awareness and contact with self, others, and the environment. It embraces the centrality of the therapeutic relationship (Buber, 1937/1970) and underscores the here-and-now, process over content, and the use of creative, experiential techniques. The key theoretical concepts of Gestalt therapy are grounded in (a) gestalt psychology (field theory and figure/ground); (b) organismic theory (organismic self-regulation, interruptions to awareness and contact); (c) interpersonal and Reichian psychoanalysis (layers of the personality, inauthentic self, and social influences); (d) Eastern philosophy (Zen Buddhism and Taoism); and (e) the creative arts (music, art, and movement). It integrates aspects of these concepts to create a unified and unique approach to psychotherapy (Perls, 1973).

Figure and Ground

Figure/ground is a theoretical explanation for how the self develops and organizes experiences as it interacts within the environmental field. The field is differentiated into figure (foreground) and ground (background). People organize the field into meaningful patterns in which one element emerges as the figure of interest (the dominant need at a given moment), while the other elements recede into the ground. As soon as the need is met or interest is lost, it retreats into the ground and a new figure emerges. All behavior is organized around emerging needs and their satisfaction (Perls, 1973).

Organismic Self-Regulation

Organismic self-regulation is a natural growth process whereby a person is continually disturbed by the emergence of a need and strives to restore equilibrium by reorganizing and adapting to changing circumstances. It has been operationalized into a cycle known as the Cycle of Experience: (a) awareness of sensation, (b) figure formation, (c) mobilization, (d) action, (e) contact, and (f) withdrawal (Figure 2.1). This cycle provides a way to understand health and dysfunction as well as guide therapeutic process interventions.

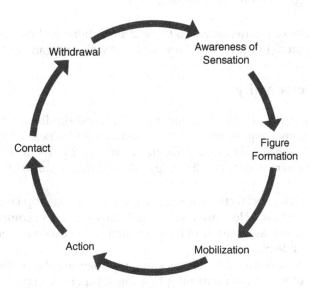

FIGURE 2.1 CYCLE OF EXPERIENCE
diagram.

- Awareness of sensation—commences the cycle and identifies feelings, drives, or perceptions that emerge from within the self or in response to environmental stimuli.
- Figure formation—organizes sensation into a meaningful want or need in relationship to the environment.
- Mobilization—the surge of energy that impels the figure formation into action.
- Action—the movement that brings the person into contact with self or an environmental object.
- Contact—the meeting of self and other at the boundary to either assimilate or reject the object.
- Withdrawal—the disengagement and fading of figure into background and closure of the Gestalt.

Organismic self-regulation can be viewed as a developmental process of growth toward wholeness and integration. When the process is interrupted, the person disowns parts of self and becomes stuck in dysfunctional and rigidified adaptations.

Interruptions to Awareness and Contact

Interruptions to awareness and contact are dysfunctional processes, developed early in life, that people employ in an attempt to meet their needs. These dysfunctional processes interrupt healthy figure/ground formation and completion as well as organismic self-regulation. Some examples include (a) introjection, (b) projection, (c) retroflection, (d) confluence, and (e) deflection.

- Introjection—to uncritically accept others' beliefs and standards without discriminating and assimilating what belongs to self and eliminating what does not.
- Projection—to disown certain unacceptable aspects of self by ascribing them to other people or the environment.
- Retroflection—to turn back onto self what is meant for someone else.
- Confluence—to blur the differentiation between self and the environment where there is no clear demarcation between internal experience and outer reality.
- Deflection—to distract in order to diminish the intensity and sustained sense of awareness and contact (Polster & Polster, 1973).

Gestalt therapists bring awareness to these interruptions and create experiments to lessen them and restore figure/ground formation as well as organismic self-regulation.

Layers of the Personality

Layers of the personality are the changing, persistent, and rigidified adaptations of self to the expectations and requirements of the external world. These adaptations disrupt natural organismic self-regulation and result in disowned parts of self and four *inauthentic* layers of the personality: (a) cliché, (b) role, (c) impasse, and, (d) implosion.

- Cliché—the ordinary social chitchat and the most superficial, top layer of the personality such as: Question: "How are you doing?" Answer: "Can't complain."
- Role—a part a person assumes in an interpersonal context such as: the "kind person" or the "invulnerable person."
- Impasse—a layer of confusion and stuckness representing the conflict of moving to a deeper layer of self versus returning to a more superficial layer. The client often

experiences the impasse layer as an image: "I am swirling in an abyss" or "I am walking through a foggy cemetery."
- Implosion—the death or paralyzed layer where a part of self has been interrupted and disowned: "Everything is dark."

There is a fifth layer of the personality known as the explosion layer. This is the deepest, *authentic* layer where contact with the genuine self occurs and feelings of joy, grief, anger, or orgasm explode into awareness. During therapy, specific interventions by the therapist help the client move through the layers to contact the authentic self (Perls, 1973).

▪ DEFINITION OF MENTAL HEALTH AND PSYCHOPATHOLOGY IN GESTALT THERAPY

Psychological Health

People are psychologically healthy when they are self-regulating and have few interruptions to organismic self-regulation. There is a natural flow of figure formation and completion. They move through the cycle of experience in a rhythmic, sequential fashion with awareness, excitement, and aliveness. Healthy people are self-aware. They have an understanding of their past and look toward the future with vigor and aliveness. All parts of self are integrated and available. Healthy people are able to respond adequately to their wants and needs and are capable of realistically evaluating situations and responsibly initiating behaviors accordingly. They live in the here-and-now, have sufficient self-support, make rich contact, and move with excitement toward higher levels of growth (Perls, 1973).

Psychopathology

Psychopathology exists when people do not have a flow of figure formation and completion. There is a loss of awareness and contact. Organismic self-regulation is interrupted by the dysfunctional processes of confluence, introjection, projection, retroflection, and deflection (Polster & Polster, 1973). Gestalts remain incomplete and clamor for attention. These incomplete gestalts usurp the full attending powers for meeting new situations and dampen the ability to be fully present. People have diminished energy and a reduction of vitality and aliveness. Unfinished business and disowned parts of self are abundant. People live within inauthentic layers of existence (cliché, role, impasse, and implosion). Authenticity is dimmed and reified patterns occur as individuals cling to selves that are inauthentic. Self-support is limited and excessive environmental support is sought through manipulation. Instead of growth, there is stagnation (Perls, 1969/1992).

▪ THERAPEUTIC GOALS IN GESTALT THERAPY

The goal of Gestalt therapy is to assist clients in restoring excitement and growth. The title of the first Gestalt therapy text reflects this goal and is called *Gestalt Therapy: Excitement and Growth in the Human Personality* (Perls et al.,1951/1994). Clients reclaim awareness and return to their natural state of organismic self-regulation. New gestalts emerge and are brought to completion with fluidity. Clients reintegrate disowned parts of self, complete unfinished gestalts, and work through inauthentic layers of the personality (Perls, 1973). They become integrated and return to a state of aliveness and growth. Clients are able to make rich contact with self and others and live a more authentic, vital, and responsible life (Perls, 1973).

■ PERSPECTIVE ON ASSESSMENT IN GESTALT THERAPY

Assessment is a discovery process that allows for understanding the phenomenological experience of clients while recognizing factors that hinder awareness, contact, and organismic self-regulation. It is approached with respect for figure and ground movement, allowing clients to bring to the foreground what is deemed important, rather than a linear questioning procedure. Collaboratively, clients and therapists come to a shared understanding of what is poignant, salient, and relevant for exploration. An agreed upon case formulation and goals are determined; these are tentative and always take second place to the flow of experiencing in the moment (Watson, Goldman, & Greenberg, 2007).

Process factors are figural in Gestalt therapy assessment and include how the client relates to the therapist, the manner in which the narrative is told, the level of awareness and contact, interruptions to awareness and contact, and nonverbal behavior such as body language, voice tone, mannerisms, posture, and energy level. Process diagnoses such as retroflected anger or deflected sadness during a session are identified and later serve as a guide for interventions. Content factors are background and include information such as the precipitating problem, symptoms, stressors, psychiatric, developmental, and family history, substance use, physical health history, current social situation, mental status, and personality characteristics. Content factors are important and help in selecting the type of experiment to employ in addition to determining the pacing and timing of the work. Assessment occurs during the initial session and is ongoing throughout the course of psychotherapy (Knight, 2013).

■ THERAPEUTIC INTERVENTIONS IN GESTALT THERAPY

Gestalt therapists are interested in what is emerging in the moment and in making the past, present, and future come alive in the here-and-now. The here-and-now is the place where change occurs. Gestalt therapists closely track the client's process and content with moment-to-moment awareness in order to understand what is immediate and to tailor appropriate interventions. Two critical therapeutic skills for the Gestalt therapist are the ability to establish an authentic, I–Thou relationship and the ability to craft creative experiments (Perls, 1973; Zinker, 1977/1998).

I–Thou Relationship

The I–thou relationship is an authentic, nonjudgmental, carefully nurtured dialogic relationship between the client and the therapist (Buber, 1937/1970). It is an encounter where both persons are subjects, rather than one being subject and the other object. The client is not "talking to" an aloof expert, but rather "communicating with" a therapist who is aware, authentic, vulnerable, and fully human. The therapist strives to understand the client's phenomenological field by experiencing his or her own reactions to the client and the therapeutic process, while also attending to the client's thoughts, feelings, and behaviors. It requires suspending preconceptions and bracketing anything that may interfere with an ability to attend to immediate experience. It also requires an attitude of openness and humility and to approach the client with genuine interest, curiosity, and profound respect for his or her way of experiencing the world. It further requires the therapist to create a safe environment where the client feels understood without fear of criticism or judgment (Yontef, 1993).

Creative Experiments

Designing and implementing carefully tailored, creative experiments to heighten awareness, promote the expression of emotionally laden material, support contact, and create moments of healing are the cornerstones of Gestalt therapy interventions. They help restore organismic self-regulation, reintegrate disowned parts of self, complete unfinished gestalts, and work through inauthentic layers of the personality (Perls, 1973). Experiments are spontaneous and emerge from the dialogic interaction between the client and therapist (Zinker, 1977/1998). Creating experiments requires the therapist to be very aware and attend to the nonverbal as well as the verbal content of the client's narratives in order to understand and focus on what is alive and immediate (Knight, 2013).

Experiments are unlimited. Gestalt therapists bring their unique life experiences and skills to the creation of the experiment; thus, each Gestalt therapist's work is different. For example, in reviewing the experiments in my case study, I note that I pay close attention to the body, noticing rate and depth of breath as well as volume, timbre, and tone of the voice. I also pay close attention to the syntax, fluidity, and meaning of language. I frequently have clients tell me what they are experiencing in their body. I often use the technique of exaggeration to heighten awareness. I use metaphor and imagery, especially when working with the impasse layer. I use focusing to bring attention to alien aspects of self. I work with dreams to help integrate disowned parts of self. I often ask clients to use the language of responsibility in order to increase awareness and contact. I use empty chair dialogues to heal splits in the self and complete unfinished business with others. I especially like to use music and other creative arts to bring forth and concretize moments of healing. My choice of experiments depends on the characteristics and developmental readiness of the client, the stage of the relationship, and my creativity in the moment (Knight, 2013).

- **Body awareness.** Clients frequently have blocked body energies, which may be manifested by speaking in a restricted voice or fidgeting fingers. I may ask, "What are you experiencing right now in your body?" or "Go inside and see what is emerging in your body now."
- **Exaggeration.** Clients may be asked to exaggerate a body movement where energy is blocked. For example, I may ask a client who is moving one foot back and forth to "Do it more" or "Exaggerate the movement."
- **Metaphor and imagery.** Clients may be asked to allow a metaphor or image to emerge when at the impasse layer. For example, I asked a recent client to create an image when she was stuck at the impasse layer. She imaged seeing herself scuba diving in the Atlantic Ocean off the coast of New Jersey. She described herself as "anchored"—not being able to get back into the boat nor to take the plunge into the dark, cold water.
- **Focusing.** Focusing may be used to make contact with alienated aspects of self (Gendlin, 1981). For example, if I notice shallow, restricted breathing, I might ask the client to bring his or her attention to the breathing and describe what he or she is experiencing.
- **Dreamwork.** Gestalt therapy views dreams as disowned parts of self that need to be reintegrated; thus, I may ask clients to assume different parts of the dream and tell it

as if it is happening in the here-and-now, using present tense rather than past tense (Perls, 1969/1992). I may have clients dialogue with different parts of the dream that appear most poignant and salient.

- **Language of responsibility.** This technique is useful to increase the intensity of awareness and contact by using the first-person pronoun. For example, if a client says, "It's hard for many people to feel sadness," I may ask him or her to say, "It's hard for me to feel my sadness."
- **Empty-chair dialogues.** Empty-chair dialogues may be used to integrate two conflicting aspects of the self (L. S. Greenberg, 1979) or to complete unfinished business with a significant other (Paivio & Greenberg, 1995). For example, a recent client revealed that part of her wished to express anger while another part was not so sure. An empty-chair dialogue took place: First, "Put your anger in the chair and tell it that it is not OK to be expressed and must be held inside." Then, "Tell it that it is OK to be expressed and roar out like a wildfire." Dialogue continues until the conflict is resolved.
- **Moments of healing.** I especially like to use music and other creative arts to bring forth and concretize moments of healing. For example, I played the song "Lullabye" by Cris Williamson (Joel, 1990, track 17) at the exact moment a recent client made contact with her authentic sadness over the loss of her mother, who was compromised by illness.

These are merely a few examples of the many types of experiments used in Gestalt therapy. Gestalt therapists pay close attention to the client's process and create experiments based on the client's needs that emerge in the moment (Knight, 2013).

■ CASE STUDY

Background

I first met Donna at my private practice 3 years ago, when she was referred to me by her neurologist. At that time, she was 33 years old and had been recently discharged from a general hospital where she was hospitalized for 3 days after having a grand mal seizure. She was diagnosed as having a psychogenic nonepileptic seizure (PNES), also known by the older term of *pseudoseizure*. PNES is categorized as a Conversion Disorder in the Fifth Edition of the *Diagnostic and Statistical Manual of Mental Disorders* (*DSM-5*; American Psychiatric Association, 2013). This was the second time she had a seizure. Her first was 8 years prior when she was 25 years old. Both were grand mal seizures with severe muscle contractions and loss of consciousness. In both cases, all laboratory and diagnostic tests were normal. These seizures do not represent excessive cortical activity as in epileptic seizures, but instead are caused by psychological factors.

Unlike many patients with this diagnosis, Donna was relieved that the seizures were diagnosed as psychogenic, for she believed she would have more control over them and could eliminate them with psychotherapy. As a result, she came to therapy to work on the underlying psychological causes of her seizures. Donna has been my patient for 3 years and I have had 140 individual Gestalt therapy sessions with her. Some important data culled from my initial assessment notes reveal the following:

Donna is an attractive, married, 33-year-old, Caucasian female of German and Polish descent who works as director of marketing at a pharmaceutical company. She is open and cooperative and interacts in a warm, responsive, and thoughtful manner. She has never been in psychotherapy, but has always toyed with the idea of trying it out and believes it might be of some benefit. Other than the grand mal seizures, she has no medical problems, but did report that, as an adolescent, she had frequent dizzy spells and even fainted a few times when under stress. Her physician thought they were "growing pains."

Donna hails from a small town in New Jersey. She grew up in an intact family system, which she describes as stable, loving, and predictable with clearly defined, traditional roles. She is the middle child of three, having an older and younger sister, each spaced 5 years apart. Her sisters are married with children and have professional careers. They live nearby and she enjoys a good relationship with them. Her parents have been married for 38 years. Her father, of German descent, owns an electrical business. Donna describes him as strong, loyal, and loving, but emotionally bereft. Her mother, of Polish descent, ended a career in teaching after the birth of her first child, and is a homemaker. Donna describes her as caring, smart, and anxious. She was diagnosed with a panic disorder with agoraphobia after the birth of her third child. Both parents work hard and instilled in Donna a strong work ethic, a value of education, and a sense of community responsibility. There is no history of substance use.

Donna states that her early years were uneventful. Her developmental milestones were reached within typical expectations. She did well academically, had many friends, and was involved in a number of school activities. Donna states she had some difficult experiences during adolescence but these were not out of the ordinary, and deflects with a laugh. After high school, she went to college and majored in business. While at college, she met her husband, Toby, and they married soon after graduation. They have been married for 13 years. Toby works as an industrial hygienist. They have two daughters who are 9 and 10 years of age. She does not think she is in love with her husband and sometimes thinks about ending the marriage, but would not do so when her daughters are still so young. She laughs as she tells me that although her husband has some positive qualities, he is also lazy, boring, and addicted to television. She sometimes calls him "Toby Television." They live in an upper-middle class neighborhood in a spacious home. Donna has a large support system of family and friends.

Her mental status is normal in all major areas and she reveals no psychological symptoms. She has a good vocabulary, her fund of knowledge is excellent, and her level of intelligence is estimated in the above average range. Her sleep, appetite, and energy level are good and there is no indication of suicidal or homicidal ideation. Her insight and judgment are good. Her DSM-5 diagnosis is Conversion Disorder, with seizures and with psychological stressors.

Gestalt therapy process assessment reveals a woman who lacks awareness and contact. Her organismic self-regulation is frequently interrupted by the use of retroflection (energy directed inward by biting her lip and picking at her cuticles) and deflection (awareness and contact is diminished by the use of laughter and humor). She is very matter-of-fact and glosses over difficult situations when retelling her life narrative. Nevertheless, it is noted that at these times, her breathing will change and she will develop a red rash on her neck, indicating a lack of awareness of her inner experience. She speaks about feelings in an intellectual fashion and does not experience them; thus, her feelings are disowned. She has unfinished business related to the emotional reactions she had prior to the seizures that replicated past events from her childhood. She lives within an inauthentic role of competent, smart, hardworking, and funny, having no use for the polar opposites of these characteristics.

My initial plan with Donna was to build a safe and trusting therapeutic relationship and to restore organismic self-regulation by reducing her interruptions of deflection and retroflexion. I also hoped to reintegrate disowned parts of self (her feelings) and to complete unfinished business from the past. I hoped to work through her layers of the personality, in particular her inauthentic roles, allowing her to become more authentic and integrated and take control of her life. I did not plan to focus on her seizures per se, as these were merely symptoms of dysfunctional psychological processes.

Transcript of Gestalt Psychotherapy Sessions

The transcripts were selected from segments of the beginning, middle, and final phase of therapy.

BEGINNING PHASE

The early part of our work concentrated on developing a trusting relationship, developing the narrative, understanding the client's phenomenological experience, and conducting beginning level awareness work. The work was slow and mainly focused on events in her current life. Donna was able to speak about her current family and work situation in an intellectual and humorous way; however, she was fearful of experiencing her feelings and her inner world. She gradually began to notice bodily sensations and retroflected feelings, such as shallow breathing and cuticle picking. Donna employed humor to deflect from difficult situations, which I frequently brought to her attention. Donna needed an abundance of safety and trust to begin to explore her inner landscape. In week 16, we had a major breakthrough that she often referred to as *The Rediscovering Joy and Excitement Session*. The following is part of the session:

APPN:	This is our 16th session and I want to start by asking you how you think our therapy is going?
Donna:	Slowly *(laughs)*.
APPN:	Say more about that.
Donna:	I know I come in here and drone on and on about my minutiae of the week *(laughs)*.
APPN:	I notice you laugh when you say that the therapy is going slow and that you drone on about your weekly minutiae. What does the laughter say?
Donna:	Well, I think it's a laugh of embarrassment. I know that I frustrate you—not deliberately of course—but, you try to have me go deeper and I resist you—I really resist myself—it's not you.
APPN:	I'm wondering if you could create an image of this resistance.
Donna:	I don't know what you mean.
APPN:	A representation—a graphic picture of how you resist yourself.
Donna:	OK. Let me think *(pause)*. It's like driving down a two-lane road and a school bus is coming toward you on the opposite side and then stops to let off some school children—you see the display of flashing lights and the STOP signal arm comes out of the side of the bus.
APPN:	Uh huh.
Donna:	Well, that's how I resist myself. It's like I have a STOP signal arm that won't let me pass—in my case, to go deeper into myself—my unexplored abyss *(laughs)*.
APPN:	That's a powerful image—your unexplored abyss.
Donna:	*(laughs)* Yes. A deep chasm—a bottomless pit.
APPN:	So, if you went into the pit, what might happen?

Donna:	I might encounter things I don't want to see.
APPN:	What might you see?
Donna:	I don't know. And, I may not get out. I may go crazy—even die.
APPN:	Uh huh. That's a scary thought.
Donna:	Yes.
APPN:	Do you experience that anywhere in your body?
Donna:	I can feel my stomach tightening up.
APPN:	Would you put your hand on your stomach and take some slow deep breaths and visualize your breath moving into that area?
Donna:	*(follows instructions)* I feel more relaxed now—less tight.
APPN:	So, the thought of going deeper with our work scares you.
Donna:	Well, not as much as when I first started coming here, but yes it does.
APPN:	If things become too scary, we can stop and do some grounding work.
Donna:	Well, I know how to do that now *(laughs)*.
APPN:	I wonder what you are laughing about?
Donna:	Well, we have spent a lot of time doing grounding work, so I know what to do if I become overwhelmed.
APPN:	Terrific. Would you be willing to do an experiment?
Donna:	Sure?
APPN:	I was wondering if you could imagine a dark chasm in front of you, knowing you have the choice to decide how close you get to it.
Donna:	I can do that.
APPN:	OK. So, close your eyes and imagine you're walking in a safe place. See the environment around you *(pause)*. Hear any noises and smell any scents *(pause)*. In front of you is a chasm. You approach it and take it in. Allow yourself to experience the chasm and just notice what happens. Keeping your eyes closed, speak in first-person present tense, as if you are experiencing this right now.

Commentary: *Speaking in the first-person present tense heightens awareness and brings the work into the here-and-now, which is the place of healing.*

Donna:	I am walking on a path in a meadow. There are spring wildflowers around me. I smell their beautiful aroma. I am safe. I see in front of me there's a large hole in the ground. It looks like an old-fashioned well, but maybe three times the diameter. I go close to it and examine it, but still at a safe distance so I won't fall in. It's dark, but filled with water—dark, black water. I feel afraid of the water, but, something in me wants to go into it.
APPN:	Just stay with the image and breathe *(about 2 minutes pass)*.
Donna:	I make a decision to jump in, but I can't do it. I feel like I did when I was 8 years old jumping off a high diving board at a pool club for the first time. I need to give myself the confidence to jump. I tell myself: "You will be OK. You will not die."

APPN: *(silence)*

Donna: I am going in now. I jump. I am slowly sinking. I can't stop myself from sinking. A white rope line appears and I grab it. It looks like an anchor line—the type used when scuba diving, so you can safely return to the starting point when visibility is poor. I feel safe knowing I have the support of the rope *(pause)*.

APPN: What's happening now? *(I notice she is smiling and looks pleased)*

Donna: Oh my! The water has turned into the Caribbean. I see angel fish, sea anemones, coral reefs, yellowtails, black sea urchins. Oh, my goodness— it's heavenly!

APPN: Just stay with it.

Donna: *(after about 3 minutes she opens her eyes).* Oh my God. It was blissful. I didn't want to return.

APPN: What are you experiencing Donna?

Donna: Pure, unadulterated joy!

APPN: Be with your joy as long as you like.

Donna: *(after about 2 minutes)* What the hell just happened?

APPN: What do you think happened?

Donna: I was at a well, I jumped in, I was sinking, a rope line appeared, I grabbed it, and the water turned into the Caribbean. I was in sync with the rhythm of the water and looked at all the underwater beauty. I felt as if I was breathing and moving in synchrony with the sea anemones and underwater flora. It was incredible!

APPN: You are so excited!

Donna: Yes. And, joyful.

APPN: *(I stay present with Donna, silently witnessing her excitement and joy)*

Donna: What does all this mean psychologically?

APPN: What is your sense?

Donna: I don't really know, but it seems as if I moved to a deeper place—no pun intended *(laughs)*. Can you put it into psychological terms for me? Give me a psychological explanation of what happened. I need to understand . . . .

APPN: I would describe it as moving to a deeper layer of your personality. You were at a stuck place, resisting movement. In Gestalt terms, you were at an impasse. And, when I asked you to create an image, you came up with a well with a large diameter. You eventually went into the water and started to sink and then the rope appeared and you grabbed onto it, which gave you support to go even deeper. I would say that you felt safe and as you sank, you moved into the death layer, often called implosion—the part of yourself that was dead or cut off. As you experienced the death layer, you moved into the life layer, often called explosion. Here emerged joy and excitement—feelings that at one time were cut off.

Donna: Oh my. Are you saying that I cut off happy feelings and found those in the abyss *(laughs)*? I thought I would only find anger and sadness and pain there.

APPN: You find whatever needs to appear at the moment. The body knows what needs to emerge.

Donna: Well, for my first dive I'm glad I found angel fish and not barracudas! Maybe I'll go into the abyss again *(laughs)*.

Commentary: This was a breakthrough session. I found it so interesting that feelings of joy and excitement emerged for Donna. These were the first feelings that she experienced in session. In Donna's family, both positive and negative feelings were invalidated, so she learned to disown all feelings. The only time she was able to feel was when she listened to music or when she watched a movie, but, in these cases, she was able to keep them at a distance, for they did not belong to her, but belonged to the musician or actor. For a client like Donna, who was so fearful of feelings in general, it seemed like the perfect entry into the deeper parts of self—from the impasse, to the death layer, and finally to the life layer of joy and excitement.

MIDDLE PHASE

The next 2 years of our work focused on decreasing interruptions, completing unfinished business, reintegrating parts of self, and restoring organismic self-regulation. Once Donna began to access the deeper parts of self, she would come to session with a clear figure to work on. Although she still retained her sense of humor, she became more serious during her sessions. The following is part of session #69:

Donna: Well, here we are again.

APPN: Yes. Welcome.

Donna: Did you ever hear the Van Morrison song, "Till We Get the Healing Done"?

APPN: Yes. I think so.

Donna: Well, it came on the radio as I drove here today. And, it is so true.

APPN: Say more.

Donna: Well. It's a long song and it just hit me hard. I actually had to stop the car and pull over for it made me cry. I googled the lyrics and sang along.

APPN: Very powerful words. What are they for you?

Donna: That's what it feels like—like I am trying to heal—get rid of the poison inside and live in the land of the sun and right here-and-now.

APPN: That's really poignant.

Donna: Anyway, you are my guide to get the healing done *(laughs)*.

APPN: *(smiles)*

Donna: I was thinking this week about a story my father told me as a child—and told with some frequency. His mother was killed by a drunk driver when he was around 5 years old. He was sent by his father to an orphanage for about a year. There was no one to watch him as he was not yet in school, and his father needed to work long hours. The plan was that in a year when he started school, his father would come get him and he would move back home. My father had two older sisters, but they were in school and had after-school jobs. Anyway, the owner of the orphanage was a woman named Mrs. Booker. According to my father, she was very mean to the children—a Mrs. Hannigan type figure. One day when his father visited, my father told his father how mean she was and that he didn't want to stay there—my father said that he cried like a baby as he told his father. Well, his father was naturally very upset and confronted Mrs. Booker. His father asked her to be nicer to my father for he was so young and had just lost his mother. Well, according to my father, when his father left, Mrs. Booker punished him—made my father kneel on hard, uncooked corn kernels for several hours—a harsh punishment that would now be considered child abuse. My father proudly would say that he took his punishment and didn't cry a teardrop, for she would never get the best of him again. He would end his story by saying: "I learned my lesson from Mrs. Booker. Hide your feelings and keep them to yourself, for showing them gets you nowhere in life."

APPN: That certainly is a powerful introject. I'm wondering what you experience as you tell me the story of Mrs. Booker and your father. What is it like for you?

Donna: *(after a few minutes)* I feel sad for my father that he had to cut off his feelings and I guess sad for me and all of us in the family.

APPN: Can you say, I feel sad for me.

Donna: I feel sad for me *(tears in her eyes for a few seconds)*. That's enough. Let's move on.

APPN: Just notice for a moment that you felt some sadness and have some tears.

Donna: Are you going to make me kneel on corn kernels *(laughs)*?

APPN: It's hard for you to stay with your feelings.

Donna: Yes. I took it in and believed it. I wanted to be like my father. I modeled much of my personality after him. He had the power in the family. He was also positive and energetic—just fun to be with. My mother was so anxious.

APPN: Say more.

Donna: *(silence)* I just had a thought about the first seizure I had.

APPN: Uh huh.

Donna: Remember I told you that before the seizure, I spoke to my mother on the phone?

APPN: Yes. I do remember, but that was as far as you wanted to go with the story.

Donna: Well, I was in Bermuda for 5 days . . . *(her voice trails off)*.

APPN: What are you experiencing now?

Donna:	I want to give you some information about my mother before going right into what happened—to give some context.
APPN:	I wonder why that's important? I noticed your eyes darted back and forth. I'm not sure what's going on.
Donna:	I just want you to understand some things about her before I tell you the specifics of that day—give some background—set the stage, so you don't think she's all negative . . . *(her voice trails off).*
APPN:	So, it's important to you that I understand who she is and perhaps not judge her.
Donna:	Yes.
APPN:	So, are you taking care of your mother or yourself?
Donna:	Probably both. I just need to set the stage, so you get me and get the situation.
APPN:	I'm wondering if you feel I misunderstand you?
Donna:	That's always been an issue for me. Actually, I think you do understand me, but I still need to make sure and set the stage.
APPN:	OK. *(I am aware that Donna does this frequently, i.e., spends time giving detailed information about the context, so she's not misunderstood. I make note of this but move on, for I realize this is a form of self-support that is necessary for her.)*
Donna:	Well, my mother has a college degree in education and taught before she had my sister. As soon as she was born, she stopped working and never returned to the paid workforce—never worked outside of the house. Her role as wife, mother, and homemaker defined her existence. I would describe her as a quintessential traditional woman. She sacrificed her life for her children, living through their achievements—she seemed unfulfilled as a woman. She was determined that her children be successful—reading stories to us, quizzing us as if we were Jeopardy contestants, helping with homework, and rewarding achievements. But, what was unspoken in our home was her high level of anxiety.
APPN:	How did her anxiety affect you?
Donna:	I was frequently disappointed and gradually withdrew from her.
APPN:	Can you recall a situation when you were let down by her?
Donna:	Well, I was not let down all the time. She was often there for me.
APPN:	I am aware that when something negative is said about your mother, you find it difficult, and bring forth something positive.
Donna:	You got me. I guess I am loyal *(laughs)*. OK. I do remember feeling disappointed.
APPN:	Go on.
Donna:	I remember an event in third grade. I was 9. My teacher invited mothers to come to class for the day—one at a time. We picked the rotation out of a hat. I remember, I was #10 in a class of about 15 students. On the

day she was scheduled to visit, I was excited. But she didn't come. My father came instead.

APPN: What was that like for you?

Donna: I don't know. I want to make a joke. He was good looking and my teacher flirted with him and she liked me more after that *(laughs)*.

APPN: What was it *really* like for you?

Donna: I was embarrassed that my mother didn't come and that my father came. OK. I was probably sad, but I remember feeling embarrassed. Let me go back to the story. I don't think I would let myself feel sad *(becomes tearful)*.

APPN: *(silence)*

Donna: I'm feeling sad now.

APPN: Yes *(silence for a few minutes)*.

Donna: I remembered something else. A few years after the classroom incident—I was around 11 and in fifth grade. My Brownie Girl Scout troop was having a spaghetti dinner and we were going to receive the badges we earned through the year. I was going to receive a lot of them and was excited and proud. Our parents were invited and my father had to work, so just my mother was going to come. The troop was to arrive an hour before the dinner for rehearsal. My uncle dropped me off and my mother was home getting ready. She was supposed to return in about an hour for the dinner. So, I waited and searched for her as all the other parents arrived. And, she never came . . . .

APPN: I notice that your neck is very red and your breathing has become very shallow. What are you experiencing?

Donna: Nothing. I'm experiencing nothing.

APPN: Just close your eyes and put your right hand on your chest and your left hand on your abdomen and take some deep, slow belly breaths so that your left hand rises and see if you can go back to that night.

Donna: *(follows the directions)* I am back there and I feel very scared and alone and disappointed. I make an excuse to the troop leader that my father is working and my mother is sick. I ate some spaghetti, got my badges, and my uncle picked me up and took me home. My mother was waiting for me and apologized for not being there and said she was too anxious.

APPN: What did you say to her?

Donna: I said, "Don't worry about it. It wasn't anything great anyway."

APPN: What did you do then?

Donna: Oh, I probably went to my room and listened to "Only the Lonely" on my little CD player. We had a lot of 60s music in our home *(laughs)*!

APPN: What do you need?

Donna: Nothing then and nothing now. I am self-sufficient and don't need anything from anyone *(laughs)*. I guess I learned how to take care of myself, which can be a good thing, right?

APPN:	What do you think?
Donna:	Well, some self-sufficiency is good, but I guess I needed a mother. After this, I think I withdrew from her. I remember spending a lot of time in my room—reading and listening to music. For a few summers, I won a prize at the local library for reading the most books. Not a bad thing *(laughs)*.
	In my teen years, my mother became agoraphobic—she was too anxious to drive. She would only go out of the house and shop at times when the stores were empty. And, my older sister would drive her. I don't remember her driving a car for many years. She stopped socializing. She took anti-anxiety medication and was always scared of becoming addicted, so she would cut them in half and take them only when she had to leave the house. She was like a "wounded deer." I felt bad for her. If I tried to talk to her about my problems, she would become more anxious and overwhelmed. So, I learned to keep things to myself and not share anything with her. I withdrew from her and had a superficial relationship with her for the rest of my life, although I always loved her and wished it was different. I think her anxiety was from not feeling—and probably my seizures were the same.
APPN:	So, you were unable to have much authentic contact with her because of your fear of overwhelming her. I wonder how you dealt with teenage problems?
Donna:	For the most part, I kept them to myself and listened to music. I always liked songs that were about strong women . . . .
APPN:	Such as?
Donna:	I like the old ones where the lyrics are clear—like, Helen Reddy's "I Am Woman" or Pat Benatar's "Invincible."
APPN:	Yes. I know both of them. What attracts you to these songs?
Donna:	Well, I am woman I am strong—no one's gonna keep me down—and I can do anything—I am strong—I am invincible . . . I can't afford to be innocent and need to be invincible.
APPN:	I notice invincible is a theme in both of these songs.
Donna:	Yes. I needed to be invincible to survive my teenage years.
APPN:	I notice it's close to the end of our time. We have 5 minutes left.
Donna:	Yes. And, I never got to what happened before the first seizure. Really quick—OK? Three minutes. I was in Bermuda and my mother was watching my two daughters who were very young. She was great with infants and toddlers. My first night there, I called her and she was extremely anxious and said one of the kids had a fever and diarrhea and she didn't know what to do. She was very anxious and overwhelmed. I calmed her down and when I hung up, I was furious. She let me down again, when I needed her. I was with my husband and two friends and all of them said, "No reason to be angry—we can't do anything about it here, so don't worry about it." I shut up. I remember I had diarrhea several times during the evening. It was like a volcano erupting inside. The next day, after an hour or so on the beach, we walked into town to get lunch and I was feeling weak and then I had

a grand mal seizure. I woke up in a hospital in Bermuda a few hours later.

APPN: That is a powerful story told at the very end. What do you experience?

Donna: A little anger. I can see the connection with holding in my feelings—especially the anger. It's like a circuit breaker that blew—I sort of imploded on myself.

APPN: We have to stop. If you need to sit awhile and process or write a journal entry before you leave, you can go into the office next door—it's empty.

Donna: OK. See you next week. Same time, same place.

Commentary: This was one of many powerful sessions where Donna would make contact with early traumatic memories and reexperience her disowned feelings—and then, relate them to her seizures.

FINAL PHASE

During the final phase of therapy, existential themes emerged. In this third session from the end (session #137), themes of freedom, responsibility, awe, letting go, life, and death emerged.

APPN: Hi.

Donna: We have two sessions left after today. This is our 137th session. I counted them all up *(laughs).*

APPN: Yes. We agreed to have six termination sessions and this is our fourth one. So, two more after today!

Donna: I had a dream a few days ago and I would like to work on it. I saved it for the session.

APPN: So, tell me the dream—in the first-person present tense of course.

Donna: "I am getting on a helicopter to skydive alone for the first time. I don't know where I am and I don't know the helicopter pilot, but I know I am going to do it. I am scared to do this solo. The helicopter is going up, up, up. And, I am getting ready to jump. I take a deep breath, jump out, and free-fall at a very fast speed. I like this feeling, but know I must pull the ripcord or I will die. I pull the cord and the chute opens. I am floating through the air for a long time and I feel beautifully relaxed and at one with the universe. I am getting closer to the ground. I see greenery below and know I will land safely sometime soon. I don't know where I am. I wake up."

APPN: What are you experiencing?

Donna: Awe—a sense of amazement and wonder.

APPN: Stay with that.

Donna: *(she closes her eyes and then opens them)*

APPN: Are you willing to be the parts of the dream?

Donna: Yes. I would like to work it. There's me, the helicopter, the ripcord, the parachute, the green land below. I'll start with being the helicopter.

"I'm the helicopter. I'm strong and powerful. I lift off up into the sky with my revolving rotors. I move in all directions—up and down, back and forth. I am free to go where I choose." *(Donna sits very erect as she takes on the role of being the helicopter.)*

APPN: What's that like for you?

Donna: Feels good. I'm going—don't know where, but I'm very strong and powerful.

APPN: Stay with that for a while.

Donna: I like feeling strong and powerful.

APPN: Is any other part of the dream important?

Donna: The ripcord.

APPN: OK. Be the ripcord.

Donna: "I'm the ripcord. If I'm pulled, the parachute will open and the descent will slow down. If I'm not pulled, the descent is a free-fall. I notice Donna is free falling at an exhilarating speed and, then, I am pulled and the parachute opens and the descent is slowed. I slow Donna down and allow her to see all of the beauty."

APPN: So . . . .

Donna: I can be excited and exhilarated or I can go slow and appreciate all that is. I don't know where I am going, but I am safe.

APPN: Go on . . . .

Donna: I want to be the land.

APPN: Go ahead.

Donna: "I am the green land. My soil is rich. I am fertile and can grow anything. I am alive."

APPN: Stay with that experience of being alive.

Donna: *(after a few minutes)* This is an amazing dream. I think I have found all those parts of me in my work here. "I'm strong and powerful. I don't know where I am going, but I'm going somewhere. I have support and am in control of whether I want to go fast and feel the excitement or go slow and see the beauty. And, I'll land on something rich, fertile, and full of life. I'm full of life. I'm alive."

APPN: Very profound.

Donna: Thinking about the dream now makes me think of how I was when I started here. I had had two grand mal seizures and was a disaster. I always see the seizures as an overloaded electrical system that blew a circuit breaker. I imploded on myself. We spoke about this before. I think in many ways I was dead. I was living a life and doing a lot of things, but I was dead inside. And, over the years, I wound up realizing that at the root of the seizures were feelings—and even thoughts—that I cut off from myself. Most of the time, I was not even aware of my feelings. I would move away from them and do something instead. It made me

	fairly successful in many ways, but inside I was dead, like an empty husk.
APPN:	Go on.
Donna:	What's so remarkable to me is that I got a lot of healing done. Who knows if there will be more work in the future, but for now I'm happy. I can access and express my feelings and get out of situations when I'm not getting my needs met. My divorce should be final in a few weeks and I look forward to starting a new life.
APPN:	So, you have access to your feelings and can let go when your needs aren't being met.
Donna:	I realize there will always be difficult life events. No one knows what lies around the next corner. Yet, I believe I have the tools to handle things. I trust my feelings and know they serve as a guide to know what I need to do next. I don't believe I will have any more seizures.
APPN:	What makes you say that?
Donna:	It's not only being aware of my feelings and processing, but it's not allowing myself to be in situations that trigger intense feelings. Like not hooking up with people who cannot be there for me—narcissists or people who have so many needs themselves, they cannot be there for me. And, I continue to select female friends who are empowered and secure within themselves. I realize I have the power and freedom to choose who's in my life and I'm responsible for those choices. I also believe that I use my discriminatory powers more. I feel more like the ebb and flow of an ocean wave.
APPN:	How are you like the ebb and flow?
Donna:	The ocean is constantly changing and moving—ebbing and flowing—and I need to ebb and flow with it and not get stuck, like I did before—stuck with friends that couldn't be there for me, stuck with colleagues who are negative and incompetent, stuck with a partner who doesn't and never could meet my needs. By healing many old issues and cultivating awareness of my feelings and using them to guide me, my life feels more like the ebb and flow of a wave.
APPN:	I'm also wondering if the dream is representative of our relationship in any way.
Donna:	Well, I'm bailing on you—leaving therapy very soon *(laughs)*.
APPN:	Yes, you are.
Donna:	I'm jumping out of the helicopter and pulling the ripcord and going slowly. I do have two more sessions *(laughs)*.
APPN:	I think we should look more closely at our relationship in the final sessions. Would that be OK?
Donna:	I'd like that.

Commentary: I have found that clients frequently have dreams in the final phase of their therapy. Often the dreams are symbolic of what is both happening in their lives as well as what is happening in the therapeutic relationship. Themes of termination are very apparent in this session: freedom, responsibility, awe, letting go, life, and death.

Commentary

I spent 3 years in weekly psychotherapy with Donna and had a total of 140 individual psychotherapy sessions. The therapeutic approach was guided by Gestalt therapy concepts of figure/ground formation and completion, decreasing interruptions to organismic self-regulation, completing unfinished business from past traumas, and reclaiming disowned parts of self. We developed a strong I–thou relationship. I created many Gestalt experiments, some of which were illustrated in the transcripts such as using images to move through the impasse layer, heightening awareness, and dream work.

The therapy with Donna was very rewarding. She was a client who was in serious distress when we started therapy, having had two grand mal seizures. Donna, early on, realized that prior to each seizure, a life situation had occurred that replicated a traumatic experience from her childhood and involved her inability to express her feelings. She had many disowned parts of self, in particular her feelings. She had many issues that were not worked through because of her tendency to interrupt her feelings and move on—usually doing some sort of task. This made her successful in her life, but also prevented her from meeting her needs and kept her stuck in unfulfilled relationships.

The therapy with Donna was successful. As well as experiencing no further seizures during the 3 years we worked together, she made much progress on integrating trauma memories and completing unfinished business from her childhood. She regained awareness of self and contact with others by decreasing her interruptions and restoring organismic self-regulation. Her ability to access and express her feelings was one of her more significant accomplishments, especially because feelings were not allowed in her family of origin. Toward the end of the therapy, she decided to file for a divorce from her husband and became very aware of how she wanted to have a relationship with someone with whom she had more in common and with whom she could be emotionally connected.

DISCUSSION QUESTIONS

1. Listen to the Van Morrison song, "Till We Get the Healing Done". What areas of your life can you identify that need to be healed?
2. What interruption to organismic self-regulation do you use?
3. Remember a dream you had recently. Speak the various parts of the dream in the first-person, present tense. What do you discover about yourself?
4. Are there moments in the therapy sessions that you would have worked with differently? How would you have worked these moments differently?

REFERENCES

American Psychiatric Association. (2013). *Diagnostic and statistical manual of mental disorders* (5th ed.). Arlington, VA: American Psychiatric Publishing.

Brownell, P. (2008). *Handbook for theory, research, and practice in Gestalt therapy.* Newcastle, England: Cambridge Scholars Publishing.

Buber, M. (1970). *I and thou.* New York, NY: Scribner's Sons. (Original work published 1937)

Clance, P. R., Thompson, M. B., Simerly, D. E., & Weiss, A. (1994). The effects of the Gestalt approach on body image. *The Gestalt Journal, 17*(1), 95–114.

Feder, B., & Ronall, R. (Eds.). (1980). *Beyond the hot seat: Gestalt approaches to group.* New York, NY: Brunner/Mazel.

Fodor, I. (2015). A female therapist's perspective on growing older. *Journal of Clinical Psychology*, *17*(11), 1115–1120. doi:10.1002/jclp.22221

Gagnon, J. H. (1981). Gestalt therapy with the schizophrenic patient. *The Gestalt Journal*, *4*(1), 29–46.

Gendlin, E. (1981). *Focusing*. New York, NY: Random House.

Gestalt Review. (1997). Research in gestalt therapy. *Gestalt Review*, *1*(1), 1–2.

Greenberg, E. (2015). Group therapy with borderline, narcissistic, and schizoid adaptations. *Gestalt Review*, *23*(2), 129–150. doi:10.5325/gestaltreview.23.2.0129

Greenberg, E. (2019). Surprise: A new look at the treatment of schizophrenia from a Gestalt therapy perspective. *Gestalt Review*, *19*(1), 2–7. doi:10.5325/gestaltreview.19.1.0002

Greenberg, L. S. (1979). Resolving splits: The two-chair technique. *Psychotherapy: Theory, Research and Practice*, *16*(3), 310–318. doi:10.1037/h0085895

Harman, R. (1984). Gestalt therapy research. *The Gestalt Journal*, *7*(2), 61–69.

Herera, P., Mstibovskyi, I., Roubal, J., & Brownell, P. (2018). Researching Gestalt therapy for anxiety in practice-based settings. *Revista Argentina De Clinica Psicologica*, *27*(2), 321–336. doi:10.24205/03276716.2018.1066

Joel, B. (1990). Lullabye [Recorded by C. Williamson]. On *Best of Cris Williamson* [medium of recording]. Washington, DC: Wolf Moon Records. https://www.criswilliamson.com/index.php/music/the-best-of

Knight, C. (2013). Humanistic-existential and solution-focused approaches to psychotherapy. In K. Wheeler (Ed.), *Psychotherapy for the advanced practice psychiatric nurse* (2nd ed., pp. 369–406). New York, NY: Springer Publishing Company.

Kolmanskog, V. (2014). Gestalt approaches to gender identity issues. *Gestalt Review*, *18*(3), 244–260. doi:10.5325/gestaltreview.18.3.0244

Matzko, H. M. G. (1997). A Gestalt therapy treatment approach for addictions. *Gestalt Review*, *1*(1), 34–55. http://explore.bl.uk.proxy.library.nyu.edu/primo_library/libweb/action/display.do?tabs=detailsTab&gathStatTab=true&ct=display&fn=search&doc=ETOCRN031411350&indx=1&recIds=ETOCRN031411350

Nevis, E. (1987). *Organizational consulting: A gestalt approach*. New York, NY: Gardner Press.

Oaklander, V. (1978). *Windows to our children*. Moab, UT: Real People Press.

O'Leary, E. (2013). *Gestalt therapy around the world*. West Sussex, England: Wiley.

Paivio, S. C., & Greenberg, L. S. (1995). Resolving "unfinished business": Efficacy of experiential therapy using empty-chair dialogue. *Journal of Consulting and Clinical Psychology*, *63*(3), 419–425. doi:10.1037/0022-006x.63.3.419

Perls, F. S. (1992). *Ego, hunger and aggression: A revision of Freud's theory and method*. New York, NY: Gestalt Journal Press. (Original work published 1942)

Perls, F. S. (1992). *Gestalt therapy verbatim*. New York, NY: Gestalt Journal Press. (Original work published 1969)

Perls, F. S. (1973). *The Gestalt approach and eyewitness to therapy*. Palo Alto, CA: Science.

Perls, F. S., Hefferline, R., & Goodman, P. (1994). *Gestalt therapy: Excitement and growth in the human personality*. New York, NY: Gestalt Journal Press. (Original work published 1951)

Polster, E., & Polster, M. (1973). *Gestalt therapy integrated: Contours of theory and practice*. New York, NY: Vintage Books.

Resnikoff, R. (1995). Gestalt family therapy. *The Gestalt Journal*, *18*(2), 55–76. http://explore.bl.uk.proxy.library.nyu.edu/primo_library/libweb/action/display.do?tabs=detailsTab&gathStatTab=true&ct=display&fn=search&doc=ETOCRN001960283&indx=1&recIds=ETOCRN001960283

Root, R. W. (1996). The Gestalt cycle of experience as a theoretical framework for conceptualizing the attention deficit disorder. *The Gestalt Journal*, *19*(2), 9–50. http://explore.bl.uk.proxy.library.nyu.edu/primo_library/libweb/action/display.do?tabs=detailsTab&gathStatTab=true&ct=display&fn=search&doc=ETOCRN022925908&indx=1&recIds=ETOCRN022925908

Roubal, J., Brownell, P., Francesetti, G., Melnick, J., & Zeleskov-Djoric, J. (2016). *Towards a research tradition in Gestalt therapy*. Newcastle upon Tyne, England: Cambridge Scholars Publishing.

Serok, S. (1985). Implications of Gestalt therapy with post traumatic patients. *The Gestalt Journal*, *8*(1), 78–89.

Watson, J. C., Goldman, N., & Greenberg, L. S. (2007). *Case studies in emotion-focused treatment of depression*. Washington, DC: American Psychological Association.

Wheeler, G. (1991). *Gestalt reconsidered: A new approach to contact and resistance.* New York, NY: Gardner Press.

Yontef, G. M. (1993). *Awareness, process and dialogue: Essays on Gestalt therapy.* Highland, NY: Gestalt Journal Press.

Zinker, J. (1998). *Creative process in Gestalt therapy.* New York, NY: Vintage Books.)Original work published 1977)

Zinker, J. (1994). *In search of good form: Gestalt therapy with couples and families.* San Francisco, CA: Jossey-Bass.

Person-Centered Therapy: A Client With Postpartum Depression

Laura Kelly

■ PERSONAL EXPERIENCE WITH PERSON-CENTERED THERAPY

As a fledgling therapist in the late 1980s, amid significant changes to the payer system in healthcare and a move away from long-term-ongoing psychoanalytical therapies to shorter problem-focused approaches, I set out to "find my way." Despite my education at Rutgers University in the theoretical orientation of interpersonal psychoanalysis through the works of Hildegard Peplau and Harry Stack Sullivan, I found myself more aligned with the humanistic approach of Carl Rogers and his Person-centered therapy (PCT).

It may have been my own anxiety specific to my therapeutic skills that initially drew me toward a framework where the therapist would have a more supportive, nondirective approach rather than the directive, interpretive approach of psychoanalysis. My supposition that PCT would allow me to relax and not do too much work was soon dispelled. Creating Rogers' core conditions of genuineness/congruence, unconditional positive regard, and accurate empathic understanding necessitated an extremely high level of presence and concentrated listening as well as an awareness and understanding of myself and the client, moment-to-moment during the therapy sessions. It required that I track the client's narrative by carefully following the sequence of events and staying on topic without interrupting or changing directions in order to truly understand the client's phenomenological experience. It demanded fostering a deep client–therapist connection that allowed for an attuned responsiveness based on sensing the client's experience. It necessitated the utilization of facilitative communication skills that carefully matched the client's experience. And, it required the delivery of a judicious response at choice points that emerged during a session. This was not easy and required a great deal of therapeutic skill as well as my own personal self-growth work.

In the years that followed, I spent countless hours reading the works of Carl Rogers and those that followed in his footsteps. I watched numerous videos of his work and attended many conferences, workshops, and training programs in the humanistic approach. As I honed my skills, my naïve understanding of his theory matured and my utilization of his techniques, along with other types of humanistic therapies, helped a multitude of clients in relatively brief periods of time.

As a PhD student in nursing during the late 1980s, and the only psychiatric advanced practice nurse in the program, there was little place for qualitative research. I struggled trying to wrap my qualitative mind around the quantitative world that I had entered. Rogers, in contrast, was utilizing qualitative methods. He was one of the first scientists to test the underlying hypotheses of his theory on the process and outcome of psychotherapy. His work helped me broaden my understanding of the possibilities for psychotherapy research.

As an educator, Rogers' theoretical framework also guided my teaching. Rogers' publication, *Freedom to Learn*, based on student-centered teaching (Rogers & Freiberg, 1994) and the many modern works on the topic that were birthed from his seminal concepts, have assisted me in developing my teaching skills and creating person-centered learning environments.

PCT techniques are an ideal modality when working with women during their reproductive years. My practice is primarily treating women before, during, and after pregnancy. Many women seek my services while desiring to become pregnant and have been told by their current providers that psychopharmacologic treatment during pregnancy is not possible. Other women come because they are pregnant and experiencing psychological symptoms that interfere with their optimal level of functioning. Still other women come in the postpartum period often experiencing anxiety and depressive symptoms that are not familiar to them, and are therefore causing significant disturbances in their lives.

As a prescribing practitioner, some of my interventions are more directive. Nonetheless, PCT allows me to frame directives in a way that makes it clear, regardless of my input, that clients can oversee their own decision-making and I will be present and supportive regardless of the decisions they make. My stance as a clinician is nonjudgmental and empathic.

I have been practicing reproductive psychiatry as an advance practice nurse for the last 15 years and have had the opportunity to work with women over time and through numerous pregnancies. This has allowed a lifelong relationship with numerous women with many points of contact and comfortable transitions as psychotherapy care was required.

■ FOUNDERS AND LEADERS OF PCT

PCT, originally known as Client-centered therapy, was developed in the 1940s by Carl Rogers (1902–1987). Rogers, considered to be the most influential psychotherapist of the 20th century (Cook, Biyanova, & Coyne, 2009), published three seminal books that are foundational in most psychotherapy programs. The first, *Counseling and Psychotherapy* (Rogers, 1942), challenged the authoritative role of the therapist seen in psychoanalysis, and focused on the necessity of creating a nondirective atmosphere during therapy using facilitative communication techniques such as reflecting, clarifying, exploring, and focusing. In this book, he presented the first verbatim transcript ever published of an entire course of therapy, which was revolutionary at a time when no one knew what actually happened during a therapy session. His second book, *Client-Centered Therapy* (Rogers, 1951), described the necessary conditions for effective therapy: genuineness/ congruence, unconditional positive regard, and accurate empathetic understanding. The book also focused on the importance of understanding the client's phenomenological experience and utilizing actualization as a positive force for change. His third book, *On Becoming a Person* (Rogers, 1961), focused on the importance of the therapeutic relationship and the therapist and client being "true to self" in order for the therapy to be successful (Knight, 2014).

Rogers had a profound influence on psychotherapy in other ways as well. He was one of three therapists who demonstrated their psychotherapy approach in the two iconic psychological film series, *Three Approaches to Psychotherapy*. In these series, an actual client was filmed while engaged in therapy with three extraordinary therapists: the client *Gloria* received therapy from Carl Rogers, Fritz Perls, and Albert Ellis in the first series in 1964, and the client *Kathy* received therapy from Carl Rogers, Everett Shostrum, and Arnold Lazarus in the second series in 1977 (Shostrom, 1965, 1977). These classic films are considered to be essential viewing for students studying to become psychotherapists (Knight, 2014).

Rogers and others have applied PCT to many other types of therapy including group therapy (Rogers, 1970), expressive arts therapy (Rogers, 1993), and play therapy (Axline, 1947/2002). PCT is also a major component in motivational interviewing (Miller & Rollnick, 2002) and emotion-focused therapy (Greenberg, 2011), two contemporary, humanistic–existential psychotherapy approaches. Rogers' work has been applied to parenting, education, and industry (Kirschenbaum, 2009), and his facilitative communication skills are an integral part of undergraduate and graduate psychiatric nursing curriculums (Knight, 2014).

In the last decade of his life, Rogers facilitated PCT workshops throughout the United States and the world. He was devoted to applying PCT concepts in areas of social conflict and worked for peace in Northern Ireland and South Africa. He was nominated for the Nobel Peace Prize in 1987. His influence continues today, with over 200 organizations and training centers worldwide (Kirschenbaum & Jourdan, 2005). Howard Kirschenbaum, an internationally known expert on Rogers, has authored his biography in the book *The Life and Work of Carl Rogers* as well as a documentary about Rogers' life and teachings (Kirschenbaum, 2009).

▪ PHILOSOPHY AND KEY CONCEPTS OF PCT

PCT views human nature in an optimistic way and assumes that people are trustworthy and essentially good. Human development is viewed as consistent with positive growth and change and a movement toward self-actualization. Individuals are thought to have the capacity for self-awareness, the potential for self-understanding, and the ability to find personal meaning and purpose in their lives (Rogers, 1961). PCT believes that individuals are capable of coping with a wide range of thoughts, feelings, and behaviors and have the ability to direct their own lives. It assumes that individuals seek to resolve their own conflicts and inner tensions that exist between the existential concepts of freedom and responsibility (Corey, 2017).

PCT posits that positive growth and change occur as a function of our relationships with other people. In a therapeutic context, clients experience positive growth and change when the facilitative conditions of unconditional positive regard, genuineness, and empathic understanding are present and when the therapeutic relationship is trusting, collaborative, and respectful. Therapists understand as much as they can about their clients, to be present and help the clients accept who they are despite their shortcomings. When clients can accept who they are, they can change (Rogers, 1961). According to Rogers (1957), there are six conditions that lead to therapeutic change:

- The therapist and client need to have psychological contact. This level is not met simply by the client and therapist being in the same room. Rather, there must be a collaborative relationship allowing the therapist and client to work as effective partners and thus have an impact on each other.

- The therapist needs to be congruent, genuine, and authentic. This requires that a therapist has experienced many hours of personal growth work. The therapist must be aware of self, responsive to the level of communication with the client, and spontaneous and open in the relationship.
- The therapist must show unconditional positive regard, also known as a nonjudgmental stance. The therapist does not establish any conditions of worth. Positive and negative judgments can be disruptive of change.
- The therapist experiences and expresses empathy to the client. The ability to demonstrate an emotional understanding of and sensitivity to the client's experience is essential to effective therapy.
- The client perceives the empathy and feels accepted by the therapist. Without the client experiencing empathy and acceptance, the therapy is less likely to be successful.
- The client must be experiencing incongruence, which is defined as a lack of alignment or a discrepancy between the real self and the ideal self. Without incongruence, change is not possible.

■ DEFINITION OF MENTAL HEALTH AND PSYCHOPATHOLOGY IN PCT

In PCT, the client is treated as an entire human being, a movement away for the medical model of psychopathology (Haugh, 2018). Rogers did not use the terms *mental health* or *mental illness*; instead, he used the terms *adjustment* and *maladjustment*. A person is considered adjusted if there is a congruence between the ideal self (what one wants to become) and the real self (what one actually is). An adjusted person is fully functioning, open to new experiences, and lives life with freedom, authenticity, and a natural movement toward self-actualization (Rogers, 1961).

In contrast, a person is considered maladjusted if there is an incongruency between the real self and the ideal self that leads to living an inauthentic life and an interruption to the natural flow toward self-actualization. The maladjusted person cannot be true to self, which leads to distress in daily living and impedes the self-actualizing process. The feeling of incongruence starts when a person encounters *conditional worth*—when worth is dependent upon what he or she does or does not do. These feelings often manifest as anxiety, which the person attempts to relieve through denial and defensiveness (Frankel, Johnson, & Polak, 2019). Rogers believed that the therapist must assist the client in achieving congruency by getting behind the masks that are worn and which develop during the process of socialization. The client comes to recognize that contact with self has been lost by using facades; during therapy, the client begins to access his or her authentic self (Corey, 2017).

■ THERAPEUTIC GOALS OF PCT

The cornerstone of PCT is the view that the client, in a relationship with a facilitating therapist, has the capacity to define and clarify his or her own goals. Accordingly, goals are set by the client and the therapist has little role in goal setting (Elliott, Bohart, Watson, & Greenberg, & Watson, 2011).

There are overarching hopes that the PCT therapist has for the client that are in tune with the overall philosophy of PCT. These include having the client become a fully functioning and congruent person, who can live life authentically, cope well with life's problems, and be engaged in the process of self-actualization. The PCT therapist hopes that the client develops an internal evaluation of self, replaces conditional positive regard with unconditional positive regard, develops the ability to be self-directed rather than looking to others, and be willing to continue growing even after therapy ends (Raskin, Rogers, & Witty, 2008).

■ PERSPECTIVE ON ASSESSMENT IN PCT

Therapists practicing from a PCT approach generally do not find traditional assessment procedures such as taking a psychiatric history, using psychometric tests, and formulating a diagnosis useful because these procedures encourage an external and expert perspective of the client (Elliott et al., 2011). These procedures give the client the message that the therapist is the expert who provides the solutions. In a PCT approach, the client is not considered a sick patient in need of treatment, but a person who is prevented from realizing his or her potential. Rogers believed that diagnostic constructs are inadequate, prejudicial, and often misconstrued (Rogers, 1942). If providing a diagnosis is necessary, a collaborative approach is used in which the client and therapist together formulate the diagnosis (Bohart & Watson, 2011). Rogers saw therapy as collaborative—the client and therapist working together to formulate the ongoing issues in therapy.

The therapist begins the assessment by asking the client where to begin and what issues to work on. The client's phenomenological experience, rather than the presenting problem, is the focus. The therapist is genuine, empathic, and caring and sets aside preconceptions in an attempt to understand the inner world of the client. The therapist creates an understanding atmosphere that encourages clarification and reflection of present feelings and experience (Knight, 2014).

■ THERAPEUTIC INTERVENTIONS IN CLIENT-CENTERED THERAPY

In PCT, each session is considered fresh and unpredictable. Structured techniques and process interventions beyond facilitative listening are avoided. The therapist honors the wisdom of the client and the ability of the client to determine the direction of therapy. This encourages greater self-exploration and improves self-understanding (Knight, 2014). The therapist creates the following facilitative conditions that enhance the therapeutic relationship (Rogers, 1961):

■ NONDIRECTIVENESS

Nondirectiveness, the primary technique used in PCT, is much different than most therapies that use directive techniques such as setting an agenda, reviewing homework, engaging in interpretation, and determining the flow of the session. With nondirectiveness, the therapist uses a discovery-oriented approach and encourages the client to talk freely and direct the session in the way he or she chooses. The therapist is an equal collaborator, rather than someone who directs the client toward a specific goal (Rogers, 1942).

Unconditional Positive Regard

Unconditional positive regard occurs when the therapist accepts and cares for the client as the client is in the moment. This does not necessarily mean that the therapist must like the client or agree with the client, but the therapist does not judge the client. It is essential that the client feels valued by the therapist.

Congruence

Congruence is a match between one's inner and outer experiences manifested by genuineness and authenticity. The client usually enters therapy struggling with a sense of incongruence. The therapist exhibits congruence by openly expressing thoughts and feelings as well as reactions to the client in a well-timed, constructive fashion. As the client experiences the congruency of the therapist, pretenses drop, allowing the client to model the authenticity and genuineness of the therapist (Knight, 2014).

Empathy

Empathy is a very deep understanding of the client. It requires moment-to-moment attunement to the client and an accurate understanding of his or her subjective experience. Showing empathy requires understanding the client's feelings and reflecting them back to the client to help him or her understand these feelings (Elliott et al., 2011).

Affirmations

Affirmations are a form of encouragement and can be verbal or nonverbal. An open, accepting body language (e.g., nodding, leaning forward toward the client) all indicate an open, accepting, safe environment that tells the client the therapist is interested in what he or she has to say.

Active Listening

Active listening is listening with all senses and without exhibiting judgment (either through tone, body language, or verbal responses). The therapist fully concentrates on what is being said rather than just passively hearing the message of the client.

Reflection

Reflection is a restatement of what the client says, which allows the client to hear himself or herself. It is not directive and not advice giving. When the therapist uses reflection, he or she shows an understanding of the client's situation and displays empathy (Seligman, 2014). Reflection is not simply just repeating what the client has said, but sensing the underlying thoughts and feelings as well as the deeper meanings that are communicated (Knight, 2014).

■ CASE STUDY

Background

Pseudonyms and minor changes have been made to protect the client's identity. Rivka is a married Orthodox Jewish woman who came to see me initially at the age of 28 after the birth of her sixth child. She had been married for 9 years at that time. Her children's ages were 8, 7, 5, and 3 years, 15 months, and 6 weeks. She came to see me for psychotherapy. She stated, "I've just not bounced back to myself and I am already 6 weeks post-partum—something is just not right."

Rivka is a client that I saw initially for 18 sessions. She worked on identifying and expressing her feelings, finding her voice, and validating herself rather than punished

herself for having these feelings. She returned to therapy 4 years later to work on assertiveness skills in decision-making. Rivka was someone who did not feel safe in identifying or sharing her feelings for fear of being judged. She worked very hard and made
significant strides in her work in therapy.

She recently reentered therapy and is currently pregnant with her 11th child. She has
weathered many difficulties since her first entrance into therapy, but has been able to
accept and express her feelings and not judge herself too critically. Last year, her sixth
child, the one whom she had right before entering therapy the first time, was diagnosed
with neuroblastoma. The 10th child was 8 months and when she reentered therapy, she
had just found out she was pregnant with her 11th baby.

Transcripts of PCT Sessions

The transcripts selected here were selected from segments from the beginning phase,
middle phase, and final phase of therapy. Also, there is a reentry into therapy phase.

Beginning Phase

APPN:	Hi Rivka. Welcome, please make yourself comfortable. Tell me, what brings you here?
Rivka:	Gosh. I'm not sure where to begin. I just know something is off—not right. I have not bounced back the way I usually do after a baby (*quiet and looking down at her hands*).
APPN:	Umh, hmm (*sits quietly waiting*).
Rivka:	Well, I mean I don't feel present. I feel like I am looking at myself out-side of myself (*looks up*). Does that make any sense to you? Have you ever heard of such a thing?
APPN:	Tell me more, I want to understand.
Rivka:	(*Long pause*) My baby, he is just delicious, I mean the other children they are crazy over him, and he is such a good baby. He only cries when he wants to eat (*looks up at me and down again*). But something is wrong. I don't feel like he is mine, like I am not bonding with him like I did my other babies. I just feel not present, that's the only way I can explain it (*cries softly*).
APPN:	(*Hands client a box of tissues*) And this makes you sad. Does it bring up other feelings as well?
Rivka:	Scared. I think I may be going crazy. Or that maybe, I don't know, maybe because of how I was feeling while I was pregnant, I caused this, this terrible disconnection.
APPN:	Umh, hmm.
Rivka:	(*Long pause*) I'm afraid to even say out loud how I was feeling during the pregnancy. I am afraid to utter the words. But the baby on top of him, my 15-month-old, he was, ah is, such a hard, demanding baby. Gosh, he is an infant himself, and he has all sorts of gastrointestinal (GI) problems. He is allergic to everything, he has tube feedings to supple-ment so he gains weight. He is a terrible sleeper (*cries, dabs tears, and looks at me*). I am a horrible mother, I can't believe that I thought during

this pregnancy that I wished I would miscarry and now God has given me a perfect child—I don't deserve him (*cries more*), especially since I didn't even want him, and now he is so good and I don't think he is mine. And no one knows how I felt, not even Moishe (*her husband*), because a mother should never feel that way about a child (*cries more*). I feel so alone and now I am going crazy. I can't connect with him. I am going through the motions day by day, but I don't feel anything.

APPN: It seems like you are saying these negative feelings during your pregnancy had been so hard for you and that you have had to keep it to yourself because you don't think any mother would feel this way about her unborn child.

Rivka: Yes, right, exactly. What kind of a mother wants her baby to die?

APPN: If you'd like we can explore that. Tell me about yourself as a mother. Perhaps if you would like, describe how you are feeling on a typical day.

Rivka: OK. Yesterday, for instance. Let's see. I got up to feed my baby at 6. Then he went back down and I showered. My husband was already getting the three oldest ready and giving them breakfast. I went in to take care of Yehuda. He's my baby that needs to be tube-fed. I usually have to bathe him again in the morning because sometimes the tube feedings give him diarrhea. So, I was busy with him. He also is not walking yet, so I must carry him everywhere. Once he is all dressed my husband takes the three oldest and Yehuda out the door and then goes directly to the Yeshiva where he learns all day. I quickly got some breakfast and then fed my newborn, Zvi, again. My 3-year-old is generally awake and hungry by now so I feed her, dress her, and then the three of us set off. We only have one car, so I bundle the newborn and my Chana and we walk to the sitter to drop off Zvi. Then Chana and I walk to my work. I am an assistant in a day care. I teach in a 3-year-old class so she can come with me. At 3:30 I leave the day care, pick up Zvi, and walk home. By then it is 4:00 and my husband arrives home with the four children. He has to leave to go back to Yeshiva, so I am now needing to take care of all six kids. This is the hardest time because usually Zvi needs to eat and Yehuda is cranky because he is also hungry. They won't tube-feed him at the babysitter and he is a terrible eater. My 3-year-old is also kvetchy because she is tired, but my 8-year-old is so good with her, and she will usually color with her so I can take care of Yehuda. And little Zvi swings patiently in his swing (*long pause, looks down*). After I get caught up, I make dinner for the others, and then baths and more time with Yehuda. He gets OT so I am working with him on his exercises; he is making good progress and he should be walking soon! He almost stands on his own. And that Zvi is swinging or sleeping, never a peep. Sometimes I almost forget he is there (*looking down, tearful*). By 7:30 my husband gets back home and gets the older kids to bed. He then leaves again by 9 and is home for the night by midnight. We try to eat a quick dinner before he goes back out. Once all six kids are quiet, I then throw in laundry, make lunches, call in a grocery order, and clean up. I am not a neat nick—my house is lived in, but I don't like dirt. I usually feed Zvi one more time and get to bed by 1 a.m. Yehuda usually gets up twice, but my husband and I take turns soothing him or giving him a little food. Then before you know it, time to do it all over again!

APPN:	You described a very busy day. However, I didn't hear you describe too much about how you were feeling, only what you were doing.
Rivka:	(*After a pause*) Hmmm, I didn't even hear you ask me how I felt, I thought you wanted to know what I did. Hmm. How was I feeling? (*Cries and long pause*)
APPN:	Yes.
Rivka:	I am afraid to feel. I am afraid that if I let the feelings come in, I will lose control and how will I care for my family? What if this causes me to go crazy?
APPN:	Crazy? Tell me more about what you mean.
Rivka:	I mean crazy. Like I will need to be locked up in a hospital. Like my children will be taken away. I'm not sure I can do this. Is there a pill to help me? Get rid of this feeling? This disconnection. Or maybe I am being punished. God knows what I thought (*crying*).

Middle Phase

Rivka and I saw each other 18 times over 10 months. This session was a little more than midway through the 18 sessions. She just found out she was pregnant with her seventh child. While she had become much better at owning her feelings and sharing them with her husband, this session illuminated the work she still needed to do in understanding where her feelings came from.

Rivka:	I know I told you last time that I thought I might be pregnant again—well I am, only a few weeks but the pregnancy test was positive last Sunday. Funny you know, since I decided against an intrauterine device (IUD) I knew it would happen. And I can honestly say that I am not feeling ready and I am scared and disappointed. I was hoping it would take a little longer (*to get pregnant*) but I know we will all manage (*long pause*). Much different than the dread and anger I felt while pregnant with Zvi (*laughs*). Listen to me admitting out loud that I was angry! So angry I wanted a miscarriage!
APPN:	In the beginning you carried the feelings within you, such a secret. A dark place for you.
Rivka:	It was amazing. Once I started saying how I was feeling out loud, that disconnected feeling went away. Slowly at first. I told Moishe about the pregnancy and how I was disappointed that it happened so fast. I asked how he felt and he said he felt the same. He also told me he appreciated that I could be honest with him about how I felt. I am still sad about Zvi. I was so absent in his first months of life—I mean absent emotionally. I wonder how this will affect him in the long run, especially now that we are adding another baby—seems like Zvi has not gotten what the others had—a happy, present mother from the beginning.
APPN:	I know I didn't know you before Zvi was born, but I think what I am hearing from you is that when you look back you perceive a very different mother before Zvi. I am wondering if the birth of Zvi just illuminated what was already going on with you in a way you couldn't see prior to that. Just curious what you think about that?

Rivka:	Gosh I have thought about that. You are right. I never expressed my feelings out loud, unless I thought the feelings were what others expected. When I think back to my first babies, they were all good—just like Zvi. It was not until Yehuda that things became more difficult—he needed so much. He still does. You know he is making progress, but it is so slow. He is still needing supplemental feedings. And he is still not walking (*long pause, then she became tearful*). Oh no, I just realized something, it's not that I am angry and disappointed and afraid about being pregnant—I am mad that Yehuda isn't better. And somehow having more babies is a reminder that he is not progressing and I do resent that he needs so much from me. Why can't he just be normal? (*crying*)

Final Phase

This was Rivka's 18th session, her last of her first time in therapy prior to reentering 4 years later. Here she reviews the connections she has made and speaks about the deeper understanding that she has about herself and how she is able to cope better with her feelings now that she has an understanding about where they come from.

Rivka:	Remember how I told you that I was thinking about my mother and her expectations of me? You know, she was really good at not stating directly, "Rivka I expect that as the oldest you will do so and so . . . ." Instead she would say things like, "You are so good at getting yourself and your sisters breakfast, it's amazing that you don't need me to help you." By that time, I probably had three sisters and I was only 6! One of my sisters was just a real picky eater and I remember giving her candy for breakfast, just so I could tell my mother everyone ate. I knew this was not a good idea, but I could not imagine my mother being disappointed in me. And now I am thinking how clever she was—she was probably feeling completely overwhelmed herself, she had 15 children—so she needed me to be a helper. If she convinced me that I was doing a great job, I guess it would be highly unlikely I wouldn't strive for perfection. I certainly don't blame her, but gosh I was 6 . . . and I have been thinking a lot about myself as a mother—do I do that to my oldest kids? (*pause*) I mean, I was only 6.
APPN:	Am I hearing a little resentment toward your mother? You did an awful lot to please her.
Rivka:	Yes, for sure. Boy I would never have admitted that in the beginning. I didn't even realize it in the beginning. I love my mother so much, but now I realize, much of the way I respond to others—especially those that I perceive may judge my skills as a mother, wife, friend, whatever, I just respond in a way that I think I should. It never mattered how I actually felt, only how I thought I should feel. And now I see why I used to be so mean to my sister right below me—she was always easy going, never a care, never a worry, the perfect kid . . . (*pause*).
APPN:	Perfect like Zvi?
Rivka:	Yes exactly. Easier to be angry toward someone who could take it. Now I see when Yehuda was born, with all his problems, he messed up the flow. Not his fault of course, so how could I possibly be mad at him? So, I recognize now that feelings I often have may be misdirected—so they

don't feel "right," they are, well, prohibited. So, I think the disconnection that I was feeling when I started was a defense mechanism against feeling these prohibited feelings (*pauses*).

APPN: And instead carrying them deep inside you?

Rivka: Yes, yes. Because I could not trust myself. I didn't even know how to feel and once I let myself feel then I started to realize that the feelings I was having were often misguided. Targeted often at the wrong person or situation. Oh my . . . what a mess this is!

APPN: You've been meeting other peoples' expectations of you for your entire life. It's a lot to unpack in less than a year. What do you think of your progress?

Rivka: Hmmm . . . well, I have an awareness now that I never had before. I don't need to feel happy and carefree all the time. I can feel angry, frustrated, anxious, sad, or any other feeling. I now also take the time to look at the situations and try to figure out what I am really feeling about. I have become so reflective! Moishe teases, he says, "I know you need time to think about how you feel and then we can talk about it!" He has been a blessing, such an understanding husband. We are all works in progress.

Commentary

We did not have a formal termination, but instead had discussed the difficulties we had in meeting regularly as she had a very busy schedule. However, no matter how many weeks had gone between sessions, Rivka always came back, having given a lot of thought to her feelings and behaviors, and making a lot of connections. She truly wanted congruence. At the end of this session, we had decided to wait until after the fall holidays to set up another appointment. I did not hear from her again for 4 years. However, as I ended every session with "I am here for you whenever you need to come back," she felt comfortable in reaching out and returning to a place where she felt safe and not judged.

REENTRY INTO THERAPY AGAIN: Rivka returned to therapy 4 years after our last session.

APPN: I am so happy to see you again.

Rivka: You remember me? (*laughs*)

APPN: Of course, I remember you. I remember a woman who worked very hard identifying and expressing her feelings. Tell me, what brings you back?

Rivka: Well, my 10th baby is now 8 months old. Remember Yehuda? He is big and gaining weight and eating on his own—no more feeding tube for years! I hardly remember those times. And I just found out yesterday I am pregnant again. I made this appointment before I knew. Lots of stuff going on—which is expected when managing a big family. I was hoping when I made this appointment that I could work on my assertiveness skills—I really want to have an IUD put in—obviously it will be after this pregnancy, but I think my family is big enough (*pauses*). Zvi was diagnosed last year with neuroblastoma. He is doing well.

Just finished his sixth round of chemo. Moishe and I realized when he was diagnosed that we needed to divide and conquer and Moishe has been wonderful. He oversees Zvi and getting him into and out of the city for care. Moishe also handles all the doctor's appointments and then he and I review the plans and options and make decisions. Oh, so I am here because I realized that while owning and expressing my feelings are very important—and I am no longer afraid to feel them—I also need to be able to assert myself in situations that in the past I felt like I had no control over. One of these areas is spacing my kids.

APPN: Mhm . . . hmm. So, are you saying that understanding how you feel and being able to express that to others in your life doesn't necessarily change situations that you would like to change? That you would like to have some control over changing?

Rivka: Yes exactly. I need to be able to do both. If something makes me mad or overwhelmed or unhappy or happy or angry or resentful or whatever, just feeling it isn't enough. Neither is just expressing it! It's been like "thanks for sharing but this is how it is." Now I realize that it is only step one. I need to be heard, yes, but I also need to be able to make changes. And up until now, I have not, I still feel afraid. I feel like a little child who let's big decisions get made by others.

APPN: Because making big decisions might make others unhappy or make them judge you?

Rivka: Yes, I think so. I guess I was also thinking that if I explained to my husband or the rabbi or my mother how I was feeling then they would make the decisions needed to make me feel better. This is crazy, isn't it? I am still not taking responsibility for myself. It took me 4 years to figure this out? Really?

APPN: You sound surprised. But you spent your entire life until 4 years ago never even letting yourself feel. Change does come in steps. The fact that you have made this recognition and now want to do something about it is a big step.

Commentary

I continue to work with Rivka. She is at the end of her 11th pregnancy. Her son Zvi is not doing well and will likely succumb to his disease as his treatments have not stopped the progression. Dealing with the anticipatory grief and all the feelings she is discovering through this ordeal has been a lot, but she is asserting herself in some ways—one example was choosing not to continue treatments that are not working and giving Zvi some time to "just enjoy" without the side effects of the chemo that have been very difficult for him. She and her husband agreed with this decision, but she did receive some negative responses from the community. She stated that in the past this would have probably made her change her mind, but she and her husband have stuck by their decision and although it is very painful to deal with a dying child, she is content that this is the right decision for him. As the therapist, being an active listener, providing unconditional positive regard, and providing Rivka a safe place to explore her emotions in depth with no consequences to outside relationships were the key components in my role. Rivka is the driving force of each session. My key role is to do my very best to be present, nonjudgmental, and understanding.

DISCUSSION QUESTIONS

1. Would you be able to be present with Rivka without being more directive or active in your techniques?
2. What do you mainly hear Rivka saying throughout the sessions?
3. Are you able to empathize with Rivka and enter her experiential world?
4. What are your personal reactions to Rivka?
5. Are you able to accept the decisions that Rivka has chosen for her son Zvi? Do you accept her decision of doing nothing to avoid pregnancy?

REFERENCES

Axline, V. (1947/2002). *Play therapy*. New York, NY: Ballantine.

Bohart, A. C., & Watson, J. C. (2011). Person-centered psychotherapy and related experiential approaches. In S. B. Messer & A. S. Gurman (Eds.), *Essential psychotherapies: Theory and practice* (pp. 1–38). New York, NY: Guilford Press.

Cook, J. M., Biyanova, T., & Coyne, J. C. (2009). Influential psychotherapy figures, authors, and books: An Internet survey of over 2,000 psychotherapists. *Psychotherapy: Research, Practice, Training, 46*(1), 42–51. doi:10.1037/a0015152

Corey, G. (2017). *Theory and practice of counseling and psychotherapy* (10th ed.). Belmont, CA: Brooks/Cole.

Elliott, R., Bohart, A. C., Watson, J. C., & Greenberg, L. S. (2011). Empathy. *Psychotherapy, 48*(1), 43–44. doi:10.1093/acprof:oso/9780199737208.003.0006

Frankel, M., Johnson, M., & Polak, M. (2019). Inter-personal congruence. The social contracts of client-centered and person-centered therapies. *Person-Centered & Experiential Psychotherapies, 18*(1), 22–53. doi:10.1080/14779757.2019.1571435

Greenberg, L. S. (2011). *Emotion-focused therapy*. Washington, DC: American Psychological Association.

Haugh, S. (2018). The handbook of person-centered therapy and mental health: Theory, research, and practice. *Person-Centered & Experiential Psychotherapy, 17*(2), 188–190. doi:10.1080/14779757 .2018.1431565

Kirschenbaum, H. (2009). *The life and work of Carl Rogers*. Alexandria, VA: American Counseling Association.

Kirschenbaum, H., & Jourdan, A. (2005). The current status of Carl Rogers and person-centered approach. *Psychotherapy: Theory, Research, Practice, Training, 42*(1), 37–51. doi: 10.1037/0033-3204.42.1.37

Knight, C. (2014). Humanistic-existential and solution-focused approaches to psychotherapy. In K. Wheeler (Ed.), *Psychotherapy for the advanced practice nurse* (2nd ed., pp. 369–393). New York, NY: Springer Publishing Company.

Miller, W. R., & Rollnick, S. (2002). *Motivational interviewing: Preparing people for change* (2nd ed.). New York, NY: Guilford Press.

Raskin, N., Rogers, C. R., & Witty, M. C. (2008). Client-centered therapy. In R. J. Corsini & D. Wedding (Eds.), *Current psychotherapies* (8th ed., pp. 141–186). Belmont, CA: Thomson Higher Education.

Rogers, C. R. (1942). *Counseling and psychotherapy: Newer concepts in practice*. Boston, MA: Houghton-Mifflin.

Rogers, C. R. (1951). *Client-centered therapy: Its current practice, implications, and theory*. Boston, MA: Houghton Mifflin.

Rogers, C. R. (1957). The necessary and sufficient conditions of therapeutic personality change. *Journal of Consulting Psychology, 21*, 95–103. doi:10.1037/h0045357

Rogers, C. R. (1961). *On becoming a person: A psychotherapists' view of psychotherapy*. Boston, MA: Houghton Mifflin.

Rogers, C. R. (1970). *Carl Rogers on encounter groups*. New York, NY: Harper & Row.

Rogers, C. R., & Freiberg, H. J. (1994). *Freedom to learn* (3rd ed.). New York, NY: Pearson.

Rogers, N. (1993). *The creative connection: Expressive arts as healing*. Palo Alto, CA: Science and Behavioral Books.

Seligman, L. (2014). *Theories of counseling and psychotherapy: Systems, strategies, and skills* (4th ed.). Upper Saddle River, NJ: Pearson Education.

Shostrom, E. (Producer). (1965). *Three approaches to psychotherapy I: Parts 1–3* [Film]. Corona del Mar, CA: Psychological & Educational Films.

Shostrom, E. (Producer). (1977). *Three approaches to psychotherapy II: Parts 1–3* [Film]. Corona del Mar, CA: Psychological & Educational Films.

4

Existential Psychotherapy: An Older Adult Client at a Crossroad

Candice Knight

■ PERSONAL EXPERIENCE WITH EXISTENTIAL PSYCHOTHERAPY

When I was a psychiatric-mental health graduate student in the early 1970s, existential psychotherapy was the major theoretical orientation in my program at Hunter College. Our key textbook was Joyce Travelbee's *Interpersonal Aspects of Nursing* (1966). Travelbee's approach, which she called the Human-to-Human Relationship Model of Nursing, is an application of the existential work of Søren Kierkegaard and the logo therapy of Victor Frankl. Travelbee's approach emphasizes free will and the search for meaning in our clients' experiences of pain, illness, and distress (Travelbee, 1966). She saw psychiatric advanced practice nursing as a way to help clients find meaning in their experience of suffering. Although Travelbee's work was very important during the late 1960s and early 1970s, her untimely death at the age of 47, after a brief illness in 1973, precluded her work in the existential approach to further develop. Nevertheless, this initial introduction to existential psychotherapy had a major influence on my therapeutic approach. Throughout the next six decades, I attended numerous seminars and training programs in existential psychotherapy and trained with some of the giants in the field, including Irvin Yalom, Will Kouw, and Kirk Schneider.

Existential psychotherapy is very effective when working with older adult clients, the largest constitute of my current private practice. Twenty years ago, I completed a 1-year, full-time internship program with older adult clients at a large psychiatric hospital and nursing home. In the years that have followed, I have also worked with older adult clients in assisted living facilities and in my private practice.

Older adults frequently come into psychotherapy with a variety of comorbid psychiatric and medical disorders. Common psychiatric disorders include anxiety disorders, substance use disorders, depressive disorders, suicidal ideation, insomnia, and neurocognitive disorders such as Parkinson's disease and Alzheimer's disease. Common medical disorders include cardiovascular disease, cancer, respiratory disease, diabetes, and arthritis (American Psychiatric Association, 2013; Cassidy & Rector, 2008; Center for Disease Control & Prevention, n.d.).

Many older adults seek psychotherapy, not just for psychiatric or medical disorders, but for psychological issues that are developmentally common to this age group. The most frequent psychological issues are loss and role change. Loss may entail the death of a friend or family member or the loss of a job due to the prejudice and discrimination of ageism in our society. It may include a loss of meaning and purpose in life, a loss of one's youthful appearance, or loss of physical stamina common to aging and illness. In addition, loss may entail impending death and loss of life due to a terminal illness. The role changes commonly seen in older adults include retirement, a decrease of income, a change in living situation, and a decrease of social support. Also common to older adults is an awareness of life regrets that often emerge during this developmental stage (Agronin & Maletta, 2011).

Erik Erikson, in his Developmental Stage theory, identified the last stage of life for those over the age of 65 as *Ego Integrity versus Despair*. He found that if individuals successfully complete this stage, the outcome is the ego strength of *Wisdom* (Erikson, 1950). To help navigate this stage, clients can do an introspective life review in which they celebrate their life successes and work through their life regrets; this leads to a sense of satisfaction and contentment in this last stage of life. Meaning and purpose may also be restored and death is not feared, but rather accepted as a normal phase of life. Unsuccessful navigation of this stage may result in despair with a sense of regret, bitterness, depression, and meaninglessness; death is typically feared and unaccepted (Haight & Haight, 2007). An introspective life review is incorporated into my existential approach when working with older adult clients.

■ FOUNDERS AND LEADERS OF EXISTENTIAL PSYCHOTHERAPY

The formal beginning of existential psychotherapy in the United States can be traced to 1958 with the publication of the book *Existence: A New Dimension in Psychiatry and Psychology* by May, Angel, and Ellenberger (1958). Although many people helped shape the existential psychotherapy movement, Rollo May (1909–1994), Viktor Frankl (1905–1997), and Jim Bugental (1915–2008) were the leaders who played an early role in developing and promoting existential psychotherapy, while Irvin Yalom (1931–) and Kirk Schneider (1956–) are the contemporary leaders involved in further developing this approach.

Rollo May, a psychologist often referred to as the father of American existential psychology, was concerned with the importance of anxiety for self-growth as well as themes of freedom and responsibility. May believed that psychotherapy should be concerned with the problem of *being*, rather than problem-solving (Bugental, 1996). Viktor Frankl, a physician and philosopher interned at a concentration camp when Hitler came to power during World War II, wrote *Man's Search for Meaning* (1963) based on his experiences. This compelling book introduced Frankl's logotherapy, an existential therapy that translates into *meaning therapy*. Logotherapy supports the view that people have the freedom to choose their attitude in any given set of circumstances and discover meaning (Frankl, 1963). James Bugental, a psychologist, focused on living an authentic and responsible life (Bugental, 1965). He contributed a great deal to the practice of therapeutic presence, rather than therapeutic techniques, in conducting existential psychotherapy (Schneider & Greening, 2009). Irvin Yalom, a psychiatrist, addressed the four *givens of existence*: freedom and responsibility, isolation, meaninglessness, and death (Yalom, 1980). Yalom's existential application to group therapy, seen in his widely employed and respected book *The Theory and Practice of Group Psychotherapy* (Yalom, 2005), has solidified an enduring presence for existential therapy in the group therapy modality. Kirk Schneider, a psychologist and contemporary spokesperson for existential–humanistic psychotherapy, is well known for his development of the existential concept of *awe*, and how to cultivate awe in existential psychotherapy (Schneider, 2009). Schneider, cofounder of the Existential–Humanistic Institute in San Francisco, has been integral in fostering a global dialogue of existential themes in psychotherapy, a framework for psychotherapy integration, and a link between existential theory and postmodernism (Schneider & May, 1995).

▪ PHILOSOPHY AND KEY CONCEPTS OF EXISTENTIAL PSYCHOTHERAPY

Existential psychotherapy is a philosophical approach to psychotherapy. It addresses the large, universal themes of life. These themes, considered to be the *givens of existence*, create a focus for existential psychotherapy. They include meaning and purpose, awareness and responsibility, choice and freedom, authenticity and genuineness, connection and aloneness, fear and anxiety, transience and death, belief and faith, love and hate, and awe and wonder (Corey, 2011). Most important to older adults is the theme of meaning and purpose as well as transience and death (Knight, 2013).

▪ DEFINITION OF MENTAL HEALTH AND PSYCHOPATHOLOGY IN EXISTENTIAL PSYCHOTHERAPY

In existential psychotherapy, mental health exists when the existential themes are worked through and resolved. For example, it is important for older adults to give meaning to their life and reduce their feelings of meaninglessness. Older adults may ask questions such as, "Will what I did be forgotten once I am gone?" "Has my life had meaning and purpose?" "Were the choices I made the best they could be?" Mentally healthy older adults accept their mortality and are able to overcome inordinate fear of death. Awareness of death is the terrible truth and must be faced before one can truly live (Schneider & May, 1995). It is also important for older adults to embrace the human condition of aloneness, accept their physical limitations, and take responsibility for their life choices (Knight, 2013).

Psychopathology exists when clients have unresolved existential themes. Clients may not be able to find purpose and meaning; hence, they live a meaningless life. They may not accept the anxiety of being alone or may blame others and not take responsibility for their life. They may also fear death (Bugental, 1987).

▪ THERAPEUTIC GOALS IN EXISTENTIAL PSYCHOTHERAPY

The goal of existential psychotherapy is to help clients face the anxieties of life, freely choose their life direction, take responsibility for their choices, and create a meaningful and purposeful existence. Clients are encouraged to face the anxieties generated by freedom, choice, aloneness, and death. Existential psychotherapy can also help clients recognize how they are not living fully authentic lives, and hence, make choices that will lead to living life authentically (Corey, 2011).

▪ PERSPECTIVE ON ASSESSMENT IN EXISTENTIAL PSYCHOTHERAPY

In existential psychotherapy, the emphasis of assessment is on creating an authentic therapeutic relationship and gaining a phenomenological understanding of the subjective world of the client rather than employing traditional assessment procedures and diagnostic constructs. The existential psychotherapist focuses less on the client's past; instead, the emphasis is on the choices to be made in the present and future. Preconceptions are bracketed in order to be present with the immediate experience during the therapy session (Knight, 2013).

The first few sessions are extremely important for building the therapeutic relationship and understanding the client's values and assumptions about the world. The therapist attempts to understand the client's current life situation as well as the existential themes of awareness, authenticity, freedom of choice, meaning and purpose, potential for meaningful change, and expectations for therapy (Corey, 2011).

Once a strong therapeutic alliance is formed and the phenomenological experience understood, a detailed life review is completed. This is a timeline, from early childhood to the present, which is completed during an early psychotherapy session. This timeline identifies life successes and life regrets and allows the client to reflect on his or her experiences in order to celebrate life successes and work through life regrets (Haight & Haight, 2007). I typically use a simple timeline and offer a sheet of paper with the sequential time periods as shown in Figure 4.1. In each age period, I ask the client to identify one or more successes and regrets.

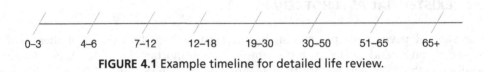

| 0–3 | 4–6 | 7–12 | 12–18 | 19–30 | 30–50 | 51–65 | 65+ |

FIGURE 4.1 Example timeline for detailed life review.

■ THERAPEUTIC INTERVENTIONS IN EXISTENTIAL PSYCHOTHERAPY

Existential psychotherapy does not identify with a specific set of designated therapeutic techniques, but rather employs a set of guidelines for the therapeutic encounter. The existential psychotherapist is free to draw on techniques from other orientations, but places them in an existential psychotherapy framework (Schneider, 2008). Interventions are based on an understanding of what it means to be more fully human. Guidelines can be grouped into three categories: the therapeutic use of self, presence, and experiential reflection.

Therapeutic Relationship

Existential psychotherapy places a high premium on the therapeutic relationship as a healing agent. This relationship is an authentic, I–thou encounter between the client and therapist. It is characterized by mutuality, authenticity, openness, immediacy, and dialogue (Buber, 1937). The use of the therapeutic self is central to the development of an authentic, I–thou relationship; thus, the therapist needs to be mature and have a personal philosophy that is congruent with the theoretical underpinnings associated with the existential psychotherapy approach. It is essential for the therapist to have grappled with the complexities and paradoxes of the human condition and examined and worked through his or her own universal themes of life as well (Schneider & Greening, 2009).

Presence

The existential psychotherapist cultivates the quality of presence. Presence is a subjective experience of being "here and now" in the relationship and participating as fully as he or she is able. It is attending, at a very deep level, to the client's immediate inner flow of experience (Schneider, 2008). Bugental (1987) wrote that the therapist needs to maintain full presence to the client's experience in the moment and to closely attend to the client's immediate inner flow of experience. "Be there!" and "Insist that the client be there!" were well-known mantras of Bugental's existential approach (Schneider & Greening, 2009).

Experiential Reflection

The existential psychotherapist asks in-depth questions about universal themes in order for clients to become aware and experientially reflect on how their life is being lived in the present (Corey, 2011; Schneider, 2008). The client is challenged to grapple with complexities and paradoxes of the human condition and to face the givens of existence. Experiential reflection, through in-depth questioning, addresses the "how and what" of life. It helps clients live more authentically, recognize the range of alternatives and life choices, remove obstacles to freedom, find meaning and purpose, and take responsibility to decide a life direction (Yalom, 1980). For example, a question such as, "How is your freedom impaired?" seeks to bring awareness to the client's obstacles to freedom. Other prototypic questions include:

- "What is the purpose of your life?"
- "What is the source of meaning for you?"
- "You want to live an authentic life, yet you stay in a relationship and a job that gives you little satisfaction. How are you keeping yourself stuck?"
- "What might be accomplished in therapy with me that would help you live a more authentic life?"

■ CASE STUDY

Background

I met Margaret 30 years ago, when she first came to me for psychotherapy. She had a doctoral degree in social work and was teaching presocial work courses at a community college. She had two teenage daughters. She was 41 years of age and contemplating ending her 21-year marriage to her husband. Although she was clear she wanted to leave the relationship, she was unable to make it manifest, and was struggling to solidify the final decision. My work with her entailed identifying and working through the blocks that prevented her from leaving the marriage and living an authentic, fulfilling life. These blocks included unworked through trauma that she experienced during her first 2 years of college, including a rape that resulted in an unwanted pregnancy and consequent abortion. She met her husband shortly after these events occurred and married him that summer after completing her sophomore year of college. She did not deal with the trauma she had experienced, and had decided to *"just leave it in the past and move on with my life."* Over the course of 1 year of existential therapy (48 weekly sessions), she was able to work through the traumatic events of her life and ask her husband for a divorce. She understood that her fear of ending the marriage was based on the semblance of safety he had provided for her when she was unable to muster it for herself as a 19-year-old college student. Soon after the divorce occurred, our therapy terminated.

I enjoyed working with Margaret. I found her to be a thoughtful and motivated client who also had a good sense of humor. After some initial resistance, she was willing to work on her traumatic events and she made a considerable amount of progress in self-awareness and identifying the blocks to her freedom of choosing an authentic life.

Thirty years later, at the age of 71, Margaret returned to therapy for the following reason: "I can't make up my mind whether or not I should retire." She is now remarried and in a healthy relationship with a clinical psychologist. They live in New Jersey. Margaret has one child with her current husband. All three of her children are adults and live independently, although her youngest is still in graduate school and returns home with some frequency. Margaret's parents are both deceased—her father died of pneumonia and her mother from complications due to Alzheimer's disease. Her two brothers are living and doing well. Her older brother, who was a businessman, is retired and lives in Maryland. Her younger brother, who is a physician, is still working and lives in New Jersey. Margaret has no medical or substance use disorder. She was never diagnosed with a psychiatric disorder and never took any psychotropic medication. She currently is a full professor and teaches graduate level social work courses at a university in New Jersey.

When you've been in private practice for a number of decades, it's very common for clients to return after many years, when they encounter difficulty with significant life issues. Clients age with you, and as the therapist, you bear witness to their lives over time, which is very rewarding. This case illustrates this phenomenon.

Transcript of Therapy Sessions

The transcripts presented here were selected from segments of the beginning, middle, and final phase of therapy.

Beginning Phase

The early sessions focused on building the therapeutic relationship and understanding the client's phenomenological experience.

APPN:	Welcome.
Margaret:	Hi. It's good to see you again, I haven't had a session with you in how long, about 20 years, or has it been 30 years?
APPN:	Yes, it's been awhile. It's actually closer to 30 years.
Margaret:	I'm thinking about a clinical instructor that I had years ago who told me: "Never throw away an old chart," so I wonder if you still have my old chart?
APPN:	I do and I reviewed it before you came today.
Margaret:	Great! Well, that's good to hear.
APPN:	I'm going to start with, "What's close to the surface?"
Margaret:	Two things emerge. A part of me wants to tell you what I've been doing for the last 30 years, but then another part just wants to start with what's going on with me now.
APPN:	I'd like you to speak the importance of each part.
Margaret:	(*Speaks to one part of self*) "If I tell her what happened over the past 30 years, she'll know where I've been and what I've been doing. Furthermore, she's probably curious and wants to know. And, I want her to know that I had a good life."

APPN: And, speak the other part . . . .

Margaret: (*Speaks to other part of self*) "I'm here to work on something specific, so why waste time? Time is money."(*laughs*) Well, I think a good place to start is what is going on in my life now. And, what happened over the past 30 years will come out anyway sooner or later.

APPN: That sounds like a great place to start. So, what's going on for you right now?

Margaret: Well, let me just think for a minute. What brings me back here? I guess what really brings me back, what's closest to the surface is, I can't decide what I want to do about my job. And, I'm 71 years old now.

APPN: Uh huh.

Margaret: My mother developed Alzheimer's at 75, and that disease has a pretty strong genetic component. That doesn't mean of course that I'm going to get it. I'm not even thinking I am, but at 71 . . . I'm thinking maybe it's time to retire.

APPN: Uh huh. So, what does that bring up for you?

Margaret: It would be retiring from my teaching position, and a long academic career.

APPN: Uh huh.

Margaret: When I think back, I realize that I actually started teaching in 1975. I had a little hiatus in the 1990s—but, probably, all and all, I've been teaching for almost 45 years of my adult life, 25 years in undergraduate programs, and 20 years in graduate programs.

APPN: Most of your adult working life.

Margaret: Exactly. As well as having a small private practice about the same amount of time.

APPN: Quite an achievement.

Margaret: Thank you. Yes, I feel like it's an achievement, and at this stage of life, most of my friends are retiring. And, the thing that makes me not want to retire is that I really do enjoy what I'm doing, and, I also like the perks that I get. I like the money and there is nothing specific that I would like to do with more free time.

APPN: So, you like what you are doing and the perks you get. And, there is nothing you can think of doing with extra free time.

Margaret: Right, and 71 feels like it's not that old. You know 71 is the new 61! (*laughs*)

APPN: You've named several things that certainly would be in the pro-column.

Margaret: Yes.

APPN: So, you're young, you like what you're doing, and you particularly like the perks and having money.

Margaret: And, I think most important is that I enjoy what I am doing.

APPN:	That's pretty powerful. Could you come up with some things commensurate on the other side of the argument?
Margaret:	Well, when I look back on my life, at times when I wasn't working as much, there's a few go-to things that I do. I exercise more, I play piano, I read challenging books, and I cook gourmet style. I like doing all these things, and when I'm working as hard as I'm working, I don't do them as much. And, when I do read, now, it's usually lightweight books just to relax. And, I just cook the basics now.
APPN:	So, these things you enjoy doing fall by the wayside—exercise, playing the piano, reading difficult books, and cooking more sophisticated, complicated meals.
Margaret:	Yes.
APPN:	So, you engage in more personal care and have more fun when you are not working as much.
Margaret:	Yes, absolutely.
APPN:	And, when you're teaching, you're caring for your students and your mind.
Margaret:	Yes. That's right. In retirement, it's more personal care and more fun.
APPN:	Uh huh. So, those are some compelling considerations.
Margaret:	Yes. And, going back to the other side of the argument, I think my identity is wrapped up in my position as well. I view myself as somebody who is a professional person. I don't view myself as a retired person. I have a lot of negative connotations about that. You know, retired people are supposed to play golf, live in an over 55 community, and get ready to die.
APPN:	Well, your excitement decreases when you think of retirement in these negative ways. You don't seem to like the notion of it.
Margaret:	Right, I don't like the idea of retiring.
APPN:	You seem animated when you talk about cooking and exercising.
Margaret:	Right, and I'm sure there are other things I would also like to do. I'm not somebody who likes to go to my grandchildren's soccer games.
APPN:	What else would you like to do?
Margaret:	Go to more cultural events and travel. I do travel, but I might travel a little differently. Like now, if I travel, it's for a week to 10 days, and maybe if I wasn't working, I would travel for 2 to 3 weeks at a time. I don't like being away from home that much. I can't see myself taking off for 3 months and being a snowbird or even taking a month to travel around Europe. I'd miss my dog and my cat too much.
APPN:	Uh huh. I have an experiment. I'd like you to take both sides of the argument and convince me first why you shouldn't retire and then also convince me why you should. Give me your most vivacious arguments. Speak as if you are giving yourself advice.
Margaret:	OK. (*Speaks to part of self that should not retire*) "Well, you really should not retire. It's totally ridiculous. You're making a good salary. You're in

the marketplace. You're constantly learning. You enjoy it. It's fun. Yeah, there's always a little downside with administration. You don't always get along with administrators. And, you always have to deal with that stuff. But, for the most part it's a very small part. And, the money is really great. It's nice to have that money. You've always liked money. Ever since you were a young kid you always liked your money. And, you were always ready to work for it. You always liked to buy whatever you want. You don't like to scrimp and save."

APPN: It's really hard to talk yourself into retiring after that. You think you can sway yourself to the other side. Have you finished your first argument?

Margaret: No. (*Continues to speak to part of self that should not retire*) "What's the point in retiring? Are you going to go on a spiritual journey? Go to India? Go to some Ashram? You know—it's old. Twenty years ago, you had to climb Machu Picchu. Who needs to climb it now? How many primitive sites have you seen already? You were over in Jordan and rode through the desert of Wadi Rum, had tea with a Bedouin tribe, walked through the rock-carved city of Petra."

APPN: You've had a lot of adventures.

Margaret: Yes. Enough actually. (*Continues to speak to part of self that should not retire*) "You saw the Pyramids in Egypt. You kissed the Blarney Stone in Ireland. You visited the Vatican, Pompei, and took a gondola ride through the canals of Venice. You climbed the Mayan ruins in Mexico. You certainly don't need to see Machu Picchu. African safari? That used to light your fire, but no more."

APPN: Its sounds like you have had quite enough adventure.

Margaret: There are certainly places I want to see, but they are mainly cities. I'd like to go to some cities I haven't gone to—like Prague, Budapest, Vienna, Moscow, Sydney.

APPN: I'm not sure if you are starting to sort of argue the other side or whether that was just an addendum. I'd ask if you could argue the case for retiring.

Margaret: I actually can't think of any good reason to retire. My husband's not retiring. So, what am I going to do? He likes to work. He's younger than me. Oh, OK. (*Speaks to part of self that should retire*) "I say to you, retire! You would read more, exercise routinely, play the piano, and cook gourmet meals. And, you know that sometimes you have to let go of things and enter the fertile void before something new and exciting can emerge."(*Significant silence*)

APPN: Another thought. Sort of an addendum experiment. [Suppose] I were to tell you that you have 5 good, healthful years to live. That's it. From this day forward. Would that affect your decision at all?

Margaret: That's a good question. What would I do?

APPN: I imagine you're counting on living a few more years than that.

Margaret: Right. But, that's a good one—5 years—if I had 5 years. Well, first off, I would get all my affairs in order—get all my pictures together and give a lot of items away to the children rather than put the things in a will.

That's the practical side of me. But I don't think I would move. Would I work if I only had 5 years left? That's a good question. (*Significant silence*)

APPN: It seems as if you're struggling with this experiment.

Margaret: I think what I am afraid of is that if I leave my academic position—where I make six figures—if I give that up, would I then have to worry? (*Speaks to self*) "You can't go out to dinner tonight for the budget doesn't provide for that. You can't go on vacation, for you need to save up a little money for that." I think that is probably the biggest thing. A fear of being constricted. My position gives me money and gives me freedom to do what I want. Financial success has always been important to me. It gives me freedom, which is an important part of my life.

APPN: Say more about that.

Margaret: It is a strong part of my personal history. As you know, I grew up in a solidly middle-class family where my parents both worked hard. And, they were able to live comfortably. They worked hard, but lived comfortably. We would go to dinner usually once or twice a week, we had a cleaning woman, and we always had a nice vacation. I never heard, "Do we have the money?" They were not extravagant and were in fact rather frugal in some ways. Many of my friends' parents lived from paycheck to paycheck and struggled with money. When I was a child, I would do chores for my relatives and save most of the money. My parents got me a bank account when I was 6 years of age and I put money in the account every week. I worked part time as a teenager and all through college—paying it off as I went along with the help of some scholarships. And, since then I've worked full time and did well.

APPN: And, you continued that. You've worked very hard. And, you've been frugal and you've also purchased what you wanted to. It makes sense that that would be a continuing ethos for you.

Margaret: Uh huh. I guess in many ways, I am like my parents and learned from them. I never wanted the stress of not having money to pay my bills and purchase what I want and need. My husband and I own our house and we have a few vacation properties as well.

APPN: So, that gives you a sense of freedom.

Margaret: Yes. Plus, the subjects that I teach are very interesting and keep me updated and in the marketplace. I have all my lectures put together. And, it's really quite easy for me to teach. It's just a matter of going in, teaching my classes, having some fun, and leaving. And, I'm good at it!

APPN: I hear that you enjoy it and get paid well and that you are good at it. I'm wondering what is the most essential source of meaning for you in your position?

Margaret: It's like when you raise children. You try your best to do a good job. But you realize when you get older that you made a lot of mistakes.

APPN: Uh huh.

Margaret: And, you can't redo it unless you have a new batch of children, but most of us do not have that luxury! But, when you're teaching, each year I have a chance to perfect those mistakes. So, each year, it's a new group of social work students. And, what mistakes I've identified, I can correct. And, that's kind of interesting.

APPN:	It's very interesting.
Margaret:	I don't think there are many things in life that you can do that with.
APPN:	True.
Margaret:	And, with good students, they return again and again to remind you of the effect I've had on them. And, the bad ones fade into the woodwork. And, I think what I do is kind of important. It gives me a sense of meaning and purpose that they—the students—are going out into the world to make positive changes.
APPN:	So, a sense of legacy I suppose. Something you are leaving behind.
Margaret:	Definitely. I'm old enough to know that you're forgotten after a few generations—unless you're the president of the United States and you have a library built. Or, maybe if you're a famous singer and you have a song that goes on forever or a star with a movie that lives forever.
APPN:	Well, as far as that's concerned, I think being a professor over decades of time is one of the best hedges against mortality I know of. In terms of if how we exist, we exist in the minds of those we've touched, you've touched a lot of people.
Margaret:	True.
APPN:	So, that has lent your life a lot of purpose and meaning.
Margaret:	Yes. But I think there is more to my conflict than meets the eye.
APPN:	Yes. I agree. We have to bring the session to a close now. We touched on your conflict of retirement as well as themes of freedom, purpose, and meaning. In the waning moments of the session, is there anything else you want to say?
Margaret:	No, this gives me a lot to chew on during the week and I will see you next week.

Middle Phase

The middle sessions focused on completing a timeline and identifying and working through existential issues. Because I had worked with this client in the past, we were able to move more quickly into the middle phase of therapy.

Margaret:	It's good to see you again.
APPN:	One of the tasks I like to do as we begin the deeper part of our work is to complete a timeline. It's important to look at your life and identify your successes and regrets at different time periods. Sometimes, that helps in getting to the deeper issues that prevent you from solving current conflicts.

Margaret:	Yes. Of course. Who was it? Erik Erikson and his ego integrity versus despair? (*laughs*)
APPN:	Yes. That's correct.
Margaret:	Well, I'm not very despairing, but I actually think I have a lot of regrets and I don't want my issue around retiring to be one of them. I remember interviewing my father shortly before he died (I have him on videotape) and I asked him about his regrets. I just thought of this now. He said, he wished he didn't work as hard as he did and had more fun. Do you believe that?
APPN:	Yes. That's powerful that you remember that and you have him on tape.
Margaret:	Well. Let's do the life review.
APPN:	(*APPN gives Margaret a sheet of paper with time periods as a guide to complete.*)
	So, can you write down your successes and regrets? I think they can be a pathway to the question you asked. (*Spends 10 minutes completing timeline*)
Margaret:	Well, when I look back at all different stages, I had a pretty stable childhood. I spent a lot of time in physical therapy for the first 4 years of my life and then had surgery for a birth injury. But, that's more of a trauma and not really a success or regret. And, I worked a lot on that issue in previous therapy and don't have a lot of energy around it.
APPN:	Yes. I see.
Margaret:	One regret that comes to my mind is between the ages of 20 to 41 and staying married to my first husband for 21 years. I married him at the age of 20 and divorced him at the age of 41.
APPN:	So, if you could encapsulate the outcome of what that regret is about, having spent all that time with him, what did it take from you?
Margaret:	Well. In general, just time. Time that could have been spent doing other things. I taught during those years at a community college. I think if I had a partner who was more functional and competent, I would not have stayed so long in that job. I would have moved on to teach at a graduate school. But I felt like I had to be closer to home and to be present more for my children. He was a very incompetent person—an incompetent male. I was in therapy with you when I talked about this person and finally made the decision to divorce him. After that, I moved on with my life, but I never worked through my regrets with staying married to him for so long. He was someone who I had to push and take care of—and shore-up up a lot. He came from a very poor, dysfunctional family—alcoholic father who left the home when he was around 3 years old and a neglectful mother who worked all the time or was out with her friends. He had no healthy parental role models— no one pushed him or studied with him or expected anything from him. He would see his father weekly at a bar and his father was always drunk, and would give my ex-husband a 50-dollar bill. So, he didn't really know how to be a husband or parent appropriately. So, as a result of that, there was a lot of ineffective parenting and he could never be the *bad guy* and set limits. And, I was always trying to get the kids back

on track—to do what I knew had to be done in terms of good parenting. So, I could see all the problems. But yet, I wasn't able to prevent the problems from happening. Some I did, but a lot I didn't.

APPN: Go on.

Margaret: The regret I have is why I didn't get out of the marriage sooner. I knew on my honeymoon that it was a mistake. But, rather than leave, I tried to change things. "Why? Why did it take me so long? With the maturity I have now, I believe a lot of it was introjects of the time—you know, "Till death do us part." So, rather than just ending it and cutting my losses, I attempted to make it work and put a lot of energy into making it work. And, because there was a fair amount of dysfunction, which impacted the kids, there was a lot of cleanup there. So, there was a lot of time and energy wasted. I look back and I say, "Was there anything you learned?" It's sort of like . . . . When I first started working in the mental health field, I remember working at a rape crisis center. After clients would do much of their work, I remember asking, "Well, was there anything you learned from this experience? What meaning did you garner?" Of course, we can garner meaning from anything. So, you can say to me: "What were the pros and what were the cons of staying married for 21 years? What did you learn?" And, yeah, I can come up with things. But I do feel a lot of regret that it was such a long time. Yeah, I could say I achieved some goals. I learned what it was like to be in a dysfunctional family system and what that means. So, when I teach family therapy, I have some reference points to go back to (*laughs*). But it would have been much better if I was in a healthy family system.

APPN: Well, you've provided a vignette of a regret. And, what I find interesting is that you search for meaning in a difficult situation, and you have done this with your clients as well.

Margaret: Yeah.

APPN: I'm wondering if your search for meaning in a difficult situation may actually be a way to avoid feeling.

Margaret: Could be.

APPN: Would you be willing to close your eyes and go inside to deepen the process and see if you have any felt sense in your body about staying in the marriage for such a long time?

Margaret: Yes. I feel tightness in my chest.

APPN: Stay with that.

Margaret: (*Cries for several minutes*) I think there are a lot of tears under that search for meaning!

APPN: Yes.

Margaret: I am so sad that I had such an awful life for 21 years. I was so unhappy and sad but never would let myself fully experience those feelings.

APPN: Stay with the sadness.

Margaret: (*cries*)

APPN: What do you notice?

Margaret:	I feel better. That was enough for now. I'd like to move on now.
APPN:	Then, I'd like to try to pull some of these strands together as we are approaching the end of our time.
Margaret:	Yes.
APPN:	What I heard from you is that you lacked the awareness of your sadness and instead tried to make a situation work, rather than leave. And, that caused you to stay in a situation much longer than you would have liked to stay.
Margaret:	Right.
APPN:	And, you were always a person who would try to fix something. "How can you fix it? How can you make it better?" You were not a person who would abandon something that needed fixing.
Margaret:	Exactly.
APPN:	I'm wondering if there is a connection between that and now. Are you wisely using the time you have left or are you avoiding retirement for there are things left to fix or you just can't let go?
Margaret:	Yes. I see what you mean.
APPN:	So, I'm offering that as sort of a bookend to the session.
Margaret:	Umm. I think that is a nice bookend. I spent 20 years in a marriage where I wasn't getting much out of it. So, a good bookend is to ask myself, "Do I want to spend—if I say I will only have 5 really good active years left—that doesn't mean to say that I won't have more—but assuming—Do I want to stay doing what I am doing now? Will I have regrets? Is my inability to leave my job part of a dysfunctional pattern that may not be meeting my needs?"
APPN:	Like continuing to try to refine and fix rather than . . . .
Margaret:	Yes. Yes.

Final Phase

The final sessions focused on the existential themes of meaning and purpose and living a more authentic life. This is an excerpt from our last session.

Margaret:	I had success this week. Remember, I told you that I never walk out of a movie. Even if it's horrible. I think to myself, "Well, you paid good money to see this movie. You can always find some meaning in it. So, stay and mine something out of it."
APPN:	Yes. I remember.
Margaret:	Right, Right. Well, my husband and I went to see this movie, *Bad Moms*—it was a genre like the *Hangover* movies. It was so self-indulgent and preposterous that I became angry and I felt my anger. Then, I walked out after watching it for only about 20 minutes. And, I didn't worry about mining meaning out of the movie or how much I paid to see it. I just felt my anger and walked out and it felt great.
APPN:	That was a great victory!

Margaret:	Yes. And, my husband was thrilled, for he usually stays with me when I insist upon watching a movie to the bitter end (*laughs*).
APPN:	You found the movie a waste of time and were angry and you just said to your husband, "This movie is preposterous. We're leaving." And, you got up and left.
Margaret:	Exactly.
APPN:	The movie was not a judicious use of your time.
Margaret:	Yes.
APPN:	You were wise enough to know that there was nothing there for you and even if you could mine something small, it was not worth your time and energy.
Margaret:	Precisely.
APPN:	(*Significant silence*)
Margaret:	And, I also have come to a decision. I am going to retire. I have decided to write a letter to the administration that I will retire in June of next year. That will give me 1 last year to teach and get my things in order. I can't tell you how relieved I feel. I realize that I have enough money and that no matter how many times I change my lectures, they will never be perfect. And, that I have done my work. I also realize that I have to let go to see what's next. If there's no room in my life, nothing can emerge. I feel really good about the decision.
APPN:	What do you notice now?
Margaret:	I feel a sense of completeness and certainty.
APPN:	Stay with that awhile.
Margaret:	(*Significant silence*)
APPN:	So, I want to invite you—as we are very close to the end of our time—Is there anything else?
Margaret:	This is a good place to stop. No need to guild the lily.
APPN:	Very good.

Commentary

Margaret had been a client of mine three decades ago at which time we worked on her leaving a marriage. My current work with Margaret was for 24 sessions over an 8-month time period. In the early sessions, I worked on understanding her phenomenological experience and developing a new and mature therapeutic relationship with her. Margaret was able to identify and develop her conflict about retiring. In the middle sessions, we completed a timeline and Margaret identified a number of regrets she had over her life span. There was a common theme in her regrets, which was difficulty letting go of people, places, and things that were not meeting her needs. Instead, she would stay in situations and try to make them work, thus living an inauthentic life. She identified a number of beliefs that kept her stuck, such as, "If I retire, I'll have to scrimp and budget and won't be able to do what I want to do." And, she became deeply aware of her feelings, especially her sadness and anger about staying in situations where her needs were not being met. The vignette presented in the middle phase of the therapy transcript was about her difficulty leaving her first husband of 21 years. This was merely one of many situations that she identified and processed in the middle phase of therapy. In the final termination phase of therapy, Margaret began making small behavioral changes in leaving unfulfilling situations earlier than she had previously. An example was leaving a terrible movie when she realized it was not meeting her needs rather than staying to the bitter end. And, finally, she made a decision to retire and leave her academic position in 1 year. It is hoped that with her new awareness and insight, she will continue to leave unfulfilling situations earlier and not waste time on trying to find meaning where meaning doesn't exist or on trying to change people, places, or things rather than leave.

DISCUSSION QUESTIONS

1. If you were to do a life review, what successes and regrets would you identify?
2. Can you identify a situation in your life where you were stuck and stayed too long?
3. Are there junctures in the therapy sessions presented that you would navigate in a different way as the therapist? If so, what would you do differently?
4. If a person is aware of his or her feelings, how do you think it changes life choices?

REFERENCES

Agronin, M. E., & Maletta, G. J. (2011). *Principles and practice of geriatric psychiatry* (2nd ed.). Philadelphia, PA: Lippincott.

American Psychiatric Association. (2013). *Diagnostic and statistical manual of mental disorders* (5th ed.). Arlington, VA: American Psychiatric Publishing.

Buber, M. (1937). *I and thou.* New York, NY: Scribner & Sons.

Bugental, J. F. T. (1965). *The search for authenticity: An existential-analytic approach to psychotherapy.* New York, NY: Holt, Rinehart, & Winston.

Bugental, J. F. T. (1987). *The art of the psychotherapist.* New York, NY: W. W. Norton.

Bugental, J. F. T. (1996). Rollo May (1909–1994). *American Psychologist, 51,* 418–419. doi:10.1037/0003-066X.51.4.418

Cassidy, K., & Rector, N. A. (2008). The silent geriatric giant: Anxiety disorder in late life. *Geriatrics and Aging, 11*(3), 150–156. Retrieved from https://www.researchgate.net/publication/286963396_The_silent_geriatric_giant_Anxiety_disorders_in_late_life

Centers for Disease Control and Prevention. (n.d.). *The state of aging and health in America.* Retrieved from https://www.cdc.gov/aging/data/stateofaging.htm

Corey, G. (2011). *Theory and practice of counseling and psychotherapy* (9th ed.). Belmont, CA: Brooks/Cole.

Erikson, E. H. (1950). *Childhood and society.* New York, NY: W. W. Norton.

Frankl, V. (1963). *Man's search for meaning: An introduction to logotherapy.* New York, NY: Pocket Books.

Haight, B. K., & Haight, B. S. (2007). *The handbook of structured life review.* Baltimore, MD: Health Professions Press.

Knight, C. (2013). Humanistic-existential and solution-focused approaches to psychotherapy. In K. Wheeler (Ed.), *Psychotherapy for the advanced practice psychiatric nurse* (2nd ed., pp. 369–406). New York, NY: Springer Publishing Company.

May, R., Angel, E., & Ellenberger, H. F. (Eds.). (1958). *Existence: A new dimension in psychiatry and psychology.* New York, NY: Basic Books.

Schneider, K. J. (Ed.). (2008). *Existential-integrative psychotherapy: Guide posts to the core of practice.* New York, NY: Routledge.

Schneider, K. J. (2009). *Awakening to awe: Personal stories of profound transformation.* Lanham, MD: Jason Aronson.

Schneider, K. J., & Greening, T. (2009). James F. T. Bugental (1915–2008). *American Psychologist, 64,* 151. doi:10.1037/a0014551

Schneider, K. J., & May, R. (1995). *The psychology of existence: An integrative clinical perspective.* New York, NY: McGraw-Hill.

Travelbee, J. (1966). *Interpersonal aspects of nursing.* Philadelphia, PA: F. A. Davis.

Yalom, I. (2005). *The theory and practice of group psychotherapy* (5th ed.). New York, NY: Basic Books.

Yalom, I. D. (1980). *Existential psychotherapy.* New York, NY: Basic Books.

Humanistic and Psychoanalytic Play Therapy: A Child With Attention Deficit/ Hyperactivity Disorder and Oppositional Defiant Disorder

Amelia Muir

■ PERSONAL EXPERIENCE WITH CHILD PSYCHOTHERAPY

My introduction to working with children and adolescents occurred while I was a graduate student at New York University studying to become a psychiatric nurse practitioner. I was placed at a community clinic in a low-income neighborhood in New York City treating underserved families. The children at this clinic were referred for a variety of internalizing and externalizing symptoms, and the vast majority had significant trauma exposure. This exposure most frequently occurred as a result of witnessing domestic violence, experiencing abuse (physical, sexual, psychological), systemic racism, immigration stress, having an incarcerated parent, removal from their biological parent's care, and the traumatizing effects of extreme poverty. Several research studies over the past two decades have found that children in urban areas who have been exposed to severe poverty and interpersonal violence have posttraumatic stress disorder (PTSD) rates that are more than double that of combat veterans returning from war (Kletter, Weems, & Carrion, 2009; Tanielian & Jaycox, 2008). Many of the families had intergenerational trauma and complex psychosocial stressors that created an environment of constant stress for the developing children.

While working at this clinic, I was exposed to the writing of one of the pioneers and foremost authorities in the field of play therapy, Virginia Axline. Axline was a psychologist who developed nondirective play therapy in the 1940s based partly on Carl Rogers' principles of person-centered therapy (Sweeney & Landreth, 2009). Her seminal book, *Dibs: In Search of Self* (Axline, 1964), covered her weekly sessions over the course of a transformative year with a 5-year-old boy who was initially described as "emotionally disturbed" by his teachers and parents. Axline demonstrates how play therapists can provide a corrective environment for children by providing "unconditional positive regard, empathic understanding, and authenticity," thereby allowing the individual's intrinsic drive toward "maturity, independence, and self-direction" to be realized (Axline, 1974, p. 10; Nash & Schaefer, 2011, p. 5).

With Virginia Axline's influence in mind, I was struck by how much of a child's symptoms could be reduced by nondirective play therapy alone. This occurred in the majority of cases I saw without ever discussing a child's trauma directly in sessions. One experience that particularly affected me was witnessing the transformation of one 6-year-old boy diagnosed with attention deficit hyperactivity disorder (ADHD) and PTSD who had witnessed a staggering amount of domestic violence in his life. This child struggled greatly in his functioning and displayed severe symptoms of aggression, hyperactivity, and impulsivity across settings. I initially felt that this child would only improve through immediate treatment with psychiatric medications for these symptoms, which I attributed to the ADHD diagnosis. Fortunately, my mentor and supervisor at the clinic was a very patient and perceptive psychiatrist named Dr. Adam Leczycki who encouraged me to give therapy more time.

I had initially tried the strategies that are often recommended in psychiatric training, such as behavioral modification techniques, cognitive behavioral therapy (CBT), and dialectic behavioral therapy (DBT). I might have seen modest reductions in some of his externalizing symptoms, but they were very short-lived, not present in settings outside of session, and often caused the child to become more distressed. After one particularly torturous session for us both, I decided to throw out the chart and stickers I used to encourage "good behavior" and decided to give nondirective approaches a try. This seemed to quickly reduce both of our anxiety levels and allowed more authentic connecting to occur. For most of our weekly sessions from that point on, the boy silently painted while I quietly provided reflections, emotional warmth, acceptance of his feelings, and, most importantly, tried to stay out of his way while he worked through the profound trauma of growing up around constant danger. While I often felt that we were not "doing anything" in these sessions, because the child avoided explicitly discussing the trauma he had experienced, I was awed at the improvements in his functioning and ability to regulate his emotions after just 1 year of these sessions.

Through this experiential learning, I became entranced with the subtleties of using play as a medium for therapy. I started to work with a brilliant supervisor, named Dr. David Rosenthal, who instructed me in Modern Psychoanalytic approaches in play therapy. I later went on to receive more formalized training at the William Alanson White Institute in Interpersonal Psychoanalytic psychotherapy. As a result, my approach is a blend of largely humanistic and psychoanalytic approaches.

■ FOUNDERS AND LEADERS OF PLAY THERAPY

Therapeutic play was first introduced by psychoanalysts in the beginning of the 20th century with the case study of Little Hans by Sigmund Freud (S. Freud, 1909). According to Freud, using play in therapy allowed for promotion of self-expression, wish fulfillment, and mastery of traumatic events. Reenacting traumatic events through the safety of play allows children to experience feelings of control and mastery while releasing the appropriate affect (Nash & Schaefer, 2011). Early analysts working with children viewed play as the "route into the unconscious," much in the way that dream analysis is used with adults (Levy, 2011, p. 43). Anna Freud was another psychoanalyst who later went on to use play while working with children and brought this technique into wider use (1989).

Melanie Klein (1955), also using a psychoanalytic framework, believed that play allowed the child's unconscious material to surface, which could then be interpreted. The therapist could use the interpretations of repressed wishes and conflicts with the child to help them gain greater understanding of themselves (Nash & Schaefer, 2011). Klein also saw play as a medium for children to gain mastery. Klein pioneered the use of miniatures, which is thought to allow real-world representations to be reduced to a manageable level for children. A student of Klein's, D. W. Winnicott, would go on to contribute greatly to the field of child analysis. Winnicott's theories of the "holding environment" and transitional objects are concepts widely used by therapists today (Winnicott, 1953).

Virginia Axline, a colleague of Carl Rogers, later brought humanistic approaches to play therapy through nondirective, child-centered therapy (1974). This approach involves a focus on having the child lead the way, rather than the therapist. Establishing an authentic therapeutic relationship is the main strategy in this approach without a reliance on interpreting the unconscious meaning of the child's play as is done in psychoanalytic approaches.

Another major influence in the field of child therapy was John Bowlby, a physician and psychoanalyst, who developed attachment theory. This theory describes a child's innate tendency to form attachments with caregivers, which serves an important evolutionary role in its survival (Bowlby, 1969). The relationship with a primary caregiver serves as a prototype for future relationships and is ideally a "secure base" from which children can safely explore the world. Psychotherapy serves a reparative role by providing a secure base for children to safely explore their feelings (Bowlby, 1988). Margaret Ainsworth would later build on this theory with an empirical paradigm using the famous Strange Situation procedure (Ainsworth, 1979). Ainsworth categorized an infant's attachment style as secure, avoidant, and insecure ambivalent/resistant. Disorganized attachment, which characterizes the most disordered attachment type, would later be identified by Main and Solomon (1990). Many child therapies have incorporated attachment theory as an important framework for understanding a child's way of relating to themselves and others.

■ PHILOSOPHY AND BASIC ASSUMPTIONS OF PLAY THERAPY

Play therapy is based on the assumption that play is the natural medium for children to express themselves. In much the same way that verbal communication is used by adults in therapy to process their thoughts and feelings, play is utilized to allow developmentally appropriate exploration of the child's inner and external worlds (Nash & Schaefer, 2011). Play therapy is a broad field with many theoretical orientations and approaches, such as psychodynamic, Gestalt, cognitive behavioral, filial, and child-centered (Nash & Schaefer, 2011). For the purposes of this discussion, I will focus primarily on nondirective, child-centered, and psychoanalytic approaches.

■ DEFINITION OF MENTAL HEALTH AND PSYCHOPATHOLOGY IN PLAY THERAPY

Childhood and adolescence are periods marked by immense developmental tasks. Of Erik Erikson's eight stages of development, five occur between birth and 18 years (Erikson, 1950). Trauma, in its most general definition, can disrupt healthy development and cause stagnation or maladaptation at any of the stages. Favorable outcomes for these stages include the development of a basic sense of trust, feelings of autonomy, the capacity to initiate one's own activities, the ability to apply oneself toward achievement of a goal, and a sense of individual identity.

The construct of psychopathology is generally incongruent with the conceptualization that children have an inherent tendency to move toward self-actualization in child-centered approaches (Sweeney & Landreth, 2009). Definitions of mental health by theorists in this framework typically focus on achieving congruence between a child's actual experience and the child's concept of self (Axline, 1947). Incongruence between experience and self-concept results in maladjustment, which leads to internalizing and externalizing behaviors that typically prompt a referral for therapy.

In psychoanalytic approaches, psychopathology is generally understood to involve unresolved intrapsychic conflicts that result in neuroses. When a child's psychological and emotional needs are inadequately supported by caretakers, a negative introjection of a "bad parent" develops, causing the child to view the world as dangerous and themselves as "not good enough" (Winnicott, 1971). Rigid ego defenses then develop, which "creates a psychopathology of defensive splitting of the self from the ego for preservation" (Green, 2011, p. 64). Goals of child therapy are similar to adult forms of psychoanalysis, namely by "increasing ego control by expanding consciousness" (Levy, 2011, p. 45). This helps the child to achieve equilibrium between the inner and outer worlds, leading to greater regulation of impulses (Green, 2011).

■ THERAPEUTIC GOALS IN PLAY THERAPY

For children, play is the developmentally appropriate "language" in which they can increase their self-expression and understanding, bond with another person, engage in relaxation, prepare for adult life through role-play, improve emotional regulation, and strengthen ego functions (i.e., control impulses, reality test, problem-solve, self-observe, gain a sense of mastery; Schaefer, 1993). Part of the therapeutic value of play is the safety it provides for children to have a place to dramatically act out psychologically dangerous material. It is an interactive endeavor in which the child "may develop a greater capacity for awareness of self and other, for better affect regulation, and for participating in social relationships in more satisfying ways" (Levy, 2011, p. 52).

The therapeutic frame allows children to "destroy symbolically, differentiate from, and use the therapist to advance their development" (Levy, 2011, p. 52). The therapist acknowledges the child's experiences, with the goal of integrating disavowed self-states, promoting greater complexity in the child's self-concept, and more flexibly experiencing dissociated parts of self (Saari, 1993). This process of giving voice to disavowed parts serves to differentiate affective states, distinguish feeling from acting on it, and allows for the emergence of a coherent narrative (Slade, 1994). Winnicott's view of play asserted that therapeutic play serves as a "transitional phenomena" in which the child's intrapsychic and external realities interact (Winnicott, 1971). This transitional space allows children the opportunity to internalize their relationships with primary caregivers, cocreate new representations of self and others, achieve greater acceptance of conflicting feelings, and improve capacities to relate to others (Levy, 2011).

■ PERSPECTIVE ON ASSESSMENT IN PLAY THERAPY

The initial assessment of a child necessitates not only gathering information from the child but also collecting collateral information from parents and sometimes outside parties, such as teachers or caseworkers, as children usually lack the developmental ability to provide a cohesive history. A child therapist typically gathers information from primary caregivers about how a child is functioning at home, in school, and in social domains. Clinicians also gather important developmental information, such as details of the pregnancy and birth, achievement of milestones, and quality of early bonding experiences (especially during the first year of life).

Something that is unique in working with children is that they rarely are seeking treatment on their own accord. Similarly to adults who enter treatment "by force," such as through court-mandated orders, children are usually brought by others who feel that there is "something wrong with them." In other cases, parents may be ordered to bring their children to therapy by child protective services. As a result, clients may "resist by using false and exaggerated cooperation or direct challenges and aggression" (Gitterman, 1989, p. 169). In order to engage a child who is brought to services with this idea of "imposed" treatment in mind, a therapist must identify areas of discomfort for the child that therapy may be able to alleviate, though these may be different goals than the referrer originally specified (1989). Balancing a working alliance with the adults in a child's life while also honoring the subjective needs of the child is essential to therapeutic work with children.

■ THERAPEUTIC INTERVENTIONS IN PLAY THERAPY

Play therapy may be conducted in a variety of ways, depending on the therapist's theoretical orientation. Materials utilized may also vary, but generally play therapists use toys and art supplies that a child can use projectively and symbolically (Nash & Schaefer, 2011).

Nondirective Play

In nondirective play, children are allowed the space to express themselves freely and direct the agenda with little direction from the therapist (Nash & Schaefer, 2011). Nondirective play, a humanistic approach, is based on respect and confidence that the child has the ability to direct his or her own process. It requires that the therapist maintains unconditional acceptance and positive regard for the child. There are no limits placed on the child unless the behaviors are dangerous or destructive. The therapist recognizes the feelings the child is expressing and reflects those feelings back in such a manner that helps provide insight into the behavior. The therapist helps the child identify his or her feelings in response to what is happening in the play, rather than what may actually be going on for the child in his or her life (Axline, 1974).

Therapeutic Relationship

Across theoretical orientations, the relationship between the therapist and child is an essential aspect of the treatment (Levy, 2011). In psychoanalytic approaches, the engagement of the therapist in the drama of the child's play is itself the therapeutic intervention (Levy, 2008). A safe therapeutic relationship creates a secure base in which children are permitted to explore parts of themselves that are in conflict, disavowed, or dissociated (Winnicott, 1971). During play, a child is able to act out psychologically dangerous thoughts and feelings while maintaining plausible deniability within the safety of the therapeutic relationship (Levy, 2008).

The therapist models for the child how thoughts and feelings may be freely accepted and addressed in more productive ways (Levy, 2011). Child therapists must be able to "tolerate uncomfortable states that may be painful, hard to imagine, or even repulsive" as these feelings of countertransference are seen as a form of "implicit communication" (2011, p. 52). Much of the symbolic meaning of play may never be fully understood by the therapist; thus, special attention must be paid to these feeling states to better understand the child's experience of him or herself and the world.

Holding Environment and Containment

D. W. Winnicott posited the idea of the "holding environment" (1965). Ideally, an infant develops with a holding environment in which the "good enough mother" provides comfort and emotional resonance when he or she is distressed. Winnicott argues that the primary purpose of the therapeutic relationship is to provide a corrective holding environment, which often "takes the form of conveying in words at the appropriate moment something that shows that the analyst knows and understands the deepest anxiety that is being experienced, or that is waiting to be experienced" (Winnicott, 1965, p. 240). This promotes the child's ego-strengthening and self-integration.

Wilfred Bion's theory of containment is similar to the holding environment but differs in important ways. According to Bion, an infant projects onto its mother intolerable feelings, which the mother then experiences (or "contains"), and finally gives back the feelings in a form the infant can manage (Reisenberg-Malcom, 2001). This allows overwhelming emotions to be safely experienced and integrated by the child and, in turn, reflected upon. A therapist can provide containment for the child by putting into words his or her overwhelming feelings, which can be used as "building blocks for emotional and intellectual development" (2001, p. 171).

Use of Interpretations

The use of interpretation, a cornerstone of adult psychoanalysis, is varied among child analysts. Anna Freud viewed interpretation as an essential aspect of child analysis. In her model, analysts are to use interpretations of transference and ego-defenses to help children become more aware of their inner conflicts (A. Freud, 1989). Klein also asserted that interpretation is essential in working with children as it "advances analysis by removing repression of intrapsychic material," allowing an individual insight into unconscious conflicts (Levy, 2011, p. 45).

Winnicott differed in his view of using interpretations in child therapy. His view posited that it was the therapist's participation in play that provided the therapeutic value; therefore, interpretations out of the frame of play were not required (Winnicott, 1971). This dynamic interaction creates opportunities for the child to reenact his or her relational models using the therapist and develop new configurations of self and self with others without the need for interpretations of the symbolic material.

■ CASE STUDY

Background

I first met Nick when I was interning as a nurse practitioner student at a low-income community mental health clinic in New York City. He had been receiving individual psychotherapy for about 6 months when he was referred to me for a psychiatric evaluation for diagnostic clarification and to determine if medications were indicated. Nick was a 5-year-old boy of Puerto Rican descent living with his biological mother Lisa (then aged 26), his maternal grandmother (in her early 50s), and intermittently with his maternal grandfather (also in his early 50s).

Nick was originally referred for mental health services by the principal of his kindergarten about 2 months into the school year. The mobile crisis team had been called by the school due to concerns about Nick's oppositional and aggressive behaviors. He frequently acted inappropriately in the classroom and had many sexualized behaviors, such as touching other students inappropriately, exposing his buttocks, simulating sexual acts, and using sexualized language. The school also contacted child protective services out of concerns regarding his sexualized behaviors. The case was eventually closed and there was no conclusion drawn as to whether Nick had experienced any sexual abuse or inappropriate exposure from other sources, such as viewing pornography or seeing adults engaging in sex.

One of the striking aspects of this case was the discrepancy between school and parental reports on his functioning. He was described by school staff as "constantly" in trouble during pre-K with his externalizing behaviors only worsening in severity during his kindergarten year. Lisa stated during intake that she was "not aware" of any past behavioral issues and stated that she did not have any concerns about his behavior outside of school. Teachers reported that Nick tended to form intense attachments with other students quickly but struggled to maintain friendships. He often alienated other children with his verbal or physical aggression. Lisa described Nick as "popular." She was quick to blame other children or teachers when instances of peer conflicts were pointed out.

Nick's family had an extensive history of psychiatric conditions, though his mother was somewhat guarded about full details. He last saw his biological father about a month before he was referred to the clinic and his involvement in Nick's life was very inconsistent. Nick's father had a history of serious mental health issues (diagnosed with schizophrenia or bipolar disorder, according to Lisa) and was completing an inpatient substance use program for heroin addiction at the time of referral. Nick's mother and maternal grandmother were both in treatment for depression and anxiety. Nick was named after Lisa's older brother who had committed suicide after discharge from a psychiatric facility when she was an adolescent. Of note, it was the 10-year anniversary of his death a few days prior to his referral. Nick had witnessed his maternal grandmother become dysregulated at home and throw several dishes in reaction to this anniversary, which Lisa reported made him "anxious and fearful."

Although Lisa denied having any knowledge that Nick had been exposed to anything "traumatic," it became clear from history taking that he had been exposed to unstable relationships with caregivers and a chronic level of stress in their home throughout his life. Additionally, Lisa reported that Nick had seen adult horror movies at his maternal grandfather's home. She expressed concern about Nick spending time with this grandparent after this and described him as "mentally ill." Nick's disruptive behaviors were reported to have worsened after spending time with his grandfather, but there were conflicting reports from his mother about how much time he was still spending with him. Nick had also been exposed to his father and grandfather being intoxicated in the past, but it was unclear what exactly these incidents entailed.

When I met Lisa for the first time, she appeared highly anxious and somewhat skeptical about the clinic's involvement. She was largely minimizing of Nick's behavioral issues and had little insight into the severity of his symptoms. Lisa had two prior cases with child protective services and expressed concern that "people were trying to take away [her] kid." Lisa could not recall the details of her first case but indicated that the second case was called in by her mother out of concerns about Lisa's parenting when Nick was 2 or 3 years old. Nick was connected to mental health services for the first time as a result of this case and had completed 2 years of individual play therapy for oppositional behaviors. Details of this course of therapy were largely unknown as Lisa was reluctant to share details or allow communication with past providers.

Lisa tended to rationalize his sexualized behaviors as normal childhood curiosity and was reluctant to discourage his "self-expression" or cause him to feel shame about his body. She denied that Nick had been exposed to any sexual acts in or outside of the home but reported walking around partially nude at home. She felt that the real issue was that the school did not know how to handle his provocations and was unsupportive of his needs. Lisa was reluctant to pathologize Nick's behaviors but she agreed that it was inappropriate to touch others in sexualized ways at school. She presented with an attitude that it was Nick and her against the world.

Lisa's pregnancy with Nick and his achievement of developmental milestones were described by his mother as "normal." Lisa had been living with her parents at the time of his birth and was experiencing relationship stress with Nick's father due to his ongoing substance abuse. Nick was described as being very difficult to soothe as a baby and "constantly" crying. Lisa also reported experiencing postpartum depression and anxiety in the first year of his life. Descriptions of Nick's temperament along with the presence of maternal mood symptoms raised concerns for impaired bonding and attachment in the child's early life. Extensive research on the effects of maternal depression has shown that negative effects on the child may last well after the mother recovers and raises the risk of the child developing mood disorders even into adolescence (Murray & Cooper, 1999). Additionally, children of depressed mothers have an increased risk of insecure attachment, sleep disturbances, difficulties self-regulating, separation issues, decreased empathy, and behavioral problems (Field et al., 2007; Martins & Gaffan, 2000; Stein et al., 1991).

Nick had some tactile sensitivities, difficulty with transitions, and some obsessive tendencies, but there was not a concern for autism spectrum disorder based on other assessment data. He had no known medical issues and was not taking any medications for other conditions. He was diagnosed at the clinic with ADHD, oppositional defiant disorder, and an unspecified trauma- and stressor-related disorder. It was never fully clear how Nick had come to possess such detailed knowledge of sexual acts (whether it was through abuse, exposure to pornography, or by seeing adults engage in sexual acts), but it was apparent that he had experienced chronic, attachment trauma since early infancy.

During the psychiatric evaluation, Nick's presentation vacillated between a regressive and sweet persona to hostile and provocative. He appeared eager to interact and receive validation from me while also seeming to enjoy my exasperation as he jumped wildly on the furniture. The moment that stands out the most from my first encounter with him was the climax of his dysregulation where he threw a toy with great force at my head while smiling. With the adrenaline of the moment getting the best of my therapeutic presence, I attempted to limit-set and said something sternly to him. He immediately appeared deflated and started sucking his thumb while curled up on the couch. This moment efficiently illustrates his disorganized and anxious/avoidant attachment style (Ainsworth, 1979). He clearly craved the nurturing and bonding that he was deprived of in his early development, but he was severely impaired in his ability to evoke this response consistently from others.

After Nick received about a year of therapy, his original therapist left the clinic and the case was transferred to me during my first month of working as a nurse practitioner (I went on to work full time at the clinic where I had first met Nick as an intern). I felt some anxiety going into our first session together as I remembered the intensity of aggression and oppositional behaviors that I had observed during the initial evaluation with him. Even with his outwardly "difficult" behaviors, I quickly felt a great fondness for Nick. I saw the fragile child underneath the defensive aggression who craved warmth and connectedness with others. Over the course of a year and a half of work together, Nick made significant strides in his ability to relate to others, manage his frustrations, and experience positive emotions. In the text that follows I will outline some of the nondirective approaches that I utilized in our work together and the phasic shifts in his presentation.

Transcript of Therapy Sessions

The transcripts presented here were selected from segments of the beginning, middle, and final phase of therapy.

BEGINNING PHASE

In the early sessions, Nick was frequently critical and rejecting of me, which helped me to understand how he had internalized interactions with others and some of the disavowed negative feelings he had toward himself. Our sessions always included power struggles (often over minor infractions), difficult transitions, and feelings of frustration for us both. There were many crying tantrums. Nick was highly anxious, perfectionistic, and angry during this period. The countertransference I experienced was that of being ineffective, anxious about making mistakes that would upset him, and eager for the calm moments when we felt connected (though, of course, we were connecting during negative interactions too). After our sessions, I was often left thinking, "I'm the worst therapist in the world."

A mistake I made in my early work with him was to try to name how his critical statements made me feel (i.e., "It hurts my feelings when you say that" or "That isn't very nice language to use"), which did not show that I accepted him as he was. Instead, I essentially shamed him for speaking freely in session and did not allow a holding environment for his negative feelings. This approach reinforced his feelings of inferiority, as well as his inability to relate to others.

In this following excerpt, I will show how I later shifted my approach and instead went with his resistance. Instead of trying to discourage his negativity through behavioral modification, cognitive strategies, and limit-setting, I attempted to model ego-strength by accepting his criticism and being curious about the sources of these feelings. This curiosity serves to accept the impulse or feeling behind his behaviors and plant the seed that there is a difference between impulse and action. The therapeutic goal is that he will eventually be able to talk about the feelings and not act on them. By calmly accepting his critical statements about me, I showed that one's imperfections could be accepted and even talked about. Only when I was able to demonstrate that I could accept all of him without crumbling, or enacting the common experience of rejection that he usually received from adults, did his negative behaviors eventually diminish.

(As I approached him in the waiting area, he started talking immediately.)

Nick:	You know I've been really, really good.
APPN:	Oh?
Nick:	Yeah. I've been really good so I should get something. C'mon let me show you.

(He leads me into the area where we pick out supplies for the session and started to look through a bin filled with different kinds of craft tape.)

Nick:	Look I'll show you. I've been really good for years here, right?
APPN:	What does it mean to be "really good"?
Nick:	I'm good with you. I haven't been fighting or talking back.
APPN:	It would be alright if you wanted to do that here. We could talk about it.

Nick:	I need some boy tape.
APPN:	How do we know if something is "boy tape"?
Nick:	Something with a lot of it so I can take it home.
APPN:	It's okay that you want to take home something that belongs to the clinic but you can't actually take it.
Nick:	I need this tape so I remember you between weeks.
APPN:	Ah . . . I see. So, what we need to do is find something that could help you to remember me between visits?
Nick:	Yeah. I'll forget if I don't have this. (*He tries to put a tape roll in his pocket.*)
APPN:	It's okay that you want to take home something that belongs to the clinic, but you can't actually take it. It's so frustrating when we can't have things that we want. (*He puts the tape roll back.*)
Nick:	But I really need it.
APPN:	Maybe we could make a picture of us together for you to look at in between visits? (*Nick ignored that suggestion.*)
Nick:	Alright. C'mon. Let's go. We need to get started. We don't have a lot of time. (*Nick leads the way to my office. We have to pass through a heavy hallway door that he struggles to open by himself.*)
APPN:	Here, let me get that.
Nick:	(*shouting*) Hey! Nobody asked you!
APPN:	You know, you're right. I can really get in the way sometimes. (*He gets to my office door and finds that the door is locked.*)
APPN:	Should I open the door?
Nick:	Yeah, you can open the door (*stated calmly*).
	(*We normally use a room dedicated for play sessions that does not have a desk or items that are off-limits, but today we had to use my small office instead. Nick runs in and tries to grab items from the top of my desk.*)
APPN:	Oh man . . . I brought you to the wrong office. I just realized how many things are in here that we can't play with! You need an office where you can play and you don't have to worry about things. (*I shake my head.*) I hate this. What are we supposed to do? (*Nick ignores this at first and continues to keep grabbing items off my desk.*)
APPN:	This is going to be tricky . . . I know there are things you really want to touch but they aren't for us to play with. How can I help you stay in control? (*Nick picks up my stapler.*)
APPN:	Oh man, that's one of those things we can't use. (*I say with a disappointed tone in my voice*). Should I let you know what things I have in this room that we can't play with?
Nick:	Yeah, okay.
APPN:	Okay everything behind this line is stuff we can't use, but anything on this side of the line is okay for you to touch. (*Nick does not verbally*

	acknowledge what I said to him, but he shifts tasks and starts on the craft project.)
Nick:	Okay, we're going to make a fortune teller out of this paper and tape.
APPN:	Okay, what should I do? *(Nick then proceeds to instruct me step-by-step how to complete the craft. He hovers over me and makes comments about my progress.)*
Nick:	No! You're doing it wrong!
APPN:	Oh man, really? I hate when I mess up.
Nick:	Look at this! This is totally ruined! *(He holds up a piece of paper that I did not fold perfectly in half and rips it into little pieces.)*
APPN:	Oh, I can really mess things up sometimes. Should I try it again?
Nick:	Here, start over.
APPN:	I really hope I do a better job this time.
Nick:	You're doing it wrong again! Look at this! You're no good at this.
APPN:	I guess I'm not really good at this. How did I get this way?
Nick:	You're disgusting.
APPN:	I can be disgusting sometimes. What should I do about it?
Nick:	Your breath smells.
APPN:	My breath can smell sometimes. What should I do? *(I continue to complete the craft while Nick looks over my work.)*
Nick:	Look at this! You messed up. This is disgusting. You're disgusting. *(He rips up the paper for a second time.)* Start over.
APPN:	I can really be disgusting sometimes. And, I keep making mistakes. I feel so frustrated with myself when I can't get it right.
Nick:	You're not very smart.
APPN:	That's true. I've been told that before. How did I get this way? What should I do about it? Maybe you can help me.
Nick:	Here do it this way. *(Nick demonstrates how to fold the paper correctly and becomes frustrated when it does not line up perfectly.)* This is ruined! *(Nick starts to cry loudly.)*
APPN:	What is wrong with this paper? It just won't do what we want it to do. *(We then tried completing the craft for a third time and this time he appears satisfied with the result.)*
Nick:	Okay, let's go show Mommy. *(He rushes out to the waiting area and proudly shows his mother the craft.)*
Lisa:	Oh wow, Nick. That's really nice. You did a really good job.
Nick:	*(Quietly to me)* You did a good job. *(His voice then becomes very regressive while he talks to his mother and me.)*
Nick:	I can do a flip on my bike. Really, I can! But I don't like to do it because I get scared and I don't like to show off.

APPN:	Oh, I get really scared on my bike too. (*As the three of us have a casual conversation in the waiting area while they get ready to leave, Nick wanders over to the elevator and stands in the doorway.*)
Lisa:	(*Suddenly shouting*) Don't do that! Why would you do that?! You know better than that! You could get hurt! (*The sudden shouting startles both Nick and me. He appears deflated but seems to recover quickly.*)
Nick:	Let's go put the things away. (*Nick surprises me by wanting to walk with me to return the supplies, which he normally does not like to do. As soon as his mother was out of earshot, he begins negotiating.*)
Nick:	Okay, I would really like to take home this roll of tape so I can think of you when I miss you this week.
APPN:	Oh man, I wish that you could take things home from the clinic, but these items need to stay here.
Nick:	(*Shouting in a deep voice*) You lied! You should never lie. You said that I could take it home. I can't believe you would do that! You're so stupid. Why would you do that?!
APPN:	Oh, I've let you down.
Nick:	You don't understand! Nobody's listening to me! I'm never gonna see you again! I have no friends. You're my only friend. (*He starts to cry loudly and thrash his arms.*)
APPN:	I'm your only friend and I'm letting you down. That's really terrible. I wish there weren't so many rules. (*Nick pulled his arm back as if to punch me.*)
APPN:	Hey! It's okay for you to want to hit me but it's not okay for you to actually hit me. You can tell me if you want to hit me. (*He stopped himself and lowered his arm.*)
APPN:	What if I put the tape in an envelope on my desk and save it for you to use when you come back here next week?
Nick:	No!
APPN:	Oh man, I have lots of bad ideas. (*I wrote Nick a note on a piece of paper that said, "Amelia is thinking of you," in an attempt to offer him an acceptable transitional object.*)
Nick:	(*Looking at the note briefly before throwing it in the garbage*) This isn't good enough.
APPN:	I've really let you down. We can talk about it more next time, if you'd like. It's time to go now.

Middle Phase

In the middle phase of our work together, Nick and I found more comfort with each other and he achieved more positive results across settings. Reports from his teachers indicated that he was advancing academically, having more positive peer interactions, and generally was able to follow the classroom routine and rules. He had not had any recent sexualized behaviors and had only one physical fight at school that semester, which was a significant decrease from his nearly daily incidents the year before. In session, I observed Nick as increasingly able to express positive feelings, less perfectionistic, and having fewer tantrums. While he still engaged in limit-testing, I had a better understanding of the countertransference feelings of incompetence, anxiety, and being out of control that these behaviors provoked. As a result, I was able to depersonalize his attacks and recognize them as transference feelings of unmet needs and projected or displaced hostility (Gitterman, 1989).

A critical part of Nick's treatment was the work that I did with his mother Lisa. For better or worse, Nick's mother was a fierce advocate for him. At worst, she was in denial about the significance of his impaired functioning while projecting blame onto others. At best, he had an involved parent, who clearly loved him very much, and tried to look out for him as best as she knew how.

Lisa presented as extremely suspicious for the first several months that we worked together. She could even be intrusive at times in the treatment. For example, whenever we changed treatment rooms from week to week, Lisa would ask to see the room before we started and would sit as close to the door as space would allow. She even barged into a session once when Nick was having a tantrum to scold him about it. The effect of this smothering and anxious caregiving was readily apparent in Nick. I observed the internal conflict around his desire to be treated like an infant versus his desire to be independent and separate from caregivers. I began to see the risky maneuvers that Nick would make while walking down a flight of stairs or jumping around on furniture as a way that he unconsciously tried to make me feel the anxiety he felt when he was with his mother. My ability to manage my own anxiety during sessions became an essential component of my work with Nick.

While I had observed other clinicians and school staff try to explicitly limit-set with Lisa around her intrusive behaviors and try to point out Nick's role in his troubles, I adopted a similar approach with her that I used with Nick. I accepted her fears around Nick's safety (which I surmised was part of her wish to see the treatment rooms first) and listened intently about her feelings of being misunderstood by school staff. I showed her that I accepted Nick (another one of her fears) by calmly stating that he was doing great work in session even when internally I felt defeated and anxious after some particularly trying weeks.

Nick started to request the occasional dyadic sessions where Lisa would join the two of us. I modeled for Lisa how Nick could calmly be redirected instead of using frightening threats about real and imagined danger. I did not become overly concerned when he would push limits and I demonstrated that I trusted him to keep his body safe. I noticed that over time Lisa became much less anxious and intrusive with Nick.

I believe that much of Nick's hyperactivity came from being internally overstimulated by various feelings and impulses that were too much for him to manage. The more that I followed his lead and avoided making contact unless he requested it, the less micromanaging and critical he was with me. Even giving positive feedback can be too overstimulating for some children. It may also serve to shape a child's behavior in session to be more approval-seeking from the therapist and discourage the expression of thoughts or feelings out of fear of disappointing the therapist. I learned to adopt phrases like "not bad" to convey positivity instead of more verbose or affect-laden expressions.

In the following excerpt, you will see how Nick was now able to express more positivity, garner attention from me through positive interactions, and transition more easily. These were significant gains for a child with a severe attachment disorder.

As I approached Nick and his mother in the waiting area, I witnessed a touching moment between them that demonstrated an important shift in their relationship. Nick was eating a snack and his mother gently dabbed a napkin on his face to clean him in a nurturing but not infantilizing manner. Nick smiled and seemed to enjoy the care.

APPN:	Hey guys, how's it going?
Lisa:	Hey, Amelia!
Nick:	(*Smiling bashfully and saying quietly*) I missed you.
APPN:	I missed you too, Nick. I'm really glad to see you today.
Nick:	C'mon, let's go!
APPN:	Okay, hang on one sec. Lisa, we're going to be in a room just around the corner through these doors. (*I expected Lisa to ask to see the room as she normally would do.*)
Lisa:	Okay, no problem. Nick, I'll be here and I'll see you guys when you're done.
APPN:	Okay, sounds good. We'll see you in 45 minutes.
	(*Nick and I walked back to the treatment room and passed a piece of equipment that belonged to another program. Nick ran to touch it.*)
APPN:	Oh Nick, that actually belongs to someone else. We can look at it though.
Nick:	(*Responsive to my direction*) Oh, okay. I want to show Mommy. Mommy, look! (*running quickly to grab Lisa*)
Lisa:	Wow, that's really cool!
	(*Nick and I continued on our way to the treatment room.*)
APPN:	Nick, there is something here that we can play with and something that we can't touch. How should I let you know? Would saying "red light, green light" work?
Nick:	Yeah, that's okay.
APPN:	Okay, cool. Thanks for letting me know how I can help you.
	(*We entered the treatment room, which we had never used before.*)
Nick:	Wow! Look at this! (*He hurriedly runs around the room inspecting the toys and exclaiming positively.*) This is so cool!
APPN:	Oh, I'm glad you like it. It is pretty cool in here.
Nick:	C'mon, let's make a bracelet.
APPN:	Okay, what should I do?
Nick:	Here, you sit down and I'll make you food. (*Nick proceeds to start "cooking" for me in the play kitchen.*)
APPN:	Wow, that's really nice of you. I'd love some food.
Nick:	What should I make you? Do you like fish?
APPN:	You can make whatever you'd like. Fish sounds great.
Nick:	Okay, I'll make that. (*Nick then starts to sing a kid's song and asks me to play the song on my phone.*)
APPN:	Okay, is this the song?
Nick:	Yeah, that's it! (*He then starts to sing and dance while he worked in the play kitchen.*)

APPN:	How should I make the bracelet? What kinds of beads should I use?
Nick:	Whatever you want. (*For the first time, Nick continues his activity and does not hover over me as I complete the craft.*)
APPN:	Oh, okay. How is this? (*I show him my progress and ask for his input periodically.*)
Nick:	Yeah, that looks good. Keep going. (*I stumble into an issue trying to fit certain beads onto the yarn.*)
APPN:	Oh man. I feel frustrated. I can't get this to work. (*Nick calmly walks over to inspect the issue.*)
APPN:	I'm nervous that I can't get this to work the way I want it to.
Nick:	Here, let me try. (*He struggles for a few moments, unsuccessfully.*)
APPN:	Hmm . . . maybe this will work. Would it be alright if I tried something? (*Nick silently gives me back the bracelet.*)
APPN:	Ah, here we go!
Nick:	Here, your food is ready!
APPN:	Oh, wow. This looks delicious! Not bad.
Nick:	Here, let me cut your food for you. (*Nick tenderly pretends to cut up my food for me.*)
APPN:	Thank you so much. I needed that help.
Nick:	Here, let me get the dishes.
APPN:	Should I help?
Nick:	No, you just sit and keep making the bracelet. Let's listen to another song. Can I see your phone? (*Nick grabs my phone quickly before I have a chance to respond and proceeds to put on a music video with images from various horror movies in it.*)
APPN:	Hmm . . . I don't know about this video.
Nick:	No! It's fine!
APPN:	What if we just listened to the music and didn't look at the video?
Nick:	No! Put it back on! (*Sensing a power struggle melt down, I changed tactics.*)
APPN:	You know, I think this video is a little too scary for me. I know you're old enough to watch it, but it makes me feel really scared!
Nick:	(*Laughing a little*) No . . . .
APPN:	(*I continued, playfully*) Yes! It's too scary for me! I can't watch things that are too scary. I'm going to put it over here so I can't see the scary stuff.
Nick:	Okay . . . .
APPN:	I'm almost finished with the bracelet and there's about 5 minutes left to play today. (*Nick seems to ignore the comment about time being almost over.*)
Nick:	Here, you need to make a bracelet for mommy too.
APPN:	Oh yeah?

Nick:	Yeah, she needs one. (*I quickly complete a bracelet for Lisa while Nick dances and talks about the music.*)
APPN:	Okay, it's time to go now.
Nick:	What! No! You didn't make me a necklace! You said you would!
APPN:	I did?
Nick:	Yes! You have to! (*Starting to cry loudly*)
APPN:	I feel so disappointed when we don't have enough time to do all the things we want together.
Nick:	I need it!
APPN:	I hate when we have to say goodbye. It's really hard when we're having fun. We can finish the necklace next time, though. (*Nick appears deflated but starts off toward the waiting area.*)
Nick:	Mommy! Look what we made today! (*Nick proudly showed his mom the necklace.*)
Lisa:	Wow, you guys. That's really cool!
Nick:	We had fun today! (*Nick excitedly bounces around the waiting room while Lisa and I talk.*)
Lisa:	(*Saying somewhat bashfully*) I'm sorry that we missed so many sessions . . . I tried to be better about communicating with you about when we couldn't come.
APPN:	Yeah, you really did a good job with that. That was really helpful when you texted ahead of time that you guys couldn't make it, thank you. It really helps to know ahead of time. See you next week. (*Nick gave me a quick hug.*)
Lisa:	See you next week. (*Nick calmly walked out with her.*)

Final Phase

After about a year and a half of working with Nick, he transferred to a school on the other side of the city from the clinic. Nick and Lisa always had a suboptimal attendance record to appointments, but the change in schools made it even more difficult. After weighing out some options, Lisa and I agreed that it made sense to transfer Nick's treatment to the clinic based in his school. Following is a transcript of our final session together.

	(*I greet Nick in the waiting area where he is sitting calmly with Lisa and working on his homework.*)
Nick:	Hey, c'mon. It's time to play.
APPN:	Okay, Nick. Are you ready to walk with me to our room?
Nick:	Yeah, let's go.
APPN:	Before I can open the door, I have to tell you about this room. I didn't pick the best room for us to use today! There are things being stored in here that we can't touch. What's the best way for me to let you know what we can and can't touch? Red light, green light?

Nick:	Yeah, that's okay.
APPN:	Okay, thanks for letting me know how I can help you stay in control. (*He runs into the room and starts to look quickly at all of the items in the room.*)
APPN:	This area is all "red light" but everything over here is okay. (*Nick does not respond but he listens to the directive.*)
APPN:	Nick, I think Mommy mentioned it again before you came today, but I just want to remind you that today will be our last time playing together. Is there anything you'd like to talk about right now?
Nick:	No, let's play a song.
APPN:	Okay, what should we listen to?
Nick:	"Murder on My Mind"! Let's play the video.
APPN:	Oh, that sounds like it might be too scary for me to watch! (*I say this playfully.*) We can just listen to music. But if it's too scary for me, I might not be able to listen to the whole thing. (*Nick proceeds to play the song, which is filled with inappropriate language. I allow him to play a few seconds before turning it off.*)
APPN:	Oh, this song is a little too scary for me. I wonder what it's about? What do you like about this song?
Nick:	Let's make a puppet show.
APPN:	Okay, what should I do?
Nick:	You be this guy and I'll be this guy. (*We each pick up our puppets and I wait for Nick's direction.*)
Nick:	Okay, let's have a fight.
APPN:	Okay, how should we do that? (*Nick starts to have his puppet kick and punch mine in an exaggerated manner. I follow his lead and make sound effects as our puppets fight.*)
Nick:	Now they're kissing! (*Nick starts to have his puppet simulate kissing on mine. I pull my hand back to break physical contact.*)
APPN:	Oh, it looks like they aren't fighting anymore. What was the feeling behind that kiss? Can you help me understand? (*Nick makes a joke about two boys kissing and starts to get more sexually aggressive with his puppet. I pull my hand out of the puppet.*)
Nick:	They're having sex!
APPN:	It's okay if you want to talk about sex in here. It's okay to talk about anything in here.
Nick:	Here, you be the girl puppet now.
APPN:	Okay, now what should I do?
Nick:	Let's get married (*He looks at me while saying this.*)
APPN:	Our puppets are going to get married? What do married people do?
Nick:	They have sex! Take off your clothes!

APPN:	(*I respond using the puppet.*) Oh, I don't think I want to do that with my body. I have no problem if that's how you feel. You can talk to me about it, but we can't do it. Here in therapy we're allowed to talk about everything and anything.
Nick:	(*He stops with the sexualized play and switches gears.*) Okay, we can play a game instead.
APPN:	I'd like to do that with you.
Nick:	Let's play catch.
APPN:	Okay, where should I stand?
Nick:	Here, do it like this and I'll stand over here. (*Nick and I proceed to play catch with a piece of pretend food.*)
APPN:	Ouch! That one hurt my hand.
Nick:	Are you okay?
APPN:	Yeah, I'm okay. Thanks, for asking that.
Nick:	Here, let's hit it back and forth with our hands like this.
APPN:	Ouch. This kind of hurts my hand.
Nick:	Are you okay?
APPN:	Yeah, I'm okay. Thanks for checking. I'll try to hit it with a different part of my hand. (*Nick and I keep throwing the toy back and forth with each other. He was acting very silly and tried to make me laugh as we did this. Some of his throws went a little wild as a result.*)
Nick:	Oh, I'm sorry. Are you okay?
APPN:	Yeah, that's okay. Thanks for asking. Maybe we should throw something softer so that it doesn't hurt as much.
Nick:	Okay. How about this stuffed animal?
APPN:	That's a great idea. I think that will be easier to catch. (*Nick and I play catch for a few minutes more. He continues to be very silly and starts to fall on the ground dramatically after each throw.*)
APPN:	Oh, you're making some cool moves with your body today.
Nick:	Let's play "ninja" now. Here, let me show you. I learned how to do nunchucks karate. Here, you do it like this. (*Nick starts to demonstrate some "karate moves" using two puppets. He is able to do it safely at first. He then starts to get closer to me and is more aggressive in his maneuvers.*)
APPN:	Uh, oh. I'm starting to feel afraid. This toy could hurt me. (*Nick does not respond and starts to actually hit my body with the toys.*)
APPN:	What did I do that made you want to hit me? (*Nick continues swinging the toy wildly.*)
APPN:	(*with a deeper voice*) Nick, it's okay if you *want* to hit me. But you can't actually hit me. This is starting to hurt my body. (*I say a version of this a few times, but Nick does not back off. He is more disorganized in his movements and appears very emotionally activated.*)

APPN:	Okay, Nick. I have to move over here now because my body is starting to get hurt. Can we sit over here for a minute? (*I lead Nick over to the couch where we sit down together. He quickly appears more regressed and curls his knees into his chest. He starts to suck his thumb while rubbing my thumbnail with his other hand, making the smallest bit of physical contact.*)
APPN:	We only have a minute left today. I wrote you a goodbye card. Would you like to read that together now or later when you're home with Mommy?
Nick:	. . . with Mommy.
APPN:	Okay, no problem. I just wanted to let you know how much I've enjoyed playing with you for the last few years. I think you are such a special person and I've learned a lot from you. I'm going to miss seeing you every week.
Nick:	I'll miss you too. (*Nick says this quietly and quickly gets up to leave.*)
APPN:	Okay, Nick. I'll walk you back to see Mommy now.

Commentary

Nick had made some considerable progress since he first started at the clinic, but he showed some predictable signs of regression toward the end of work together. Termination can be difficult for any client but a child with an attachment disorder is likely to have an even more pronounced response to this kind of ending. The ending of therapy can activate unconscious feelings of loss for other important figures in the client's life. In Nick's case, termination may have activated feelings of loss and complex feelings of rage and hostility about his cutoff from his biological father.

In our final session, the emotional activation of termination appears to have brought more aggressive and sexual impulses toward the surface. I demonstrate how I attempted to continue to provide a holding environment for these impulses and accept them nonjudgmentally. Even when Nick becomes more overtly aggressive and sexualized in his play, I try to respond in ego-protective ways by making comments about myself rather than Nick (i.e., "My body is starting to get hurt," versus "*You* are hurting my body"). When Nick asks to play a song during the session that is filled with inappropriate language, I allow it in order to open the conversation up about the personal meaning such a song has for him. It is clear that choosing a song with the word "murder" in its title has significance for the feelings activated by termination (i.e., feelings of anger that I am being "killed off" or a desire to think of me as "killed" as a way of coping with the loss).

As we terminate our therapeutic work together, I find that one of the changes I am most struck by is how Nick asks several times if "[I'm] okay?" during this session. This small but profound statement illustrates his growing ability to consider someone else's feelings and take ownership over his role in an interaction. There is still much to be accomplished in his therapeutic journey, but I believe that this shows a strengthening of his ego that is vitally important for his development of self and ability to relate well with others.

DISCUSSION QUESTIONS

1. What other strategies could be utilized if a child was not responsive to the therapist's attempts to redirect physical aggression toward him or her in the session?
2. How can a therapist convey understanding toward a child who does not engage verbally during play therapy sessions?
3. How can a therapist explain the usage of "play" in child therapy to a parent who insists that his or her child must "talk about his or her problems" to reach therapeutic goals?
4. How might a child therapist explain to a parent why his or her child appears to be more symptomatic during the termination phase?

REFERENCES

Ainsworth, M. S. (1979). Infant–mother attachment. *American Psychologist*, *34*(10), 932–937. doi:10.1037/0003-066X.34.10.932

Axline, V. (1947). *Play therapy: The inner dynamics of childhood*. Boston, MA: Houghton Mifflin.

Axline, V. (1964). *Dibs: In search of self: Personality development in play therapy*. Boston, MA: Houghton Mifflin.

Axline, V. (1974). *Play therapy*. New York, NY: Ballantine Books.

Bowlby, J. (1969). *Attachment. Attachment and loss: Vol. 1. Loss*. New York, NY: Basic Books.

Bowlby, J. (1988). *A secure base: Parent-child attachment and healthy human development*. New York, NY: Basic Books.

Erikson, E. H. (1950). *Childhood and society*. New York, NY: W. W. Norton.

Field, T., Hernandez-Reif, M., Diego, M., Feijo, L., Vera, Y., Gil, K., & Sanders, C. (2007). Still-face and separation effects on depressed mother-infant interactions. *Infant Mental Health Journal*, *28*(3), 314–323. doi:10.1002/imhj.20138

Freud, A. (1989). The role of transference in the analysis of children. In C. E. Schaefer (Ed.), *The therapeutic use of child's play* (pp. 141–150). Northvale, NJ: Aronson.

Freud, S. (1909). *Analysis of a phobia in a five year old boy*. London, England: Hogarth Press.

Gitterman, A. (1989). Testing professional authority and boundaries. *Social Casework*, *70*(3), 165–171. doi:10.1177/104438948907000306

Green, E. J. (2011). Jungian analytical play therapy. In C. E. Schaefer (Ed.), *Foundations of play therapy* (2nd ed., pp. 61–85). Hoboken, NJ: Wiley.

Klein, M. (1955). The psychoanalytic play technique. In C. E. Schaefer (Ed.), *The therapeutic use of child's play* (pp. 125–140). Northvale, NJ: Aronson. (Reprinted from *American Journal of Orthopsychiatry*, *25*, 1955, 223–237.)

Kletter, H., Weems, C. F., & Carrion, V. G. (2009). Guilt and posttraumatic stress symptoms in child victims of interpersonal violence. *Clinical Child Psychology and Psychiatry*, *14*, 71–83. doi:10.1177/1359104508100137

Levy, A. J. (2008). The therapeutic action of play in the psychodynamic treatment of children: A critical analysis. *Clinical Social Work Journal*, *36*, 281–291. doi:10.1007/s10615-008-0148-2

Levy, A. J. (2011). Psychoanalytic approaches to play therapy. In C. E. Schaefer (Ed.), *Foundations of play therapy* (2nd ed., pp. 43–59). Hoboken, NJ: Wiley.

Main, M., & Solomon, J. (1990). Procedures for identifying infants as disorganized/disoriented during the Ainsworth, strange situation. In M. T. Greenberg, D. Cicchetti, & E. M. Cummings (Eds.), *Attachment in the preschool years* (pp. 121–160). Chicago, IL: University of Chicago Press.

Martins, C., & Gaffan, E. A. (2000). Effects of early maternal depression on patterns of infant–mother attachment: A meta-analytic investigation. *Journal of Child Psychology and Psychiatry*, *41*(6), 737–746. doi:10.1111/1469-7610.00661

Murray, L., & Cooper, P. J. (Eds.). (1999). *Postpartum depression and child development*. New York, NY: Guilford Press.

Nash, J. B., & Schaefer, C. E. (2011). Play therapy basic concepts and practices. In C. E. Schaefer (Ed.), *Foundations of play therapy* (2nd ed., pp. 3–13). Hoboken, NJ: Wiley.

Reisenberg-Malcom, R. (2001). Bion's theory of containment. In C. Bronstein (Ed.), *Kleinian theory: A contemporary perspective* (pp. 165–180). London, England: Whurr Publishers.

Saari, C. (1993). Identity complexity as an indicator of health. *Clinical Social Work Journal, 21,* 11–24. doi:10.1007/BF00754909

Schaefer, C. E. (1993). *The therapeutic powers of play.* Northvale, NJ: Aronson.

Slade, A. (1994). Making meaning and making believe: Their role in the clinical process. In A. Slade & D. P. Wolf (Eds.), *Children at play: Clinical and developmental approaches to meaning and representation* (pp. 81–107). New York, NY: Oxford University Press.

Stein, A., Gath, D. H., Bucher, J., Bond, A., Day, A., & Cooper, P. J. (1991). The relationship between post-natal depression and mother–child interaction. *The British Journal of Psychiatry, 158,* 46–52. doi:10.1192/bjp.158.1.46

Sweeney, D., & Landreth, G. (2009). Child-centered play therapy. In K. O'Connor & L. Braverman (Eds.), *Play therapy theory and practice: Comparing theories and techniques* (2nd ed., pp. 123–162). Hoboken, NJ: Wiley.

Tanielian, T., & Jaycox, L. H. (Eds.). (2008). Invisible wounds of war: Psychological and cognitive injuries, their consequences, and services to assist recovery. Santa Monica, CA: RAND. Retrieved from https://www.rand.org/pubs/monographs/MG720.html

Winnicott, D. W. (1953). Transitional objects and transitional phenomena: A study of the first not-me possession. *International Journal of Psychoanalysis, 34,* 89–97. Retrieved from https://psycnet.apa.org/record/1954-02354-001

Winnicott, D. W. (1965). *The maturational process and the facilitating environment: Studies in the theory of emotional development.* (pp. 230–241). London, UK: The Hogarth Press and the Institute of Psycho-Analysis. Retrieved from http://doctorabedin.org/wp-content/uploads/2015/07/Donald-Winnicott-The-Maturational-Process-and-the-Facilitating-Environment-1965.pdf

Winnicott, D. W. (1971). *Playing and reality.* New York, NY: Routledge.

Group Therapy: Stages of Group Development

Richard Pessagno

■ PERSONAL EXPERIENCE WITH GROUP PSYCHOTHERAPY

I have had many group experiences throughout my graduate program. During my group practicum, I worked with a psychiatric nursing graduate faculty member in coleading a 10-week support group for recently divorced men and women. This experience allowed the faculty member to observe firsthand my development of group leadership skills, while providing me with direct supervision.

Providing another opportunity for group therapy exposure, all psychiatric nursing graduate students in my program were encouraged to join a semester-long Gestalt psychotherapy group. Led by a psychologist from the student counseling center, this group experience allowed each member to assume the role of a client. In addition, it provided firsthand experience to address personal issues as well as build cohesion among the cohort. After graduation, I joined a supervision group for new clinicians from social work, psychology, and family therapy. The supervision group was provided by a highly experienced social worker who utilized psychodrama as the group therapy approach. This was a great learning environment, furthering my appreciation for group work.

These experiences deepened my interest in group therapy. In my career, I have led a wide variety of groups, including support groups for newly diagnosed cancer patients, gay men with HIV, and individuals grieving a murdered family member. I had the opportunity to lead or co-lead short- and long-term process groups for adolescents, gay men, individuals newly diagnosed with bipolar disorder, and patients being treated within acute care psychiatric units.

Groups have been an integral component of my practice. My doctoral project examined the use of short-term group psychotherapy as an evidence-based intervention for first-time mothers with postpartum depression. The project articulated the therapeutic value of groups and highlighted how the group experience improves symptomatology.

Throughout my career, Irvin Yalow's work has served as a theoretical framework for groups I have either led or facilitated. It also provided me with greater appreciation for the groups in which I served as an educator, team leader, and team member. The American Group Psychotherapy Association is an organization that has provided opportunities for continuing education, professional networking, and a means of achieving certification as a group psychotherapist.

■ FOUNDERS AND LEADERS OF GROUP PSYCHOTHERAPY

The beginning of group psychotherapy in the United States can be traced to 1932 when Jacob L. Moreno presented his group therapy approach to the American Psychiatric Association and coauthored a monograph on the subject with Hellen H. Jennings and Ernest S. Whitin (Moreno, Jennings, & Whitin, 1932). Moreno's group approach was later called Psychodrama and included improvised dramatizations of events from patients' lives utilizing role-plays and the creativity of the group. In the 1950s, two major types of groups emerged. The first type was the T-group (training group), also known as the encounter or sensitivity group, which was pioneered by Carl Rogers (1970). It was a method where members learn about themselves and about group process through their interaction with each other using feedback and role-play. The second type was the "hot seat" group, pioneered by Fritz Perls. In this type of group, the therapist works with an individual group member on an intrapersonal issue, while the other group members remain as observers. These observers have emotional reactions to the work being done, which may be worked with later in the group; and, they are sometimes brought into the session in order to help heighten awareness and contact for the individual group member working on the "hot seat." Later, in 1980, Bud Feder and Ruth Ronall edited the book *Beyond the Hot Seat*. Here they emphasized interpersonal interactions as well as whole group interactions within a Gestalt therapy framework. Most Gestalt therapists today include intrapersonal, hot seat work as well as interpersonal and whole group interactional work in their group therapy approach.

In 1970, Irving Yalom wrote the first edition of his book, *The Theory and Practice of Group Psychothera*py. Now in its fifth edition, Yalom is considered one of the foremost experts on group psychotherapy. He has developed the concept of therapeutic factors that group therapy provides. He strongly believes that group therapy affords the opportunity for members to learn about their relationships with others; thus, much of his emphasis is on the interaction of group members (Yalom & Leszcz, 2005).

Marianne Schneider Corey and Gerald Corey have written a number of group therapy textbooks and workbooks as well as produced a number of group therapy videotapes to help graduate students in the mental health field learn how to conduct group therapy (Corey, 2016; Corey, Schneider-Corey, & Haynes, 2014; Schneider Corey, Corey, & Corey, 2018). Their method is an integration of intrapersonal, interpersonal, and whole group themes and methodically helps the student learn this powerful approach to psychotherapy.

■ PHILOSOPHY AND KEY CONCEPTS OF GROUP PSYCHOTHERAPY

A well-established body of evidence supports group psychotherapy's usefulness as a reliable and effective treatment modality. It is appropriate for a wide range of clinical issues and diverse patient populations (Burlingame, Fuhriman, & Mosier, 2003). Group treatment's effectiveness has been demonstrated in a variety of practice settings across the behavioral health continuum. The approach has been used to address many types of interpersonal issues and help individuals resolve relational problems. These types of challenges can often cause individuals to feel isolated due to the belief that their experiences are not shared by or similar to other people's experiences.

Groups provide a medium through which participants have the opportunity to bridge connections with others (Breitabarm et al., 2015). These connections can reduce the sense of isolation and affirm a shared experience. Group treatment provides members not only a means by which to identify remedies for relational challenges in the now but also ways in which to avoid problems in the future. A group modality offers individuals the opportunity to confront the obstacles that impede their ability to develop deeper and more satisfying relationships through challenging participants to identify different ways of connecting, communicating, and engaging with others. All of these are more enhanced and effective when a group has developed a strong sense of group cohesion (Steen, Vasserman-Stokes, & Vannatta, 2014).

Therapeutic Factors

Yalom and Leszcz (2005) described 11 therapeutic factors related to psychotherapy groups. Therapeutic factors can best be defined as elements or principles, which develop out of group processes. These factors come about during group therapy sessions relative to individual group members, the group as a whole, or the group leader. Therapeutic factors help or benefit members.

The Installation of Hope

Often, by the time people seek group psychotherapy, the issues with which they struggle have caused them to feel overwhelmed, leading to despair. This sense of despair creates a lack of hope. However, bringing individuals together who have similar problems and a similar sense of despair creates the opportunity for group members to witness and experience even small changes that occur in other group members, while also noting even small changes within oneself. When these changes are both acknowledged and supported by others within the group, a sense of hope surfaces. Yalom and Leszcz (2005) noted that gaining a sense of hope is an essential element that needs to occur before anything else can be achieved within the group.

Universality

Group therapy establishes a sense of universality for its members in spite of the negative personal beliefs and attitudes held by group members. For many individuals, negative thoughts and beliefs, such as having the inability to connect with others or the fear of being unlikeable, can lead to an experience of extreme isolation. Within the group experience, the acceptance of others is often able to reduce this isolation and promote a sense of connection. A major factor in group psychotherapy is the cultivation of a belief among all members in universality—essentially, that they are not alone.

Imparting Information

Within the group, information is shared and exchanged by members and the group leader. This inevitable exchange is, at times, both implicit and explicit in nature. The group leader might provide information about the symptoms associated with bipolar disorder, as well as verbalize observations or make supportive comments. When these types of exchanges occur between the group therapist and the group members, the exchanges can promote change within the group, as well as motivate group members.

Altruism

Humans are social by nature, and we tend to reach out to others who are in need or struggling. However, people who are struggling can find it difficult to accept help. Groups provide members with the opportunity to share not only personal struggles but also personal self-awareness that arises from accepting others' help. Through this self-awareness, the desire to assist and help others has therapeutic value.

Corrective Recapitulation of the Primary Family Group

Within the context of the group, members may find themselves repeating various unhealthy patterns of interaction, which were experienced within their families of origin. Group members may attempt to consciously or unconsciously work through family of origin conflicts through their interactions with other group members and the group therapist. This type of "recapitulation of the primary family group" is well suited for group therapy as it can occur and be processed effectively in a structured, safe environment.

Development of Socializing Techniques

The group can become a therapeutic space where members develop new ways of interacting while becoming aware of patterns that have created barriers to connecting with others, leading to isolation. Within the context of the group, members learn how to form healthy connections with others by challenging each other to examine social patterns that may have negatively impacted relationships. The group becomes a safe environment, not only to challenge one another, but also to offer support as members learn to create change.

Imitative Behavior

As group members strive to create change, they may copy or imitate the behaviors of other members or even the group therapist. This type of experimentation provides the opportunity to explore different ways of interacting and connecting with other people. It can also aid group members' self-exploration, which can enhance learning.

Interpersonal Learning

Groups are the ideal medium for members to learn about both intimacy and relationships. The group environment provides a supportive space for members to not only develop but also gain an appreciation for interpersonal connectedness. Through the group process, each member's self-disclosure lays part of the foundation on which other members work through their issues, such as trust. Learning through these experiences helps members gain a deeper appreciation of their own motivations and behaviors, which can promote self-awareness.

Group Cohesion

Group cohesion is one of the key therapeutic factors involved in group therapy. Through the process of building group cohesion, members can begin the work of the group. Cohesion within groups is built on establishing trust in and feeling accepted by other members. Through these elements, members experience a sense of contentment, self-worth, and hopefulness.

Catharsis

Group cohesion increases the likelihood members will share their feelings and emotions, which can lead to healing and personal growth. Thus, most people must feel safe in the group before they are willing to express deeply personal emotions. This "letting go" of emotions can be a profound experience, which is a foundational element of the therapeutic process. This type of catharsis benefits members who share their deep feelings and emotions as well as other group members, because processing shared experiences can lead to healing and growth.

Existential Factors

A wide range of struggles is inherent to the human experience, including grief, loss, and anguish. During our lives, we have a sense of our own mortality, which is inescapable. This awareness is a shared experience among humans, which can lead to a sense of oneness with other people. Responding to this knowledge with stillness and acceptance leads to a deep appreciation of life's fragility and the responsibility everyone must take for their lives (Yalom & Leszcz, 2005).

Categories of Groups

There are many types of groups. In the context of mental health treatment, groups serve a variety of purposes and functions. Depending on their knowledge, skills, and training, psychiatric nurses can develop, coordinate, and lead groups.

Psychoeducational Groups

Psychiatric nurses, when working with patients to improve knowledge or impart health-related information, frequently offer psychoeducational groups. Such groups are offered in a variety of clinical settings and facilitate the sharing of information on a wide range of topics related to physical and mental health. The purpose of this type of group is to increase knowledge on specific topics, such as medication, anger management, addiction, and self-improvement. Psychoeducational groups focus primarily on improving the knowledge of both patients and families to achieve optimal health and functioning. These groups are typically time-limited and specific topics are chosen before the groups begin. The education provided during this type of group can be formal or informal relative to how information is exchanged, using discussions, readings, and handouts.

Support Groups

Support groups are another type of group conducted by psychiatric nurses as well as lay members. These groups provide an environment in which individuals have an opportunity to share and support each other based on a common issue and shared experience. Some examples include people with a recent medical diagnosis such as diabetes, individuals who have experienced the death of a loved one, or family members who are caring for a loved one with a neurocognitive disorder, such as Alzheimer's disease. A support group is typically time-limited, approximately 6 to 8 weekly sessions lasting 60 to 90 minutes each.

Self-Help Groups

Self-help groups are a type of group that facilitates mutual self-support among its members. Typically, when people think of self-help groups, 12-step meetings come to mind. Alcoholics Anonymous (AA) and Narcotics Anonymous (NA) are two well-known examples of this type of group. Self-help groups function on the premise that members are coming together due to a common shared experience. Members share their personal experiences, successes, and failures to provide support and guidance to other members while gaining personal insight into their own struggles and reducing the sense of aloneness that often accompanies addiction to alcohol, drugs, and gambling, to name a few. While participating in self-help groups, members can gain an increased sense of responsibility, which can lead to sobriety. Twelve-step groups often employ a mentorship component, which is called sponsorship. Newer members identify with a more senior member of the group who have longer periods of sobriety and a history of active participation in the program. Through the sponsorship experience, new members have an additional source of support from the sponsor, and they can hold each other accountable for maintaining sobriety. Self-help groups are lay member–led; so, all members of the groups are responsible for participation and leadership.

Psychotherapy Groups

Unlike the previously mentioned groups, which may be led by psychiatric nurses or lay members, psychotherapy groups, also known as process groups, are led exclusively by advanced practice psychiatric nurses (APPN) as well as other graduate level prepared licensed mental health professionals. APPNs have undergone formal didactic and clinical training in group therapy, as well as received clinical supervision hours provided by a more seasoned group therapist. Psychotherapy groups can be either time-limited or ongoing. They primarily address interpersonal issues but also provide the opportunity for members to work through individual issues as well as whole group themes such as power and authority (Yalom & Leszcz, 2005).

▪ DEFINITION OF MENTAL HEALTH AND PSYCHOPATHOLOGY IN GROUP PSYCHOTHERAPY

The concepts of mental health and psychopathology are considered in the context of group composition. Group leaders screen potential group members to determine the appropriateness of group membership. Regarding mental health, it is important that members have self-regulatory mechanisms (e.g., ability to modulate emotions, ability to delay gratification, ability to tolerate conflict), for group psychotherapy is more anxiety producing than individual psychotherapy. It is also important that members have the ability to be authentic, to give support and feedback, and to set personal boundaries—characteristics of mental health. Some individuals are not suited for group psychotherapy; for example, patients who are cognitively impaired, acutely psychotic, actively using substances, or have severe social anxiety or personality disorders. These patients usually do better in individual psychotherapy or in highly structured, theme-oriented groups where anxiety is kept to a minimum.

▪ THERAPEUTIC GOALS IN GROUP PSYCHOTHERAPY

The purpose of group psychotherapy is to provide members with an environment to address interpersonal, intrapersonal, and whole group issues within the context of a group. The therapeutic underpinning of these groups focuses on providing members a medium in which to develop a deeper sense of self while navigating relational issues with other members of the group. The development of the groups provides opportunities to gain deeper insights into oneself and others, which can help members address personal challenges in how they relate to themselves and others. Groups also provide a forum where members can try out new behaviors within the group context (Schneider Corey et al., 2018).

▪ PERSPECTIVE ON ASSESSMENT IN GROUP PSYCHOTHERAPY

Prior to participating in group psychotherapy, group members are usually interviewed and screened by the group leader. The composition of the group can vary based on gender, age, or clinical diagnosis as well as the focus of the group. In addition to assessing the overall mental health and psychopathology of potential group members, other inclusion criteria necessary to assess include:

- Does the potential patient have the capacity to attend regularly and be prompt? Sometimes patients have unpredictable and hard-to-control work demands, an extremely stressful life, or are dependent on others for transportation. These patients may not be appropriate for group psychotherapy.
- Does the patient have the ability to self-disclose and reveal him- or herself to the group? Sometimes, patients are unable to self-disclose in a group setting. They may be fearful of being judged or humiliated. In some cases, these members may not be appropriate for the group.
- Does the patient have the ability to examine interpersonal behaviors? Some patients may be too defensive and lack the ego strength necessary to examine their own behavior in a group and may not be appropriate for group membership.

■ THERAPEUTIC INTERVENTIONS IN GROUP PSYCHOTHERAPY

Group Structure

Group leaders are responsible to set the structural foundation of the group for the members. Therapy groups are typically 90 minutes in length and consist of six to 10 members, but can vary. The group's meeting time, dates, and location are established. The leader determines if the group will be closed or open to new members. Issues related to, for example, confidentially and level of participation are agreed upon and managed by the group members.

Initially, the group leader is responsible for identifying and clarifying the purpose, goals, and group norms. Explicit norms are spoken openly and include time norms (e.g., what happens if a member comes late?), attendance norms (e.g., what happens if a group member is frequently absent?), confidentiality norms (e.g., what happens if issues are shared outside of group), and members meeting outside of the group norms (e.g., can members meet outside of the group?). Implicit group norms are the unspoken norms that are informal but significant for group development. These may include the expectation that members are authentic, give feedback, offer support, and self-disclose. The group leader needs to decide how norms are determined and communicated to members. In addition, the group leader decides how much input members have in creating the group norms. In group psychotherapy, norms are initially identified by the group leader and then, as the group develops, transferred to and upheld by the group members (Schneider Corey et al., 2018).

Group Process

Conducting group psychotherapy is a very complex endeavor. The leader is responsible for creating group safety and trust, developing a therapeutic relationship with each member, and fostering a sense of cohesion in the group. Every group has its own specific dynamics that the group leader needs to assess moment-to-moment. The leader is responsible for tracking verbal and nonverbal interactions, facilitating group communication, redirecting focus, pointing out group themes, and managing conflict within the group therapy sessions. Communication is encouraged in all directions and not just through the leader; thus, the group leader is responsible for providing an opportunity for everyone to contribute. The group leader needs to offer support and encouragement when needed. Further, the group leader also must confront the dysfunctional roles members may play (e.g., the monopolizer, the aggressor, or the help-rejecting complainer; Yalom & Leszcz, 2005).

■ CASE STUDY

Background

All groups progress through stages of development regardless of the type of group. These stages of group development track the group's progression and can determine the impact or outcome of the group relative to its purpose. Bruce Tuckman (1965) developed five stages of group development. These are (a) forming or orienting, (b) storming or transition, (c) norming or cohesiveness, (d) performing or working, and (e) adjourning or terminating (Tuckman, 1965). My case study includes five case vignettes that reflect these stages of group development. Pseudonyms are used in all the vignettes instead of the participants' real names in order to protect their privacy.

Forming or Orienting

In this stage of development, group participants are learning to adapt to the group. Members will often look to the group leader to provide guidance about the group's structure and boundaries. Expectations regarding important issues, such as behavioral norms and appropriate ways to interact with other group members, are established during this stage. At this point in the group's development, the members may feel uncomfortable or even apprehensive about participating. Typically, group members do not disclose much personal information about themselves until a sense of comfort and safety has been experienced.

The setting for the following example of a forming or orienting group is a community hospital where an APPN on the oncology unit has noticed that some family members of patients undergoing cancer treatment seem confused about or overwhelmed by navigating the community resources available to them. The APPN decides to offer a weekly psychoeducational group for family members on the oncology unit to help them navigate these resources. Family members whose loved one will be discharged over the course of the following week are welcome to attend.

Three family members were in attendance at the group meeting when the following dialogue was recorded. Mrs. Williams is a 65-year-old married Caucasian woman whose husband was recently diagnosed with colon cancer. Mr. Williams underwent a colon resection and now has an ostomy bag. The couple is new to the community and has limited knowledge of the resources available.

APPN: I wanted to thank everyone for coming. During this program, I will be providing you with information about resources that can be accessed after discharge that can help with a variety of things, such as support groups, meal preparation, transportation to and from appointments, and respite care options.

Mrs. Williams: Nicole, I am so happy you are offering this group. I am terrified that I am not going to know what to do for my husband when he is discharged on Wednesday.

APPN: I think this group will provide some good, basic information to everyone about resources in our community that can be accessed after discharge. I understand it can be overwhelming not to know any of the resources that can provide support and assistance after discharge.

Mrs. Williams: Are you going to show me how to take care of my husband's ostomy today? I really need to know how to clean it. (*Example of the family member looking to the group leader for guidance and expectations for the group.*)

APPN: That is a very important issue that needs to be addressed before Mr. Williams goes home; that information won't be covered in this group, but the ostomy nurse will be meeting with you and your husband before he goes home to make sure you both know how to care for his colostomy. During this group, I will provide you with information about getting assistance with transportation that can help you get your husband back and forth from his appointments with the oncologist. I think I remember you saying you were concerned about that last week. (*Example of group leader providing information about the purpose of the group, as well as clarifying boundaries and expectations of what the group will provide.*)

Mrs. Williams: Oh good, I do need to know who I can call for help with transportation.

APPN: Mr. Banks, I noticed before you came into our group that you were very upset. You haven't said much since you sat down. Can you tell me what is upsetting you?

Mr. Banks: I am sorry to be crying. I usually don't cry, especially not in front of strangers. I am not even sure if I should discuss this here, but I really need to talk to someone because I don't know if I can handle this. . . . My wife has breast cancer, and I think she is going to die. (*Example of a member feeling uncomfortable and apprehensive about participating and seeking information about expectations regarding appropriate behavior in the group.*)

APPN: Mr. Banks, that must be very upsetting for you. This isn't a support group; would you be willing to meet with me after the group? What I can do is give you some information about a local support group for family members who have a loved one who has been diagnosed with cancer. You might find the information about the support group helpful. (*Example of the group leader engaging a group member who was reluctant to talk while clarifying the focus and purpose of the group. The group leader also clarified the boundaries of the group.*)

Storming or Transition

During the storming stage, the members are exploring how they fit into the group. Tensions may increase as members explore this issue, and thus, an increase in conflict may occur. There is also an increased awareness of how the group members are similar and different. The storming phase of development is necessary for the group to grow.

The following example of a group in the storming phase involves Bart, an APPN who works in private practice. Bart was asked to lead a weekly support group for men who have prostate cancer. The group has eight participants, and eight sessions will be held. The support group is held at a local counseling center on Tuesday nights. Bart agreed to lead the group. The following is an exchange that took place during the fourth session.

APPN: Thanks to everyone for coming. It looks like the only person who isn't here is Chuck. He didn't call me, so I think he is still coming.

Drew: This is the third time Chuck has been late. It's really unfair that he continues to be late. Each week, we have to catch him up on what we already discussed during the first 15 minutes of the group because of his lateness. Does anyone else feel this way, or is it just me? (*Example of conflict being brought up.*)

Dan: I agree with Drew, it's really annoying. Bart, why don't you tell him if he can't be on time, then he can't keep coming to the support group?

Larry: I agree that it is rude for Chuck to always be late because it doesn't show any respect for the rest of us who do come on time, but I don't think Bart should tell Chuck he can't come anymore. This is just a support group. (*Example of continued exploration of tension among group members.*)

Ed: I agree with Larry. We are coming here for support and share experiences about having prostate cancer. Nobody has even asked Chuck why he has been running late. It seems unfair to be talking about Chuck when he isn't here and when nobody has even asked him why he is running late every week. (*Example of having increased awareness about other group members.*)

John: Ed is right. When we started this group, everyone knew it was only 8 weeks long. We never discussed lateness when we started; the structure of this group has been pretty flexible. We really didn't talk about or even agree on what rules we would follow. I think we should just start. You guys are taking this too seriously. I came to this group to talk with other men about having prostate cancer, not to complain about someone who runs late. Someone just needs to ask Chuck about being late. (*Example of a member exploring how he fits into the group by raising another perspective of the conflict and beginning to develop an understanding of others in the group.*)

APPN: I see there are lots of differing opinions about someone being late to group. When we started this support group, we didn't establish clear guidelines or rules. The group has been rather informal. Why don't we do this? Let's go ahead and talk about tonight's topic, and when Chuck comes in, someone can ask him about his not being here when the group starts. Is that agreeable for everyone? (Everyone agrees affirmatively.) OK, we'll start. Tonight, we are going to talk about the impact prostate cancer has on sexual relationships. (Chuck comes into the group.) Welcome, Chuck, it's good to see you. (*Example of the group leader building cohesion among group members, finding common ground among all group members, and identifying options for the group to address a member's lateness.*)

Ed: Hi, Chuck. Glad you could come tonight. Listen, before you came in, some of the guys were discussing the issue of you being late to group the last 3 weeks, so I am just going to ask, is there a reason why you haven't been able to get here on time?

Chuck: I am sorry for being late. I apologize; I didn't mean for my lateness to cause any problems.

Drew:	Some of us feel it's rude to not show up on time. (*Example of conflict and confrontation.*)
Chuck:	I guess it is rude. I have never been late for anything in my life. I am always early for everything, but things at home are hectic, and I have to wait for my daughter to come over before I can leave the house. My wife has Parkinson's, and she is wheelchair-bound. It's not safe for me to leave her alone, so my daughter has agreed to come over so I can attend this group. My daughter works downtown, and she fights a lot of traffic coming across town. (*Example of a group member disclosing information about himself to the group, which helps establish trust and provides information to the group.*)
John:	I didn't realize your wife was sick.
Drew:	I didn't realize it either. Why didn't you tell us this?
Chuck:	I didn't want to burden anyone, and it never really came up, so I didn't say anything.
Dan:	I feel like a jerk now. I had no idea. You sure are managing a lot. You have prostate cancer and your wife is also ill. It just goes to show you that you never really know someone's problems until you ask. We all come here because we have prostate cancer, but we really don't know much more about each other. (*Example of identifying differences and similarities among group members.*)
Jeff:	I am glad you told us, Chuck.
Dan:	Yes, thanks for telling us. You have a lot on your plate. I am glad you are able to come to the group.
APPN:	Thanks for letting the group know about your personal situation, Chuck. I think this gives everyone the opportunity to learn more about each other.
Drew:	It is a good opportunity. It also gives us the opportunity to appreciate that you really never know what someone is going through. I feel like I know Chuck a little better. (*Example of how resolving conflict and raising awareness of similarities and differences among group members provides an opportunity for a different level of support to be provided among group members.*)

Norming or Cohesiveness

During this stage, members of the group are more aligned with one another. This alignment among members helps the group focus on achieving its goals as members are working toward a common goal. Members of the group develop a greater sense of trust among one another, which enhances group cohesion.

The following dialogue is from an AA group meeting and is used to provide examples of norming. It begins with the introduction of Amy, a 43-year-old married, White female with three children. Amy is a recovering alcoholic who had been sober for 6 years prior to a recent relapse. At a reception following the funeral for her father-in-law, she had a glass of wine, which led to drinking five additional glasses by the end of the evening. After consuming the wine, Amy fell and hit her head. Her husband took her to the ED, where she was examined and released as no serious injuries were found. She has been attending

AA meetings at St. Anne Church. She considers this her home group, and she has a good support network of other members who also attend AA meetings at this location. The following day after her trip to the ED, Amy returns to her regular 6:00 p.m. AA meeting. It is a closed meeting, meaning only AA members or prospective members can attend. Open meetings are open to the public, and anyone can attend. The following exchange is from the meeting. The 6 p.m. meeting usually has about 15 people in attendance, 12 of whom are regular members and attend this meeting on a daily basis. The meeting opens and the members begin to take turns discussing their struggles with the group.

Amy: Hi, I am Amy, and I am an alcoholic. (The group responds, "Hi, Amy.") I have had a really bad few weeks. My father-in-law died last week, and the funeral was on Thursday. I didn't want to go, but I needed to do it for my husband. I always feel embarrassed and ashamed when I'm around my husband's family because early in my relationship with my husband, I was still drinking a lot. One night after drinking, I backed my car into my in-laws' new Porsche and totaled it. Luckily, no one was hurt, but it was a nightmare. I got sober after that incident, and I had been sober for 6 years until last Thursday. My in-laws have been trying to get my husband, Mike, to leave me since before we were married, but Mike has stood by me. His parents have never really let the Porsche incident go. They never really liked me. There has always been tension between us, even after I was sober. After the funeral, there was a reception in the church hall. I was so stressed out that I drank. I fell in the reception hall and hit my head. My husband took me to the ED, but there were no injuries, so I was released. Needless to say, my husband is furious, and my mother-in-law and my sister-in-law haven't talked to Mike in 4 days. I feel like such a failure. I really want to drink. I feel really ashamed of myself. In fact, I almost didn't come tonight because I didn't think I could face everyone. Anyway, thanks for listening. (*Example of a member working through feelings of embarrassment and shame by continuing to attend the group after her relapse. The information she shares is deeply personal, but through sharing, she allows herself to be vulnerable. As one member of the group is vulnerable in sharing her feelings, she is met with acceptance and support from other group members; her willingness to be vulnerable provides an example to other group members that being vulnerable is safe. The vulnerability of self-disclosure is beneficial to the individual, as well as others who observe her positive experience; it could make these members more likely to allow themselves to be vulnerable with the group, and this process improves the cohesion of the group as a whole.*)

Ginger: (Ginger raises her hand.) I'd like to share. I'm Ginger, and I am an alcoholic. (The group responds, "Hi, Ginger.") I can relate to what Amy said. I have been sober for 20 years, and I still worry about drinking at times. I had a very rough week too. I was told I have breast cancer. I am frightened and afraid I am going to die. Since learning of my diagnosis, I have wanted to drink every day. The temptation has been overwhelming. I came close to drinking several times but came to this meeting instead. I haven't shared my diagnosis with anyone, but I feel safe here. I know, from my past experience, I have support in this group. Thanks for letting me share. (*Example of a member trusting her home group. It illustrates how this member's goal of staying sober aligns with the group's goals, as well as how willingness to trust group members promotes a greater sense of trust among members.*)

Bonnie:	Hi, I am Bonnie, and I am an alcoholic. (The group responds, "Hi, Bonnie.") This is the only meeting I attend, and I feel really supported by everyone here. I share more with this group than I do with even my own family. I have had three relapses in 10 years, and after each relapse, I came right back to this meeting. I know these meetings work because they have gotten me through some of the hardest times in my life. This program has saved my life. Thanks for listening. (*Example of verbalizing the experience of trust in the group and the process of working the program, acknowledging the support of others in the group and how the process of sharing and supporting each other unconditionally engenders a sense of trust in others.*)
Heidi:	Hi, I am Heidi, and I am an alcoholic. I have been coming to this meeting for 10 years, and the members have supported me through thick and thin. This group has supported me through two divorces and when I was laid off from my job. If it weren't for this meeting and the support of this group, I would probably have died. (*Example of alignment with the goals of the group and others in the group. Illustrates a sense of trust in others in the group and in the group as a whole.*)
Janice:	Hi, I'm Janice, and I'm an alcoholic. (The group responds, "Hi, Janice.") This week was really good. I got a promotion at work, and I found out I am pregnant. While I am excited about being pregnant, I am worried I will screw this kid up because my mom drank, and she screwed me up. I have been sober for 4 years, and I know that if I keep working the program every day, then I can stay sober. My husband is really excited about the baby, but I haven't told him how worried I am. I appreciate having this meeting because the support from the folks in this room has helped me stay on track and continue to work my program. (*Example of deep trust in the other group members and evidence of alignment with the goals and purpose of the group.*)

Commentary: *This example of an AA group meeting illustrates that even self-help groups move through stages of development. This ongoing AA group, with its core of regular members, provides an environment where members feel safe to talk about very personal and private issues. All the group members are aligned in the common goal to stay sober. The connectedness of the group members to the group as a whole and to the individual members of the group has created strong cohesion within the group. The cohesion provides a continued sense of safety and support, which allows members to continue sharing and supporting each other.*

Performing or Working

This phase of group development does not occur in all groups. This phase of group development evidences a very high level of maturity in the group as a whole, as well as in the members. Members of the group are functioning more independently and autonomously. During this phase, a deeper sense of honesty is shared among group members. The members of the group take more ownership, and through this ownership, the group members can experience a more in-depth feeling of accomplishment.

The following dialogue highlights an element of the performing phase of group development. This long-term psychotherapy group has been meeting for 2 years. The group is composed of seven gay men, who are all original members. The group began with eight members, but one left the group due to a job relocation. In this particular group meeting, the therapist brings up the idea of allowing a new member to join.

APPN:	It's been 8 months since Jay left the group. I want the group to discuss the issue of adding a new member to the group.
Zach:	I still miss Jay not being in the group. I feel Jay leaving the group is still an issue for the group. I am not sure we are finished talking about him moving and leaving the group.
Jack:	I personally don't want to add a new member to the group. It would be too hard at this point because we all have become so bonded.
Rick:	I agree with both of you. I think we still have more to process about Jay leaving. If we add a new member, he would feel left out because he doesn't know Jay, and it might be awkward for the new guy.
Jack:	Rick, I don't think it's an issue of being ready to add a member. My feeling is we shouldn't add anyone new, period. Let's just keep it the original seven.
Jessie:	I think we should consider adding a new member. Jay has been gone for 8 months, and we need to move on. It would be good to give another guy the opportunity to participate. I really think having a new guy join would be a good experience for all of us. It's true; a new member would change the dynamic of the group, but it could also be a good opportunity for each of us to push ourselves and do something that makes us a little uncomfortable.
Rick:	The decision to add someone or not add someone has to be a unanimous decision.
Warner:	I agree. Adding someone should be something we all agree upon.
Zach:	Maybe Jack is right. Maybe we shouldn't add a new member. I know I have talked about how hard it is for me to build nonsexual relationships with guys. I finally feel completely comfortable with everyone in this group. Adding someone new would mean I have to explain this issue to him.
Rick:	Zack, I get it. That would be really hard to do. We all have shared some deeply personal things in this group. It would be hard to share all that again with a new guy, but we would continue to support each other. Maybe that might make it easier.
Jake:	I am nervous about adding someone new to the group too. I am not sure I want to retell my story to a new guy. It feels like we will have to start all over again and rebuild the trust we have established. The sense of closeness we have worked so hard to develop might be hard to reestablish. The seven of us have really shared a lot of raw emotions, and we all know each other so well. Adding a new member will be a really big shift; the group won't be the same if someone new joins.
Steve:	I agree with Jake. It took me a really long time to talk about the physical abuse I went through when my relationship with Zeke ended. I am not sure I want to rehash that again.
Rick:	You know, we haven't really thought about what it would be like for a new member to join us. I can only imagine how tough it could be. Coming into a group that has been meeting for 2 years—the experience could be really overwhelming. A new member could feel like the odd man out since we all know each other so well.

Jake:	I never thought of that aspect, Rick. You bring up a good point.
Dale:	But it could be good practice for us individually; by being vulnerable with someone new, the group could actually take on a new dimension by adding a new member. It doesn't have to be all negative. Listen, I get how challenging it has been for all of us to get to this point in the group, but adding a new member would allow us to share our stories [with someone who has] a different perspective. I think everyone has grown a lot since we joined the group in a positive way.

Commentary: *This portion of the group session provides examples of members being independent in sharing their personal feelings. It also exemplifies how the members have taken ownership of the group. The members do not seek guidance from the therapist and take it upon themselves to process how a new member would impact the group's dynamics, trust, and cohesion. Members of the group provide support and affirm each other even though some members have differing opinions. The differing opinions are respected and explored by the group members. The interaction among group members exemplifies how members can be honest and respectful of each other. The exchange also illustrates the group members' ownership of the group.*

Adjourning or Terminating

During the last phase of group development, termination, or the end of the group, is addressed and occurs. This stage of the group can often be challenging and even difficult for group members as a number of emotions and feelings may surface in relation to the group ending. This process group has been meeting for a year in the counseling center of a small liberal arts college. The group leader is an APPN, Dr. Kelly O'Shea, who works in the counseling center. The group is for students who have a history of depression and are (or have been) treated individually at the counseling center. The group is composed of freshmen, sophomores, juniors, and seniors. Mid-way through the spring term, Dr. O'Shea begins to talk about the group's termination, which will occur in 6 weeks.

APPN:	I wanted the group to start to talk about the end of the group. As you all remember, during your initial interview with me about joining the group, we talked about the fact this group would last for two semesters. Since we are mid-way through the spring term, I thought it would be a good time to begin addressing the end of the group.
Eric:	I really like this group. I didn't like coming at first, but after a few sessions, I found it was helpful to talk with other students who also struggle with depression. I am going to miss our meetings every week. This experience has really been positive. (*Group member begins to talk about what the group has meant to him.*)
Emily:	Me, too; I really like this group. I have made progress by coming to this group. I feel less alone knowing there are other people who feel like I feel. I have developed some really strong connections in the group, and I feel everyone has helped me a lot. (*Example of reaffirming another group member and articulating similarities in experiences of the helpfulness of the group.*)
Jeremy:	I don't want the group to end. Isn't there any way we can keep meeting? I have to take a summer course, and I will be on campus for the entire summer break. Breaking us up seems really unfair. Come on,

	guys; don't you feel the same way? (*Example of a group member looking for other members who share this experience.*)
APPN:	Jeremy, can you talk more about what this group has meant to you?
Jeremy:	This is the only place I feel I can be myself. The people in this group really know me for who I am. I don't pretend everything is okay all the time. This group is the only place I feel safe talking about being depressed and isolated. If this group ends, I will go back to being isolated again. (*Deeper discussion of what the group's termination means to him and being more vulnerable about the impact the group has had on him.*)
Barry:	Jeremy, I think we all feel safe in this group.
APPN:	Barry, remember to speak for yourself, not for all the group members.
Barry:	Right. I also feel safe in this group. I feel I have grown by coming to this group, and I feel more capable of managing my depression because I have participated in this group. Jeremy, I think you have made a lot of progress, too. I remember [that] for the first month, you didn't say much, but soon, you were participating a lot. You helped me by talking about your experience of being isolated. I felt the same way, but because you shared that about yourself, I began to realize lots of people have depression and that made me feel less isolated. (*Sharing a similar experience about the personal meaning of the group and acknowledging and appreciating the progress another member of the group has made over the course of the group.*)

Commentary: *Several other group members share their feelings about the group's termination, and the group ends after 90 minutes. At the following weekly meeting, the group meets and begins with all members present except for Jeremy. The group continues to talk about termination, and several members mention that Jeremy is not present at this meeting. When the group meets again the following week, all the members are present, but Jeremy is absent. The group continues to talk about the termination of the group. Halfway through the group meeting, Jeremy arrives. The discussion continues, but after a few minutes, it ends, and everyone looks at Jeremy, whose absence from the group could be directly related to his emotional reaction to the group ending.*

APPN:	I am glad you decided to come to group this evening. It's good to see you.
Fred:	Jeremy, where were you last week? (*Directly asking about Jeremy's absence.*)
Jackie:	And why are you so late tonight? We all know the group starts on time. You can't just start breaking your agreement about showing up on time. You being late is really disrespectful. Just because you don't want the group to end doesn't mean you can decide to not show up for sessions and then just show up late. (*Confrontation about Jeremy's absence and lateness.*)
Jeremy:	Jackie, get off my back. All you ever do is nag people. No wonder your boyfriend dumped you; you probably nagged him to death, and he couldn't take it anyway. (*Defensive response to being confronted about this behavior.*)

Alisha: Jeremy, stop being such a jerk. I feel the same way as Jackie. What's up with you not coming last week and not calling to let Dr. O'Shea know? (*Continues confrontation while sharing a similar experience of another group member.*)

Jeremy: I don't know. I guess this group ending is harder than I want to admit. I am not sure what I am going to do when I don't have this group anymore. It has really helped me keep it together for these past two terms. (*Begins to disclose and share his experience as it relates to the termination of the group.*)

APPN: Jeremy, I hear you saying the end of this group is hard for you, harder than you expected. Did the group ending have anything to do with you not coming last week and then showing up late this week?

Jeremy: Yeah, I am really pissed that the group is ending. I can't handle when things end. When my parents divorced, I lost it. I was so angry; I punched a hole in the kitchen wall at our house. When my roommate graduated last year, I punched the wall in my dorm room. I don't know how I am going to deal with this group ending. (*Discussing other experiences related to endings or termination. Example of disclosing a difficult emotional experience he is having related to the termination of the group.*)

Eric: Wow, I had no idea you were this pissed about the group ending. What can we do to help you?

Emily: Yeah, Jeremy, who can support you right now?

The group spends the remainder of the session processing the impact of termination on each group member.

Commentary: *Throughout my career, I have frequently used groups as a therapeutic option. Groups are a means through which those who share a commonality can be brought together. The benefit of the group for its members is interconnected with group development and the associated therapeutic values. The group's therapeutic value changes as the group moves through the various stages of development. Not all groups provide the same therapeutic value or achieve each stage of group development. The case vignettes strive to present various types of groups as they move through different stages of development. As the groups move through these stages, various elements of therapeutic value can be noted.*

DISCUSSION QUESTIONS

1. The APPN wants to refer a patient for group therapy but the patient states he "doesn't really like working in groups." How could the APPN address the resistance of this patient to join the group?
2. An APPN is leading a psychotherapy group. The group is unable to move beyond the storming phase of group development. Group members are in a state of constant confrontation with one another, and several members of the group are asserting they want to leave the group. What strategies could the APPN employ?
3. The APPN is new to the role as a group therapist and is experiencing a great deal of self-doubt and insecurity relative to group leadership abilities. How could the APPN address this self-doubt and insecurity?

4. A support group for recently diagnosed cancer patients is meeting for their eighth and final group session. At the beginning of the group, several members are visibly very upset. A group member then announces that a member of the support group died yesterday. The APPN uses the session to allow members to talk about the loss. At the end of the meeting, all group members want to have additional group sessions to continue to talk about the death. How could the APPN address this issue and what next steps could be taken as the support group was to terminate at the end of this meeting?

REFERENCES

Breitabarm, W., Rosenfeld, B., Pessin, H., Applebaum, A., Kulikowski, J., & Lichtenthal, W. (2015). Meaning-centered group psychotherapy: An effective intervention for improving psychological well-being in patients with advanced cancer. *Journal of Clinical Oncology*, 33(7), 749–754. doi:10.1200/JCO.2014.57.2198

Burlingame, G. M., Fuhriman, A., & Mosier, J. (2003). The differential effectiveness of group psychotherapy: A meta-analytic perspective. *Group Dynamics: Theory, Research, and Practice*, 7(1), 3–12. doi:10.1037/1089-2699.7.1.3

Corey, G. (2016). *Theory and practice of group counseling* (9th ed.). Boston, MA: Cengage Learning.

Corey, G., Schneider Corey, M., & Haynes, R. (2014). *Group in action: Evolution and challenges* (2nd ed.). Boston, MA: Cengage Learning.

Feder, B., & Ronall, R. (1980). *Beyond the hot seat: Gestalt approaches to group*. New York, NY: Brunner/Mazel.

Moreno, J. L., Jennings, H. H., & Whitin, E. S. (1932). *Group method and group psychotherapy*. Boston, MA: Beacon House.

Rogers, C. (1970). *On encounter groups*. New York, NY: Harper & Row.

Schneider Corey, M., Corey, G., & Corey, C. (2018). *Groups: Process and practice* (10th ed.). Boston, MA: Cengage Learning.

Steen, S., Vasserman-Stokes, E., & Vannatta, R. (2014). Group cohesion in experiential growth groups. *The Journal for Specialists in Group Work*, 39(3), 236–256. doi:10.1080/01933922.2014.924343

Tuckman, B. (1965). Development sequence in small groups. *Psychological Bulletin*, 63(6), 384–399. doi:10.1037/h0022100

Yalom, I. D., & Leszcz, M. (2005). *The theory and practice of group psychotherapy* (5th ed.). New York, NY: Basic Books.

Family Therapy: A Family Over Time

Candice Knight

■ PERSONAL EXPERIENCE WITH FAMILY PSYCHOTHERAPY

Family therapy, an approach that views psychological problems as an expression of dysfunction in the family system, is a mainstay of my practice. I have been practicing family therapy for over 40 years in a variety of settings and have received training in a number of systems-related family therapy approaches.

Initially, I was trained in Murray Bowen's Systems Family therapy approach while completing my graduate program in psychiatric-mental health nursing early in the 1970s. After graduation, I began working with families at a community mental health center in an urban environment. In that setting, I found that Bowen's approach was insufficient when working with very chaotic, unstructured families—families with confusing roles, inconsistent rules, and inappropriate boundaries. Consequently, I enrolled in a 3-year training program at the Philadelphia Guidance Center in Sal Minuchin's Structural Family herapy approach. After completing the training, I combined both of these approaches in my work with families. This combination worked well in helping families change dysfunctional patterns and reorganize into a more functional structure. More recently, I completed training in Les Greenberg and Sue Johnson's emotion-focused family therapy (EFT), an approach that focuses on reestablishing weakened attachment bonds by learning to communicate in an authentic fashion at a primary emotional level.

As a result of my depth training in these system modalities, I integrate theoretical concepts and techniques from all three approaches in my work with families. How this integration is implemented depends upon the particular family presentation. For example, if a family is very chaotic and lacks structure, interventions from Structural Family therapy take precedence, and I focus initially on family reorganization. Similarly, if family members have repeated dysfunctional patterns across generations, I focus initially on interventions from Systems Family therapy and complete a detailed genogram on each family member to highlight these patterns. Alternately, if families lack authentic, emotional communication, EFT will be the priority, and I focus foremost on reestablishing attachment bonds by helping members communicate from a primary emotional level. Thus, my integration employs the theory and techniques from all three approaches to family therapy. My case study reflects this integration.

■ FOUNDERS AND LEADERS OF FAMILY PSYCHOTHERAPY

Bowen's Systems Family Therapy Approach

Murray Bowen (1913–1990), an American psychiatrist, is the founder of Systems Family therapy, often called the Bowenian Family Systems approach. While training at the psychoanalytically oriented Menninger clinic, Bowen experienced much success with his individual clients when he brought their families into sessions. In 1954, he became the first director of the Family Division of the National Institute of Mental Health and led a research project in which he studied 18 families having a schizophrenic member over a 5-year period. From 1959 to 1990, as an academician and clinician at Georgetown University, he developed and refined Systems Family therapy. A transformative paper he presented at a professional meeting in 1967 explicated the emotional processes in his own family, which stressed the need for clinicians to work through the dysfunction in their own families if they were to be effective family therapists (Bowen, 1972). In 1969, he started the Bowen Systems Family Therapy Program, working with families and training therapists in his systemic approach. Bowen's theory and therapeutic approach are outlined in his book, *Family Therapy in Clinical Practice* (Bowen, 1978). His work has been further developed and continues with the current leadership of Philip Guerin, Thomas Fogarty, Monica McGoldrick, and Betty Carter (Carter & McGoldrick, 1980; Guerin, Fogarty, Fay, & Kautto, 1996; McGoldrick, 1995).

Minuchin's Structural Family Therapy Approach

Salvador Minuchin (1921–2017), an Argentinian psychiatrist, developed Structural Family therapy. He was an extremely creative, much loved therapist, known for his mastery of technique. Minuchin was originally a psychoanalytically trained psychiatrist who studied with Nathan Ackerman, received psychoanalytic training at the Alanson White Institute, and worked with troubled youths at the Wiltwyck School for Boys in New York City in the late 1950s and early 1960s. Realizing the limitations of psycho-analytic methods for treating these disadvantaged boys, he and a group of colleagues developed new methods for working with the boys and their families, which later evolved into Structural Family therapy. After becoming the director of the Philadelphia Child Guidance Clinic in 1965, he and his colleagues published the ground-breaking book, *Families of the Slums: An Exploration of Their Structure and Treatment* (Minuchin, Montalvo, Guerney, Rosman, & Schumer, 1967) and later his classic book, *Families and Family Therapy* (Minuchin, 1974). Under Minuchin's direction, the Philadelphia Child Guidance Clinic became one of the world's foremost family therapy training centers. In 1976, Minuchin stepped down as director of the clinic and started his own center in New York City, where he continued to practice and train family therapists until 1996. The legacy of his work continues by well-known Structural Family therapists including Harry Aponte, Michael Nichols, and Braulio Montalvo (Nichols, 2012).

Greenberg and Johnson's EFT Approach

Leslie Greenberg (1945–) and Sue Johnson (1946–), two Canadian psychologists, founded EFT in the mid-1980s. They collaborated to create the approach by reviewing videos of couple therapy sessions to identify the elements that led to positive change. Their origi-nal book, *Emotionally Focused Therapy for Couples*, outlines the theory and therapeutic techniques (Greenberg & Johnson, 1988).

Greenberg, born in South Africa, initially studied engineering and worked as an engineer before earning his PhD in psychology from York University. With his mentor, Laura Rice, who was a protégé of Carl Rogers, he began doing psychotherapy process research, attempting to scientifically define therapist–client interactions using techniques of task analysis. He later trained in Gestalt therapy and Systems Family therapy and brought elements of these approaches into EFT. Greenberg is currently professor emeritus of psychology at York University and the director of the Emotion-Focused Therapy Clinic in Toronto, where he continues to train therapists in this approach. He has published numerous articles, foundational texts, and training manuals on EFT.

Sue Johnson initially earned a BA in English followed by an EdD in Counselling Psychology from the University of British Columbia. She is currently professor emeritus of psychology at the University of Ottawa. She founded the International Centre for Excellence in Emotion Focused Therapy and has authored a number of articles, training manuals, and books on the topic for both therapists and general audiences. Johnson has trained many therapists in her approach, which has generated the development of numerous training programs in EFT throughout the United States and beyond.

Since the original publication of Greenberg and Johnson's classic book *Emotionally Focused Therapy for Couples* (Greenberg & Johnson, 1988), each has gone on to publish further texts in the area. Greenberg and Goldman (2008) have developed a variation of EFT for couples containing elements from Greenberg and Johnson's original text, but adding steps and stages related to love and power. Johnson has delved more into bonding, attachment, and adult romantic relationships. Both Greenberg and Johnson continue to write prolifically and offer training in their approaches to couples and family therapy.

■ PHILOSOPHY AND KEY CONCEPTS OF FAMILY PSYCHOTHERAPY

Family therapy, from a systems perspective, is an approach that views psychological problems as an expression of dysfunction in the family system. The family is the structure in which individuals learn what it means to be human within a particular culture. The family transmits values, attitudes, and norms, and serves as a mediator between the needs of its members and the demands of society. The family provides nurturance and support and is responsible for developing the individual's personality and socialization skills including how to express thoughts and feelings, cope with stress, and adapt to change (Nichols, 2012).

Bowen's Systems Family Therapy Approach

Bowen's approach combines the significance of the past with current patterns that maintain dysfunction. The family is viewed as a complex, self-regulating, emotional unit that strives to maintain homeostasis; a change in the functioning of one family member is predictably followed by a reciprocal change in the functioning of other family members. Key concepts include differentiation of self (degree of separation and individuation from the family); multigenerational transmission patterns (dysfunctional patterns that occur from one generation to the next); triangles (dysfunctional emotional patterns between members that manage tension); birth order (sibling positions that create certain personality characteristics); and emotional cutoffs (ruptures between family members; Bowen, 1972; Goldenberg & Goldenberg, 2012; Kerr & Bowen, 1988).

Minuchin's Structural Family Therapy Approach

Minuchin's approach posits that family problems are embedded in a dysfunctional family structure that organizes the way family members function and relate to one another. Key concepts include family structure (invisible set of recurrent patterns that organize the way family members relate to one another including roles, rules, power structures, and communication patterns); coalitions (dysfunctional alliances between two family members against a third); and boundaries (separations that serve to regulate contact, maintain individual identity, and modulate emotional closeness). Boundaries may be overly diffuse and deny family members differences and personal autonomy (enmeshed boundaries) or overly rigid and impermeable causing disconnection, limited support, and interpersonal isolation (disengaged boundaries; Minuchin, 1974; Nichols, 2012).

Greenberg and Johnson's Emotion-Focused Approach

Emotions are viewed as the primary element in the functioning of the family, for they are believed to inform family members of important needs, prepare the self for action, and create either strong or weak attachment bonds. Key concepts include primary emotions (true emotional reactions in response to a situation, such as sadness in response to a loss or anger in response to an attack); secondary emotions (emotional reactions to thoughts or feelings, rather than to the situation itself, such as feeling guilty about feeling angry); attachment style (emotional bond between members maintained by responsiveness, accessibility, and engagement, and described as secure, insecure, anxious, or vacillating); and attachment injuries (emotional injury characterized as abandonment, betrayal, or violation of trust; Johnson, 1996; Johnson & Sims, 2000; Johnson & Whiffen, 1999).

■ DEFINITION OF MENTAL HEALTH AND PSYCHOPATHOLOGY IN FAMILY PSYCHOTHERAPY

What distinguishes a healthy family is not the absence of problems, but the presence of an effective organizational structure and functional interaction patterns to handle problems effectively when they arise (Minuchin, 1974). In my integrated approach to family therapy, a functional family is defined as one that has a solid organizational structure with distinct roles and fair rules, a hierarchy of power with the top tier residing in the parents, direct and authentic communication patterns, and good decision-making functions. Boundaries are flexible and allow for good contact and healthy emotional closeness. Members are differentiated and have age-appropriate levels of separation and individuation. Healthy families are flexible and able to adapt to change. Members love, support, and encourage each other throughout their lives as well as live in relative harmony. Authentic emotions are expressed and strong attachment bonds are present.

In contrast, a pathological family is defined as one that has an unhealthy organizational structure. Roles are vague, rules are inconsistent, power is imbalanced, and boundaries are either enmeshed or disengaged. Members lack differentiation; thus, separation and individuation are thwarted. Emotional awareness and strong attachment bonds are absent. Love, support, and encouragement are limited and cutoffs from family members occur with frequency. Dysfunctional families pass down ineffective patterns through the generations (Beavers & Hampson, 1990; Nichols, 2012).

■ THERAPEUTIC GOALS IN FAMILY PSYCHOTHERAPY

The goal of my integrated family therapy approach is to help families decrease systemic factors that produce dysfunction and increase functional factors. Within an empathically attuned therapeutic relationship with family members, I emphasize moment-to-moment experiences during sessions. I strive to help family members increase self-differentiation as well as create an effective structure with distinct roles, fair rules, flexible boundaries, and productive decision-making. I help families access their authentic emotions, transform negative interactional and communication patterns, and strengthen attachment bonds, allowing members to be more accessible and responsive to each other. I aim to give families the tools needed to handle problems when they arise, for challenges emerge throughout the family life cycle. Family therapy may be short-term, taking place within 12 to 20 sessions, or long-term, lasting several years. Many families will return to therapy when a crisis reoccurs in the system.

■ PERSPECTIVE ON ASSESSMENT IN FAMILY PSYCHOTHERAPY

Assessment begins with the initial phone contact. I notice what family member initiates contact. Often this member is the healthiest member of the family. I listen carefully to how the problem is defined. If one family member is targeted as the "identified client," I try to dispel this notion as family therapy looks at the problem as an expression of dysfunction in the system. The first contact in the waiting room followed by seating in the therapy room provides clues and ideas for how to proceed and tailor opening statements and questions. For example, does the family seem resistant? Do certain members not want to be there? Where do family members sit and what is the configuration (who sits next to whom and who sits apart)? Do they seem scared or angry? Does one member seem to have a major psychiatric problem?

I typically begin the assessment session by asking each member his or her perception of the problem. I start with the parents in order to respect and reinforce the parental hierarchy, emphasizing a functional organizational structure. I empathically join with each family member, letting each one know I understand what he or she is communicating. I adjust and adapt to the family's affective style, language patterns, and energy level by emulating these aspects to solidify the alliance. In addition, I connect by making positive, confirming statements to foster the hope that change is possible. After each family member articulates his or her perception of the problem, I typically do another round and ask each member what part he or she plays in the problem. This question is often difficult, but helps me assess each member's level of awareness and differentiation; thus, unless the family is very dysfunctional, I ask, "What part do you think you may play in the problem?"

I generally use a flip chart to begin construction of a three-generational, graphic genogram during the assessment session. This interpretive tool is used to identify patterns, generate hypotheses, and obtain a significant amount of information about the evolution of family problems and the dysfunctional processes that exist and may be handed down from generation to generation. The initial genogram includes names, gender, birth dates, occupational roles, ethnicity, marriage and separation dates, and current stressors in the family. As the sessions progress, the genogram is expanded to include important life events, cutoffs, illnesses, deaths, and complex relationships between family members.

I assess the degree of function and dysfunction among members as well as the structure and emotional atmosphere of the family. Are they differentiated or undifferentiated? Are there triangles? Are there dysfunctional patterns deeply embedded within the family and, if so, how are these maintained and perpetuated? Who has the power in the system? Is the parental coalition weak or strong and do they work together? Are roles clearly defined and are they distinct and flexible, or rigid and intractable? Are the rules fair? How are tasks distributed? Do members share in decision-making, or do one or both parents make all decisions? Do the parents work together? Do members move toward resolution when problem-solving, or do they bicker and blame each other? Are there adequate boundaries and are the boundaries appropriate to age and circumstance? Is the emotional processing conflictual and reactive or is it supportive and loving? Who is close to whom? Do members feel safe? Is communication responsive and clear, or is it stifled and confused? Do members give clear messages of their wishes, thoughts, needs, and feelings, or do they expect others to magically know? Can members speak freely? Do some or all family members interrupt each other? Who talks to whom? Does one person act as the switchboard? Are perceptions accurate? Can members repeat what they have heard? Can everyone express primary feelings? How are anger and love expressed? Is there unresolved anger? Are the attachment bonds secure? Do the parents recognize normal developmental changes and are they able to renegotiate roles and rules in times of transition such as when children enter adolescence? How is stress handled and are there effective coping mechanisms? Are there signs of serious psychopathology or chronic physical illnesses that tax normal functioning?

I offer feedback throughout the assessment process. At the end of the assessment session, goals are collaboratively formed and a working plan developed. Assessment is an ongoing process. New information is continually collected and plans revised as the therapy progresses (Knight, 2013).

■ THERAPEUTIC INTERVENTIONS IN FAMILY PSYCHOTHERAPY

For the first few sessions, I like to see the family as a whole, but I may then decide to meet with family members in various configurations—individually or in different dyads. This varies with each family and decisions are made as the therapy progresses. The following are some common interventions I employ:

Empathic Attunement

In order to connect with family members on a deep level, I make contact with their subjective world, closely track their interaction patterns, and listen empathically to be sure they feel understood and engaged. I use reflective statements of deeper, primary emotions that members may be experiencing as well as evocative questions to bring forth deeper, primary emotions that are not being expressed and experienced directly (Johnson, 1996). For example, if one partner states, "She is never home and is always out with her friends," I may say to that partner: "I'm wondering if you are hurt or disappointed that she does not spend more time at home with you?" This draws attention to the deeper emotions.

Effective Communication

I assist in self-differentiation by having family members speak directly to one another, rather than to a third person (Bowen, 1978). I frequently use the communication pattern of, "Can you tell him or her that directly?" Sometimes, I will have family members shift chairs to change dysfunctional interactional patterns. I promote self-defining "I statements" by having members use first-person pronouns. I model skills of authentic communication, empathic listening, successful conflict resolution, and creative problem-solving in order that members can learn new ways of relating.

Dysfunctional Pattern Disruption

I frequently point out dysfunctional patterns by using process questions (Minuchin & Fishman, 1981). For example, I may use a statement such as, "I notice you do the tasks that your husband agreed to do but has not, and this frustrates you." I sometimes use the technique of affiliating to disrupt dysfunctional patterns, which is making a negative statement about one member while absolving him or her of responsibility for the behavior. An example of affiliating is, "You act very dependent on your spouse. What does she do to keep you incompetent?" I also ask members to try out different interactional patterns within the session. For example, I may ask a member who avoids conflict to confront someone in the family system.

Enactment Experiments

I will often do an enactment during the session. Rather than family members telling me about a difficult interaction, I will direct them to demonstrate it during the session in order to spotlight the family's structural dysfunction (Minuchin, 1974). For example, if the family describes a great deal of fighting during the week, I may ask them to choose one recent issue they fought about at home and enact it during the session. With the enactment, I notice dysfunctional patterns, such as a weak parental hierarchy, a child with too much power, or a couple involved in an unhealthy pursuer and distancer pattern. I will modify problematic interactions by creating in-session experiments to support change in the here-and-now.

Unbalancing Techniques

I try to change unhealthy boundaries and triangles in a family by using the technique of unbalancing (Minuchin, 1974). For example, a 14-year-old family member, Sally, requests more time on her computer, but is interrupted by her mother, who attempts to convince Sally that she is unreasonable, while the father sits uninvolved. I set a 3-minute timer and ask Sally to argue her point without any interruptions. I then ask Sally to leave the room and instruct the parents to come up with a solution together. After 10 minutes, I have Sally return to the session and ask the father to inform her of the parental joint solution.

Shaping Competence

I reinforce new, desirable patterns by praising family members for their success (Minuchin, 1974). For example, a couple having difficulty working together finally agrees on a behavioral plan and presents it clearly to their children. I may say to them afterwards, "That was terrific that you were able to work together and present a united front to your child" (Knight, 2013).

■ CASE STUDY

Background

I met the Thomas family, initially as a couple, 8 years ago. Carol, a 33-year-old, married, attorney in private practice, called me for a couples therapy appointment. She had been married to Tom, a 39-year-old chemist who worked for the Environmental Protection

Agency, for 12 years. They had two latency age sons, ages 8 and 9. Carol was unsure if she wanted to stay married and was leaning toward ending the marriage. Tom was happy in the marriage and did not want a divorce. Neither Carol nor Tom had therapy in the past. Our couples therapy began in 2011 and lasted for eight consecutive, weekly sessions. Carol and Tom resolved some issues in their relationship during the couples therapy, but many issues remained unresolved. Five years later, in 2016, Carol called requesting family therapy. She stated that their sons, who were now 13- and 14-year-old adolescents, were getting into trouble. They began family therapy for the next 3 years and terminated shortly after Carol and Tom decided to divorce in late 2019.

The beginning phase transcript is from the first session of our couples therapy work 8 years prior in 2011. It illustrates multigenerational transmission patterns and dysfunctional interaction styles that were apparent early in our work. The middle phase transcript consists of parts of two sessions that occurred when Carol, Tom, and their sons returned for family therapy 5 years later in 2016. It illuminates the entrenched dysfunctional patterns in the family system and the impact on the children. The final phase transcript is a session in 2019, near the end of our work together. It illustrates termination as well as the successes and failures of the therapy.

Transcript of Therapy Sessions

BEGINNING PHASE

I schedule 1½ hours for the first couple or family session in order to have enough time to build a therapeutic relationship, understand each member's experience of the problem, and construct a beginning level genogram. Typically, couples and families are eager to work on their problems during the first session, and it is not uncommon to be able to delve into issues more quickly than in individual therapy. Initial sessions are often very information rich. The following is an excerpt from my first couples session with Tom and Carol, with brief commentary included throughout the session.

APPN:	Hello, welcome.
Carol:	Hi. It's good to be here.
Tom:	(*nods yes*)
APPN:	I know from our initial phone call that you two have not been in therapy before. So, I wonder what you are experiencing now.
Carol:	Well, I'm glad to be here and to start discussing the problems we're having. As I told you on the phone, I'm thinking about ending the marriage. There are many things about our marriage that I don't like and many things have happened.
APPN:	How about you Tom? What are you experiencing now?
Tom:	I'm not sure I want to be here, but think it's necessary. I'm OK (*states flatly*).
APPN:	What do you both hope will happen in the session?
Carol:	I hope to get some clarity and figure out what I want to do.
APPN:	How about you Tom?
Tom:	I don't know what to expect. As you know, Carol is thinking of ending our marriage and I don't want that to happen. I hope to learn some ways to keep the marriage together.

Commentary: I notice Carol answers first and I have to repeat the question for Tom in order for him to answer.

APPN:	I'd like to hear from each of you what you perceive as the problems in your marriage.
	(*About 1 minute passes where Carol stares pointedly at Tom, who finally turns to look back at her, grins, and shrugs.*)
Carol:	Well, I was waiting to see if *he* would start, but *knowing* I'd have to be the one.
Tom:	I'll start if you want me to (*states reproachfully*).
APPN:	(*To Carol*) So, you believe you are the one who needs to be the initiator.

Commentary: I note there may be a dysfunctional interaction pattern of overfunctioning and underfunctioning and will assess further as the therapy progresses.

Carol:	Yes. What else is new? (*States sarcastically*) I feel the need to give you a brief history, so if OK, I will do that.
APPN:	Tom? Is that OK with you?
Tom:	Sure. OK by me (*accompanied with a sweeping hand gesture of, "Be my guest"*).
APPN:	Go ahead Carol.
Carol:	Well, Tom and I met during my last year of college and were married the following summer in 1999—thus, we've been married for 12 years. He still had one more year of college to finish, but we decided to get married anyway. For the first 6 years, we lived in apartments and either one or both of us were in college. Those years were actually pretty good. He received his BS in chemistry and I received my law degree. I started working as a lawyer in the fall of 2005, and he started working for the EPA in the summer of 2006. We bought a house in 2006 as well. It seems that soon after that, I began feeling dissatisfied in the marriage. So, it's been about 5 years now—me feeling this way. By the time we bought the house, we had two sons—one born in 2002—that's Kyle, and one in 2003—that's Todd. They are now 8 and 9 and in first and second grade. When we bought the house, the boys were 3 and 4 years old.
APPN:	A lot happened during those years between 1999 and 2006—finishing college, new jobs, having children, buying a house.
Carol:	Yes, lots of change. Our lives became very hectic with both of us working full time in new jobs, taking care of the boys, and much to do in the new house.
APPN:	Tom, would you agree with what Carol is saying?
Tom:	Yeah (*answers without enthusiasm*).
APPN:	Can you tell her that?
Tom:	I agree—those years were hectic (*states lethargically, while looking at her*).
APPN:	What's been going on the last 5 years?
Carol:	Well, it struck me a few months after moving into the house that I was the *manager* at work *and* I was the *manager* at home. And, Tom was the *helper*. And, it became too much (*bites off the final words*).

APPN:	Can you explain in more detail what you mean?
Carol:	Well, like a manager, I planned everything—kept everything in my head or on a calendar. Who had to be where when? Who had to pick up or take the boys to school? What bill needed to be paid? When did the furnace need to be cleaned? When did the boys need to go to the dentist? What groceries did we need? What vacation should we go on? And, at work, it was similar. When does the case go to court? What research needed to be done? The point I'm trying to make is that I *managed* it all and still do. And, I am sick of it!
APPN:	So, it's frustrating to be the manager at home and at work.
Carol:	Yes. It is. I'm sick and tired of doing it all! (*Sighs heavily*)
APPN:	Can you say that to Tom?
Carol:	He knows—this is not the first time he has heard it. But I will tell him again (*repeats how she is the manager and gives a spirited litany of all she does*).
APPN:	What's it like for you Tom—hearing this in session?
Tom:	Nothing new. I've heard it before (*spoken peevishly*).
APPN:	What do you *experience* when she says these things?
Tom:	I just want to leave the room (*speaks resignedly*).

Commentary: Tom has difficulty engaging in conflictual conversations and wants to flee, which makes Carol more frustrated.

Carol:	At home, he does leave the room. I usually follow him and then he refuses to engage. He shuts down. Then I withdraw or otherwise, it's like banging my head against a brick wall.

Commentary: They engage in a dysfunctional pursuer and distancer pattern of interaction.

APPN:	(*To Tom*) Are you shut down now?
Tom:	Sort of (*states noncommittally*).
APPN:	(*To Tom*) Would you be willing to engage with Carol now, rather than distancing emotionally?
Tom:	I guess so (*states half-heartedly*).
APPN:	(*To Tom*) Tell Carol what you are experiencing.
Tom:	(*To Carol*) You do plan everything, but you're better at it than me. You remember all the little details. You do a great job. And, I help you, if you ask me. I always do what you tell me to do. If you tell me it's my day to pick up the boys, I go and do it. I just don't see what the big deal is? (*Speaks with whiny tone.*)
Carol:	(*To Tom*) You do what I ask you to do, but I'm the one constantly thinking about what needs to be done. I bear the full mental load. It's exhausting.
APPN:	(*To Carol*) It sounds as if you manage a full-time job and a full-time home and are tired of being the manager in both roles. You'd like for

	Tom to share in the management—share the mental load—and not just be a helper. Do I have it right?
Carol:	Yes. You have it right (*speaks emphatically*).
APPN:	(*To Tom*) And you're OK with Carol managing and you helping. You believe she does a good job and don't really think it's a problem. Do I have it right?
Tom:	That's true (*speaks with greater conviction*).
APPN:	Tom. You look to Carol to initiate. What does Carol do to keep you as a helper?

Commentary: This technique called affiliating is to articulate a negative statement about Tom while at the same time absolving him of responsibility for the behavior.

Tom:	She is very competent. She thinks of everything. She does things well. She is on top of things. And, I'm not (*shrugs his shoulders with his palms upward*).
APPN:	(*To Carol*) What does Tom do to keep you as the manager?
Carol:	He doesn't share in the planning. He doesn't think of things that have to be done. If I don't do them, no one will. And, frankly, I'm tired and overwhelmed all the time. He tells me to slow down and relax, but there is always something to do. My life has become a hectic juggling act of doing more and more and always needing more time to fit it all in. I sometimes feel out of control. I know I need to take more time for me. I try to rearrange my priorities. Still, I get no initiation from him and it's so frustrating.
APPN:	It sounds as if you would like to have more time for yourself.
Carol:	Yes. We actually sold our house a month ago and liquidated all our assets, so if the marriage ends, it will be easy to split things up. It was my idea. We bought some property near my law office and have architectural plans to build a house. If the marriage works, we are going to move forward with these plans, and if not, we will just sell it.
APPN:	Is it less stressful without the house?
Carol:	Not really. We are in limbo, with our stuff in different places.
APPN:	Where are you living now?
Carol:	We're living with his parents temporarily and have rented a condo for the first of the month as we try to figure things out. Our house sold within 2 weeks for full price—extremely quickly—so that's why we're temporarily staying with his parents. Since our assets are liquidated, if we do move toward divorce, it will be simple—a 50-50 split. We both have good jobs and we'd split custody of the children and live near each other. If we decide to stay together, we'll rent for about 6 months and start house construction.
APPN:	You have a plan. So, the issue is, will the marriage stay together?.
Carol:	Yes.
Tom:	Yeah.

APPN: To return to one of your issues of manager and helper, you said that you have arguments about this at home frequently. I wonder if you would be willing to enact a recent argument right here.

Carol: You mean role-play it?

APPN: Yes. I would like to see how it unfolds.

Carol: OK with me.

Tom: OK.

Carol: Well, I just thought of one. It was about buying Christmas presents. This happened a few weeks before Christmas. I told Tom that I was not going to buy Christmas presents for his family this year.

APPN: Is this situation OK with you Tom?

Tom: Yeah.

APPN: OK. Let's turn your chairs to face each other (*they do so*). Who would like to start?

Tom: Go ahead Carol. You started the argument (*speaks accusatorily*).

Carol: "I have decided that I'm not going to buy Christmas presents for your family this year. I have enough to buy for my family. So, I'd like you to purchase gifts for your family" (*speaks matter-of-factly*).

Tom: "Can't you do it? You always know what to get them—especially my mother and sister. I don't know what to get them. What's the big deal?" (*Speaks defensively*)

Carol: "It's a big deal for me. I'm not going to do it. I have a lot to buy for my family and it's too much" (*speaks with irritation*).

Tom: "Alright, I'll buy for my family" (*speaks with resignation*).

Carol: "I can give you some ideas, but, I'm not going shopping for them this year" (*speaks emphatically*).

Tom: "OK. I said I'll do it" (*speaks defensively*).

APPN: (*Enactment complete*) What happened next?

Carol: Nothing. He never bought them anything, so on Christmas morning there were no gifts for them.

Tom: They didn't care, and I told them we were going to take them to dinner.

Carol: I disagree. They did care, but acted like it was OK. Typically, I would have given in and bought gifts for his family, but I was clear to Tom that I wasn't going to, so I didn't. And, he never even asked me for ideas. It's like he totally forgot about it.

APPN: What's it like for you hearing this situation reenacted?

Tom: It's OK for me. I didn't know what to get them, so I didn't get them anything (*speaks with a self-pitying tone*).

Carol: For me, I notice that I lose respect for Tom—he's like a child and needs me to do everything for him. We have a lot of experiences like this. Usually, I just give in and do it, but not anymore. I'm done (*states emphatically*).

APPN:	It sounds like you're changing this pattern of overfunctioning.
Carol:	I'm trying. The logic is that if I stop overfunctioning, he'll step up to the plate. But, it doesn't happen. He doesn't. It's one thing not getting Christmas gifts, but it's another thing not picking the boys up from their activities and having them stranded or not paying the bills and having my credit score ruined.
APPN:	I wonder what you can do at home during the week to begin to change this pattern of overfunctioning and underfunctioning? (*To Tom*) Would you be willing to initiate one thing at home this week?
Tom:	Yes.
APPN:	(*To Carol*) Can you think of one thing you would like Tom to initiate?
Carol:	Yes—to take the garbage and recycling out without me having to remind him.
APPN:	(*To Tom*) Would you be willing to do that?
Tom:	Yeah.
APPN:	OK. Let's start with this experiment for the coming week and see what happens.
Tom:	And, Carol. You don't need to remind me (*states reassuringly*).
Carol:	OK (*speaks mildly*).
APPN:	We have about 30 minutes left. It's helpful to take some time to learn about each of your families in order to better understand your current problems. I would like to diagram your families on this flip chart. Would it be OK if we did that?

Commentary: I decided to construct a genogram at this point because understanding the origin of their patterns is important.

Carol:	Yes.
Tom:	Yeah.
APPN:	Which one of you wants to go first?
APPN:	(*Silence*) How about if we start with you Tom? Tell me about your family?

Commentary: Starting with Tom will help to change the pattern of Carol being the one who initiates and overfunctions.

Tom:	OK. There was my mother and my grandmother. I have an older brother and younger sister. And my stepfather who came into the family when I was 12.
APPN:	(*Diagrams on flip chart*) I notice you didn't mention your father?
Tom:	My mother kicked him out when I was 2. As a kid, I would only see him on holidays. Now, I see him once a year on Father's Day. There's not much there.
APPN:	What happened for your mother to kick him out?

Tom:	Well, the story I was told by my mother is that he was always accusing her of cheating on him and he would threaten her. One time, they got into a fight and she hit him with a grate from the stove and he went to the hospital. She then got a restraining order and they divorced soon after. According to my father, she cheated on him and he got tired of it and left. I think he may have been a bit paranoid. Who knows the truth? My mother married my stepfather 10 years later when I was 12. I couldn't stand him—then or now—and he never liked me either.
APPN:	Give me a few adjectives that describe your mother, father, and stepfather.
Tom:	Mother—tough, controlling
	Father—strange, cold
	Stepfather—critical, wimpy
APPN:	What ethnicity are they?
Tom:	Both parents are Ukrainian and my stepfather is Czechoslovakian.
APPN:	What are their ages and birth dates?
Tom:	I don't know. I think they're all in their late 50s or early 60s. I don't know their dates of birth. We never focused much on birthdays and anniversaries.

Commentary: Typically, when a family member does not have information, the family system is more likely to be disengaged.

APPN:	What do they do for a living?
Tom:	None of them went to college. I don't think my stepfather even graduated high school. My father works at Ford Motor Company. My mother works in a pocketbook factory. And my stepfather works in a copper factory.
APPN:	How about your extended family—grandparents, aunts, uncles, cousins?
Tom:	My grandmother lived with us growing up. She died a few years back. She was born in Ukraine and came over here and worked as a housekeeper and sent her money back to her husband and daughter (my aunt) in Ukraine—with the plan that he would save the money and then she would return to Ukraine and they would buy a house there. After a few years, she found out her husband spent all her money on alcohol and gambling. She went back to Ukraine, beat him up in the middle of the street, and then returned to the United States with my aunt who was a teenager. She married again in the United States and had my mother, but he died a year later—had a heart attack. So, I never knew my grandfather. So, it was just my grandmother, my mother, and my aunt, who was much older than my mother. My grandmother and aunt never learned to speak English.
APPN:	So, your grandmother raised your mother and your aunt by herself. When your mother married your father, your grandmother moved in with them?

Tom:	My grandmother actually owned the house and my mother lived with her, so when she married my father, he moved in with them.
APPN:	What was your grandmother like?
Tom:	She was tough. She watched us when we were young for my mother always worked. She was always very old—I think in her 70s when I was a kid—so my mother did everything around the house. And, when she married my stepfather, he did nothing but work at the factory and watch television. He was lazy and useless.
APPN:	So, it seems your male role models were not very competent men and you didn't get much guidance or support from them.
Tom:	I guess that's true.
APPN:	You had a mother who worked—she and your grandmother took care of the house.
Tom:	I guess that's true. My stepfather gave my mother his paycheck, but it was not much. He never did anything around the house or outside in the yard.
APPN:	And, what about your siblings?
Tom:	I have an older brother—2 years older. We're not close, but we see each other for holidays. He's single and drinks a lot. My sister is in college now. She's my half sister—her father is my stepfather. She's 10 years younger, so we don't have much in common—again, we're not close, but I love her.
APPN:	So, what do you both experience when you hear about Tom's family?
Carol:	Well, he wasn't expected to do anything at home and like you said, he didn't have good male role models. The women did everything, so it all makes sense—the way he is.
Tom:	Yeah (*shrugs*).
APPN:	(*To Carol*) Let's spend a little time with your family Carol. We'll develop both of your families in more depth as time goes on, but I would like to hear about your family in the time we have left. So, tell me who is in your family.
Carol:	My parents and two brothers—one is 4 years older and the other is 4 years younger. My mom has a degree in business and became a stay-at-home mother when my brother was born. He is the oldest and his name is Ted. He owns a restaurant outside of Philadelphia and is married with two daughters. I don't see him that often, but feel close to him. My younger brother Geoff is an oral surgeon. He is newly married and has no children. We're close as well, but I don't see him on a regular basis. Our lives are all very busy. My father always had two jobs—one was at a chemical company and the other was his own business—an oil business. He didn't go to college and grew up on a farm in New England. His father had an oil business as well. Both of my parents are energetic and do what they do well. The roles are traditional—my father bringing home the paycheck and my mother taking care of the home. They both did a good job at parenting. Our household was structured—up at 7:30 a.m., cookies and milk after school, dinner at 5:30 p.m. There was lots of emphasis on academics, sports, and doing your best.

APPN:	What is your ethnic background?
Carol:	My father is German and my mother is Czechoslovakian and Hungarian.
APPN:	It sounds as if both of your parents were very active and hard working.
Carol:	Oh, yes. My father and mother never stopped. My father, for example, can fix anything and my mother keeps the house in good working order. They both are always doing something and enjoy keeping busy. Both my parents are very community minded and volunteer at our church. My father delivers oil at a reduced rate to people in need. They both have strong values of giving to others.
APPN:	How about grandparents?
Carol:	My father's parents live in Connecticut and are dairy farmers and are in good health. They also have an oil business, which they still operate. They both work hard. My father has two sisters who are married with children and also live in Connecticut. There are four cousins—much older than me—I don't see them much, but when I do, we have a good time. My maternal grandmother died when I was only 4, so I didn't know her well. She was a seamstress and had nine children. My maternal grandfather died a few years ago. He was very smart and was the treasurer of our church, so I always remember him quizzing me with math problems. With all my aunts and uncles, I only have two cousins on my mother's side. A number of my uncles were in the service and never married. A few married and didn't have children. It is a large extended family and we got together frequently and still do now—holidays and special occasions mainly.
APPN:	What do you both notice as you look at Carol's genogram?
Tom:	Not much new stuff here. Unlike mine, her family was *"easy street."* (He *huffs.*)
Carol:	I don't think it was *easy street*—everyone worked very hard. Their roles were traditional and there was a great deal of structure—and, everyone worked together.
Tom:	Admit it Carol. You want me to be like your father. The guy never takes it easy (*speaks accusingly*).
Carol:	That's not true. I want to be married to someone who shares the responsibility and can initiate and take charge at times. I want a partner, not a helper. There's a lot to do with work, the kids, the house. I'm not a stay-at-home mom. I want an equal partner (*states emphatically*).
APPN:	What do you think about that Tom?
Tom:	I like who I am and don't want to change. After work, I don't like to think about anything. I like to watch TV and take it easy (*states as immutable truth*).
APPN:	We need to stop now. Our 90 minutes is up. Tom, this week you are going to initiate taking the garbage and recycling out and Carol you are not to remind him. Next week our session will be for 60 minutes, starting the same time. OK?

Commentary: Carol and Tom came for seven more sessions. Minor changes occurred in their interactional patterns. The overfunctioning pattern by Carol decreased and the underfunctioning pattern by Tom decreased, but to a lesser degree. The pursuing and distancing pattern also decreased. Tom was better able to communicate his needs, but was still unable to tolerate interpersonal conflict. Carol decided to stay in the marriage. They went on a vacation to California and terminated therapy with the plan to begin construction on their house. I wondered if I would ever see them again for there was still much more work to be done.

MIDDLE PHASE

I received a call from Carol who said they needed help because her sons were getting into trouble. We made an appointment for family therapy. It was 5 years after our initial work together. Carol was now 38 and Tom 44. Their sons Kyle and Todd were 14 and 13 years old, respectively.

APPN:	Good to see you again Carol and Tom and to meet your sons.
Carol:	This is Kyle and this is Todd.
APPN:	(*To the boys*) How do you do? Is this your first time in therapy?
Kyle:	Yes.
Todd:	Yes.
APPN:	Last time I saw you, you were building a new house.
Carol:	Yes. A lot has happened in the past 5 years. We moved into the new house about a year after we finished therapy. We are still both working in the same jobs. Kyle just graduated from eighth grade and Todd seventh grade. Over the summer, they got into some trouble and are now on probation and have to each do 10 hours of community service. That's why we're here.
APPN:	(*Kyle and Todd roll their eyes and smirk*). Tom or Carol—Can you tell me in more detail what happened?

Commentary: I ask Carol and Tom, ignoring the boys' eye rolling and smirking in order to reinforce that the hierarchy of power resides in the parents.

Carol:	Yes. They have a friend Sam who was housesitting for neighbors who were away on vacation—watering plants and that sort of thing. Sam decided to invite some friends over, which turned into a party. They drank a lot of alcohol that was in the house and apparently were all drunk. They tried to clean up the mess afterward, but missed a few things. When the family came home, they saw a few things were amiss and asked Sam if he had anyone over to the house. Sam denied anything happened, so the family called the police. Eventually, the juvenile officer rounded up all the teens who were there and arrested them for criminal trespass and theft. They all had to go to juvenile court and received probation and 10 hours of community service. The case will remain open for 6 months, at which time it will be dismissed if the teens get into no other mischief. The situation has been very upsetting for me.

APPN:	(*To Tom*) What are your thoughts about what happened?
Tom:	What they did was not right, but as I told Carol, "All kids act out and will drink and it's no big deal" (*states matter-of-factly*).
APPN:	It's true that teens will usually break rules as they move through their adolescent years, but all teens do not drink to intoxication and most are not arrested for criminal trespass and theft.
Tom:	Well, I got into a lot of trouble as a teenager myself, so I guess, I don't see it as a big problem (*states defensively*).
APPN:	And, Carol?
Carol:	I am concerned that it is the beginning of more problems to come. And, I feel, we need to cut this off at the pass—before the problems get bigger (*speaks urgently*).
APPN:	Let's hear from you two—Kyle and Todd. Who would like to start and tell me what you think about the situation?
Kyle:	Sam, my friend, invited me over and I brought Todd. We didn't know it was going to turn into a big party with drinking. And, later, when the police started interviewing us all, it was scary. I told the truth though.
Todd:	I'm glad we only got probation. We're going to do 10 hours at the recycling center.
APPN:	So, you're glad you got off rather easy?
Kyle:	Yes.
Todd:	(*Shakes head yes*)
APPN:	Well, it sounds like you are both relieved.
Kyle:	Yes. And, we won't do anything like that again (*states sincerely*).
Todd:	I agree (*states sincerely*).
Carol:	I think the boys need more supervision. Tom was home the day it happened and drove them over to Sam's. I'm not saying that it's Tom's fault, but I would like him to be more attentive to what the boys are doing and ask more questions. When he's in charge, I feel that all hell breaks loose.
APPN:	So, Carol. You would like Tom to pay more attention and ask questions when it comes to dropping the boys off at someone's house?
Carol:	Yes.
APPN:	We may want to delve into this more. Today, you are here as a family, so let's take some time to look at what's going on in your family.

Commentary: I want to assess their family functioning by gathering more data and not focus on the precipitating event and parenting issues with the boys present.

Carol:	I think that Tom undermines me and makes light of things involving the boys. I can see more problems brewing and am feeling anxious.
APPN:	What are you afraid of?

Carol:	I feel the boys are getting derailed and need to get back on track. We're always fighting at home.
APPN:	Can you give me an example of a recent fight that happened at home?
Carol:	There's so many things that are problematic. Catching the school bus in the morning, for example. Both boys take the bus to school. They frequently miss it, and then one of us has to drive them to school. We each have to get to work early on some days. So, if they miss the bus, it creates a problem—rushing and getting to work late. Tom and I discussed the problem and came up with a plan with consequences for the boys if they missed the bus. Then, a few days ago, I left for work and just happened to come back home as I forgot something. I went upstairs and heard Tom say to the boys (he didn't know I was in the house), "Don't worry if you miss the bus. I can take you to school today." I couldn't believe what I heard. I felt so angry and betrayed. And, especially after we spent so long in developing a plan to help the boys catch the bus and be responsible.
APPN:	What happened next?
Carol:	I was so upset that I just left the house and didn't let anyone know I was even there. I cried all the way to work, for I realized that this probably happens all the time. He's colluding with the boys, and it's just not right.
Kyle:	(*Laughs*) Dad does that all the time.
APPN:	What do you mean?
Tom:	Go ahead Kyle. Throw me under the bus (*laughs collusively*).
Kyle:	OK. Mom doesn't like us to have a lot of sugar in the house. So, when she isn't home, Dad goes to the store and buys us junk food.
Todd:	And, then, he tells us, "Don't tell your mother I got you this."

Commentary: This is a coalition (a dysfunctional alliance between a parent and children against the other parent), which results in the children having too much power in the system.

Tom:	It's just a joke. Carol can be too strict with them (*defensively backpedals*).
APPN:	(*To Carol and Tom*) Did you two agree on a plan of no junk food in the house?
Tom:	I sort of agreed, but then, I just wanted to give the boys a little treat. You know—to make them feel good. In my family, we didn't have money to buy treats.
Carol:	The problem for me is that he agrees to something and then goes behind my back and changes it. If he would say something like: "How about if a few days a week, we buy the boys junk food for it's important to me," we could negotiate and I would be OK with a compromise and could be in on the fun as well.
APPN:	(*To Tom*) Is it that you do not agree with Carol and you want to avoid conflict? Or, is it that you want to be the good guy with the boys and have them like you? Or, is it you want to give them what you didn't have?

Tom:	I don't know. I just do what I want. It's easier that way.
APPN:	What do you boys think about this?
Kyle:	I think it's their problem. It doesn't matter much to me if I have junk food.
Todd:	I like having some junk food in the house sometimes.
APPN:	Well, these are things we can work on in family therapy.

Commentary: I thought that it was important to meet with the parents separately to work on parenting skills. If they could parent together, it would help their sons become more responsible and act-out less. Tom avoids tension with Carol by triangulating the children (e.g., "Don't tell your mother"). This dysfunctional coalition temporarily makes Tom look like the "good parent," but in the long run causes the children to have too much power and act irresponsibly (e.g., missing the school bus). When the parents argue, the children become disengaged and do what they please. Tom and Carol agree to meet for a few couples sessions. The following is an excerpt from one of the couples sessions that followed:

APPN:	I thought it important to have a few sessions so we can work on your parenting—so you can both be on the same page and hopefully help your sons.
Carol:	I think that's important.
Tom:	I'm willing to go along.
APPN:	I still have your genograms from last time you were here and I think it is important to review them again. (*I put their genograms up on flip charts.*)
Carol:	OK.
Tom:	OK.
APPN:	What do you notice?
Carol:	Well. It's the same. Nothing much has happened. I still overfunction and am too responsible and Tom never wants to take responsibility and avoids conflict.
APPN:	How does this pattern affect you?
Carol:	Well, it makes me frustrated and anxious. And, I feel alone in this marriage—like I'm holding up the fort, without much support.
Tom:	I admit that I do avoid conflict.
APPN:	What do you think your avoiding conflict is about Tom?
Tom:	Oh, I guess it goes back to my mother. If I spoke up to her, I would get hit. My mother was very tough and didn't take anything from us kids.
APPN:	So, what did you do?
Tom:	I would do what I wanted to do, but would never let her know what I was up to.
APPN:	So, you had to be *sneaky* to get what you wanted?
Tom:	You could say that. I remember a situation with my mother that involved Carol to some degree. I went into the Navy after high school. After being discharged 4 years later, I returned home and started college

on the GI Bill. My tuition was paid by the government and I received a check for about $500 each month. My mother would intercept the check, forge my signature, and cash it for groceries and bills. She would give me a small amount to get by on—an allowance. After Carol and I decided to get married, I wanted my check to buy her a ring, but my mother wouldn't give it to me. Carol was furious and said that it was my money and told me to confront my mother. I never did. Instead, I opened up a post office box and changed my address with the government, and then the check was sent to me.

APPN:	And, what did your mother do when she found out the checks weren't coming to the house?
Tom:	I don't remember. I think she was mad but there was nothing she could do.
APPN:	So, you would do things like this to avoid conflict.
Tom:	I guess so.
APPN:	And, what is that like for you Carol when you hear this?
Carol:	On one hand, I feel he did the best he could, for his mother can be like Attila the Hun, but on the other hand, I lost respect for him. I think that began happening way back then even. He never states what he wants or stands up for himself. Living with him is like connecting with cotton candy—there's nothing there. And, it's very frustrating. He does the same thing to me—except, it's not a post office box to avoid conflict, but it's always something. And then I get frustrated. And, the boys see we don't work together and it causes them to be lackadaisical. Their grades are plummeting to B's and C's, and I am afraid it will only get worse.
APPN:	Carol. Can you tell Tom directly how afraid you are?
Carol:	Tom. I'm very afraid the boys are going downhill and we need to work together.
Tom:	What do you want me to do about it? (*Stated defensively*)
Carol:	To do your part (*matter-of-factly*). I just remembered another situation regarding coming here to therapy. Tom and I agreed that we needed family therapy. We told the boys together. When they asked how many times do we have to go, I said I didn't know, but would know more after the first visit. Then, later, Todd said to me that Dad told him and his brother that they only had to go for one session. So, I asked Tom and he denied it. So, I called Todd in and asked Todd in front of Tom and Tom finally said that he might have said that to the boys, but couldn't remember and maybe he just said it to get Todd off his back.
APPN:	So. Let's look at this. What prevented you Tom from saying to Todd that we weren't sure, but would know more after the first session?
Tom:	I don't know. Maybe I didn't want to fight with Todd. He didn't want to come to therapy.
APPN:	So, you avoid conflict with your sons as well as with Carol?
Tom:	I guess so.
APPN:	Tom, how could you do that differently?

Tom:	Well, I could have just said that we will figure it out after the first session with the therapist.
APPN:	That's good Tom. Can you imagine saying that to Todd right now?
Tom:	Sure. "Todd, we don't know how many times and will figure it out after the first session."
APPN:	How was that Tom?
Tom:	OK.
APPN:	You said that well.

Commentary: Giving support to Tom, a man who avoids conflict, is important. He lacks internal support for this type of interaction.

We had many sessions in the middle phase of therapy where the couple learned to parent more effectively. Carol was always eager to change and work through issues. Tom was more resistant and often believed that he was incapable of change.

FINAL PHASE

We began the final phase of therapy approximately 3 years later. Carol asked Tom for a divorce and we had a few couples sessions to negotiate the terms of the divorce. Carol was very relieved and Tom was resigned. Both wanted the divorce and the redistribution of property to go as smoothly as possible. The following is a selection from a session that occurred late in this phase of therapy.

APPN:	Well, here we are.
Carol:	As I told you on your message tape, we have decided to divorce.
APPN:	Say more.
Tom:	Carol asked me for a divorce last week.
APPN:	How are you both doing with this?
Carol:	At times I feel sad, but for the most part I'm relieved. I know it's for the best.
APPN:	What's the sadness about?
Carol:	We have a shared history together. He knew me when I was a young woman. And, we did have some good times.
Tom:	I still wish it were different, but have accepted it.
APPN:	What do you wish was different Tom?
Tom:	I wish that I could be the man Carol needs me to be, but I can't. And, it's OK.
Carol:	Tom will remarry someone who is a better fit. I hope so (*states reassuringly*).
Tom:	Likewise (*assents in a rote fashion*).
	(*Period of significant silence*)

Carol:	Well, I guess this is it. I think we've come near the end of our therapy.
Tom:	Yes. I agree.
APPN:	What are your thoughts about our work together?
Carol:	I think the therapy helped us understand each other and what each of us were contributing in terms of the problems. I wish we could have made it work. There's just too much water under the bridge. And, we still keep having the same old issues.
APPN:	What do you mean?
Carol:	I'll give you a recent example. As you know, we're still living in the same house—separate bedrooms, but sharing expenses until the house sells. The other day, we're having two of Tom's old friends over for dinner. He and I stopped at a fish store to buy some fish to throw on the grill—to keep it simple. We went into the store together and I asked him to pick out the fish since it was his friends. And, he couldn't or wouldn't. Then he asked *me* what kind of fish *I* wanted to buy. I asked him to decide—to please decide. This went on for a minute or so and after going back and forth, I finally said: "Just get the damn salmon!" (*states peevishly*).
APPN:	Tom?
Tom:	I wasn't sure I'd pick the right fish. It's easier if Carol makes the decision.
APPN:	(*To Tom*) What would happen if you selected the fish and it wasn't very good?
Tom:	Nothing, I guess. She might say the fish isn't very good and I would feel criticized, so I try to avoid that from happening. I don't want to make a bad decision.
APPN:	Would Carol belabor the point?
Tom:	No. She's not like that, but just in case. Well. I am who I am. I don't want to change (*chuckles ruefully*). I avoid conflict and that's all there is to it. We've been over this many times before.
Carol:	And, I have come to accept this is who Tom is and I can't change him. Like the song from *La Cage aux Folles*—"I Am What I Am"—he is what he is (*laughs*).
Tom:	(*Laughs*) At least we can laugh about it a bit now.
	(*Significant silence*)
APPN:	You are both quiet.
Carol:	I was thinking about our boys.
Tom:	They're doing well. They figured the divorce was going to happen and told us they knew it was just a matter of time.
Carol:	They're now 16 and 17. They're more concerned about where they're going to live. We agreed to stay in the house for the rest of the school year until Todd finishes high school. Kyle is going to college in a few months. Then, we'll sell the house and go our separate ways. I'm still worried about them.

Tom:	They're doing fine (*states dismissively*).
Carol:	I disagree with Tom, of course. I don't think the boys are doing great. Todd was just arrested for being under the influence of alcohol at his junior prom. He and some friends created a ruckus and refused to leave when asked, so the police were called. They were arrested for being under the influence as well as for defiant trespass. I feel that I'm constantly reeling them in. Kyle barely made it through high school with all the times he was late and absent. He missed taking his SATs for he was hungover and didn't feel like going. I went to all the college meetings at the high school and hoped to be sending him off to a 4-year school, but he'll be going to community college. I hope the boys will continue to improve after the divorce, but I think it'll probably take a while. They aren't where they should be. The environment outside the family may have to provide the needed corrections, like the criminal justice system. Tom disagrees with me and feels they are fine. He always says, "Boys will be boys" (*states exasperatedly*).
Tom:	That's how I feel (*states matter-of-factly*).
Carol:	I know. We have to agree to disagree (*states calmly, but reluctantly*).
APPN:	It's been nice getting to know your family over the years and it's heartening to see that even though the marriage is ending, you both are leaving with hope for the future.

Commentary

I saw the Thomas family over a 9-year period of time—with a gap of many years in the middle of our work together. It is not unusual to see a family for a short period of time and find that they make some progress, but terminate too soon. For the Thomas family, Carol had difficulty letting go. Her parents were happily married for over 50 years. She is a hardworking woman who believed that if she just tried harder, she could make the marriage work. Tom, on the other hand, had a great deal of trauma in his childhood. He was unwilling to work on his early issues and clearly stated this in therapy. He avoided conflict, did not want to change his dysfunctional patterns, and wanted a partner who would take charge. Carol eventually reached a point of acceptance and recognized that she was helpless to make changes in their relationship patterns, and needed to let go. When Carol finally asked for the divorce and Tom agreed to this outcome, there was less tension in their relationship. Nevertheless, many dysfunctional patterns remained as illustrated in the fish story in the final phase of therapy. I worked with this family for a total of 96 sessions. At times, I was frustrated at Tom's unwillingness to work on himself, yet I understood and accepted his process. Carol was eager to change and was easier for me to work with, yet, her inability to let go was difficult even though I understood and accepted her process. In the end, I felt good about the work and hopeful for the future of all members of the family.

DISCUSSION QUESTIONS

1. Do you think the therapy was successful, even though it culminated in divorce?
2. If you were to conduct family therapy with the Thomas family, what would you do differently?

3. With which family member do you identify most, and with which family member do you identify least? State your reasons.
4. Can you identify a situation in your life where you were stuck, without getting your needs met, and stayed too long?
5. Can you identify a situation where you avoided conflict and, if so, what did you do to avoid the conflict and what were the repercussions?

REFERENCES

Beavers, W. R., & Hampson, R. B. (1990). *Successful families: Assessment and intervention.* New York, NY: Jason Aronson.

Bowen, M. (1972). Towards a differentiation of self in one's family. In J. L. Framo (Ed.), *Family interaction: A dialogue between family researchers and family therapists* (pp. 111–173). New York, NY: Springer Publishing Company.

Bowen, M. (1978). *Family therapy in clinical practice.* New York, NY: Jason Aronson.

Carter, B., & McGoldrick, M. (Eds.). (1980). *The family life cycle: A framework for family therapy.* New York, NY: Gardner Press.

Goldenberg, H., & Goldenberg, I. (2012). *Family therapy: An overview* (8th ed.). Belmont, CA: Brooks/Cole.

Greenberg, L., & Goldman, R. (2008). *Emotion-focused couples therapy: The dynamics of emotion, love, and power.* Washington, DC: American Psychological Association. doi:10.1037/11750-000

Greenberg, L., & Johnson, S. M. (1988). *Emotionally focused therapy for couples.* New York, NY: Guilford Press.

Guerin, P. J., Jr., Fogarty, T. F., Fay, L. F., & Kautto, J. G. (1996). *Working with relationship triangles: The one-two-three of psychotherapy.* New York, NY: Guilford Press.

Johnson, S. M. (1996). *Creating connections: The practice of emotionally focused marital therapy.* Philadelphia, PA: Brunner/Mazel.

Johnson, S. M., & Sims, A. (2000). Attachment theory: A map for couples. In T. Levy (Ed.), *Handbook of attachment interventions* (pp. 169–191). San Diego, CA: Academic Press.

Johnson, S. M., & Whiffen, V. E. (1999). Made to measure: Adapting emotionally focused couples therapy to partners' attachment styles. *Clinical Psychology: Science and Practice, 6,* 366–381. doi:10.1093/clipsy.6.4.366

Kerr, M. E., & Bowen, M. (1988). *Family evaluation: An approach based on Bowen theory.* New York, NY: W. W. Norton.

Knight, C. (2013). Humanistic-existential and solution-focused approaches to psychotherapy. In K. Wheeler (Ed.), *Psychotherapy for the advanced practice psychiatric nurse* (2nd ed., pp. 369–406). New York, NY: Springer Publishing Company.

McGoldrick, M. (1995). *You can go home again: Reconnecting with your family.* New York, NY: W. W. Norton.

Minuchin, S. (1974). *Families and family therapy.* Cambridge, MA: Harvard University Press.

Minuchin, S., & Fishman, H. C. (1981). *Family therapy techniques.* Cambridge, MA: Harvard University Press.

Minuchin, S., Montalvo, B., Guerney, B., Rosman, B., & Schumer, F. (1967). *Families of the slums.* New York, NY: Basic Books.

Nichols, M. P. (2012). *Family therapy: Concepts and methods* (10th ed.). Upper Saddle River, NJ: Pearson.

Cognitive Behavioral Therapy: A Grieving Client

Sharon M. Freeman Clevenger

■ PERSONAL EXPERIENCE WITH COGNITIVE BEHAVIORAL THERAPY

My introduction to Cognitive Behavioral Therapy (CBT) began in the 1980s while I was working as a psychiatric nurse in Indiana at a private for-profit psychiatric hospital. The psychologists and psychiatrists that I worked with were trained in Adlerian Psychology; and, as I observed their interactions with various clients, I was mesmerized by the way they gathered information and successfully worked with clients. I wanted to learn more about Adlerian Psychology in order to develop some of the same skills I was witnessing for use with my own interactions with clients. Adler believed that while heredity and environment had influences on personality, a third factor was as important: The individual's own choices in life (Adler, 1917). Adlerian theory influenced both my nursing and psychology graduate education training.

Adlerian psychology and CBT focus on personal life experiences in forming a person's belief system. In both theories, life experiences from the family of origin, extended family, school, and peer networks, and traumatic life changes contribute in forming a person's "schema" or "core belief" system (A. Freeman & Freeman, 2005a). A person's core beliefs, assumptions, and schemas shape his or her perceptions and interpretation of internal and external events. A photo I'm fond of demonstrates this phenomenon. It features eight women on a rollercoaster. The women in the front seat are laughing hysterically, the women in the center are smiling, and the women in the third-row seats look prim and proper with stoic faces trying to hold their skirts down. The photo caption says: "You can choose to live in the front row or the third row. . . ." The lesson of this photo reveals that the same situation has different personal interpretations of the event based on expectations, perceptions, and prior life experiences.

The experiences of my life journey directed me to earn a master's degree in psychology at the Adler Institute of Clinical Psychology (now Adler University) where I studied with Bernard Shulman, Harold Mosak, Robert Powers, Judith Sutherland, John Newbauer, Ronald Pancner, and Martin Greengrass. My journey's experiences unfolded from there, and I was honored to learn CBT and Rational Emotive Behavior Therapy (REBT) directly from Aaron T. Beck, Judith Beck, Robert Leahy, Albert Ellis, Ray Giuseppe, Stefan Hoffman, Frank Dattilio, Arthur Freeman, Christine Padesky, Marsha Linehan, Denise Davis, David Barlow, and Jeff Young, among others. I began to teach CBT at workshops and conferences with my former husband, Arthur Freeman, along with many of our friends and colleagues in the CBT world. In every experience, my own insatiable curiosity about ways to help clients heal was nourished by the hard work of each of the previously named leaders in the field of CBT.

■ FOUNDERS AND LEADERS OF CBT

The roots of CBT can be found in the philosophy of Epictetus (c. 55–135 AD), a Greek Stoic philosopher, who used logic to identify and eliminate false beliefs that led to destructive emotions (A. T. Beck, Rush, Shaw, & Emery, 1979). Years later, the Austrian psychoanalyst Alfred Adler (1870–1937), the founder of Individual Psychotherapy, also contributed to the development of CBT. Adler referred to the interrelationship of heredity, environment, and personal life choices as "soft determinism," and believed that individuals are continuously changing and evolving based on experiences and the resulting perceptions of self, others, and the world around us (Adler, 1917; Dreikurs, 1949). Albert Ellis in the 1950s and Aaron T. Beck in the 1960s, both recognized as the founders of modern-day CBT, developed their similar models of cognitive therapy. They credit the philosophy of Epictetus and the psychoanalytic theory of Adler as having a strong influence on their work.

Albert Ellis (1913–2007), an American clinical psychologist, was first trained as a psychoanalyst and was influenced by Alfred Adler, Karen Horney, and Harry Stack Sullivan. Ellis became dissatisfied by what he saw as the weaknesses of the psychoanalytic method—its passivity and ineffectiveness. He left psychoanalysis in the early 1950s and developed his own directive and active approach, which he named Rational Therapy. By helping clients understand their self-defeating thoughts (rational analysis), in light of their automatic and core irrational thoughts that led to psychological distress, clients would develop more rational constructs (cognitive reconstruction) and functional behaviors. His well-known ABCD model stated that it is not the activating event that causes the upsetting emotions, but the beliefs about the event:

- A is the activating event
- B is the self-talk or irrational beliefs about the event
- C are the upsetting emotional consequences
- D is the disputing of the irrational idea

In 1957, Ellis published his first cognitive therapy book, *How to Live With a Neurotic*, which was widely read by both therapists and lay people. From that point forward, he authored more than 75 books, many of which became best sellers. Ellis founded his own training institute for Rational Living in 1959 as a nonprofit organization to teach his approach to other therapists. The institute was chartered in 1968 by the New York State Board of Regents as a training institute and psychological clinic. In 1993, he changed the name of his therapy to REBT. Ellis was best known as a clinician, theorist, and trainer (Ellis, 1957, 1994; Ellis & Grieger, 1977).

Aaron T. Beck (1921–), an American psychiatrist, was originally trained in psychoanalysis, and was also influenced by Epictetus, Alfred Adler, Karen Horney, and Harry Stack Sullivan as well as George Kelly. Beck developed his CBT model in the 1960s after conducting research with depressed clients and discovering that their dreams did not consist of themes of anger turned inward, a common psychoanalytic concept. Rather, the dreams consisted of themes of loss, inadequacy, deprivation, and defectiveness, which led him to posit a "cognitive" element as the primary source of depression. He soon discovered that when clients identified and talked about their unrealistic and maladaptive thoughts, they spontaneously modified them in a positive direction

(Clark, Beck, & Alford, 1999). Through a series of controlled clinical trials using systematic structuring of cognitive therapy, he developed guiding principles and specific procedures for the therapist to follow (A. T. Beck, 1976; Freeman Clevenger, Miller, Moore, & Freeman, 2015).

In the 1970s he published his first cognitive therapy treatment manual as well as a number of instruments such as the Beck Depression Inventory and the Beck Anxiety Inventory (A. T. Beck et al., 1979). Originally, he focused on the client's dysfunctional automatic thoughts (spontaneously occurring verbal or imaginal cognitions) that were triggered by stimuli in the environment. He worked on changing the negative emotions and behaviors by changing the client's dysfunctional thoughts. He is known for identifying many cognitive distortions (CDs) such as overgeneralization (distorted beliefs based on a single event that is then applied to an unrelated situation) and arbitrary inferences (drawing conclusions without sufficient evidence), among others. More recently, Beck began to focus on core schemas—central beliefs about the self that are activated by situations in the here-and-now and underlie the automatic thoughts.

Traditional behavior theory focused on guided experiments to shape measurable behaviors such as fear and avoidance with little attention paid to the cognitive processes accompanying these behavioral changes. For example, fearful responses were extinguished with exposure protocols. Other researchers including Meichenbaum (1977) and Lewinsohn and his associates (Lewinsohn, Hoberman, & Teri, 1985) began to incorporate behavioral interventions within Ellis' and Beck's cognitive theoretical structures, which added context and deeper understanding to outcomes. Continuing extensive research has demonstrated significant efficacy in combining cognitive techniques (i.e., cognitive restructuring) with behavioral techniques (i.e., exposure therapy and relaxation training) into CBT (J. S. Beck, 2011). Theoretical refinement and integrated models such as Dialectical Behavior Therapy (DBT), Cognitive Processing Therapy (CPT), and Acceptance and Commitment Therapy (ACT) have been created in the past few decades, resulting in consensus that it is the interplay between thoughts, feelings, and behaviors within one's environment that results in psychopathology. Therefore, it is imperative that interventions target all three foci in order to effect sustainable changes, cognition being the pivotal point (J. S. Beck, 2011; S. M. Freeman, 2008).

■ PHILOSOPHY AND KEY CONCEPTS OF CBT

The basic philosophy of CBT is that psychological issues and psychiatric disorders are the result of distortions of automatic thoughts and core beliefs; and, these distortions are learned and reinforced through life experiences. To understand how life experience influences the development of core beliefs, consider the experience of Janice, who may have enjoyed school through the fifth grade, and then grew to hate not only school, but learning and homework in general. Janice might simply state that she had always hated school, or that not everyone likes school, or that homework is something that she never liked or completed. Upon further exploration, Janice may discover that once she moved to middle school, the new teacher was critical, discouraging, and lacked imagination in creating a learning environment. Maybe the teacher said she was stupid and unteachable and she began to loathe going to school, sought to avoid school and the homework associated with it, and fell behind in learning. If Janice fell behind enough, she would struggle with the next year's material and eventually would incorporate the idea of being "stupid" as a fact attributed to herself personally, and, therefore, feel she was unteachable. The goal of a CBT therapist would be to challenge those unhelpful beliefs by comparing distorted evidence that she is stupid and unteachable to factual evidence that she is smart and teachable. In this way, the therapist helps the client modify her belief system in such a way as to incorporate newly uncovered facts that Janice is not only smart and teachable, but that she may actually enjoy the process of learning (J. S. Beck, 2011; Dewikuea, 1949).

CBT is based on the fact that some automatic thoughts are exaggerated, distorted, mistaken, or unrealistic, and therefore play a major role in psychopathology (A. T. Beck & Weishaar, 1986). Once the core belief system is known, the therapist targets automatic thoughts and conclusions that may no longer be useful to the client. The cognitive triad that includes individual views of self, the world, and others determines emotions and behaviors. An examination of the cognitive triad in a depressed person may uncover a negative view of the self (e.g., "I'm unlovable, worthless and ineffective"), a negative view of the future (e.g., "Nothing will ever work out for me"), and a negative view of the world (e.g., "Everyone in the world is hostile"; A. T. Beck, 1989). The therapist then helps the client to examine and modify the unhelpful thoughts, resultant emotions, and behaviors, which, in turn, alters all three (J. S. Beck, 2011). For example, clients who are anxious tend to focus on "unsolvable questions" and/or symptoms, which reinforces the sense of having no control and may result in increased anxiety and panic. The symptoms of panic and anxiety may then lead to beliefs that the situation is hopeless, and/or that the client is useless. As a result, the "anxiety/panic-belief generation-anxiety/panic" vicious cycle is quickly established. The basic premise for effective CBT is based on four components: (a) the client's readiness for change must be maximized, (b) treatment must be tailored and integrated to the client, (c) both specific and general goals must be developed to guide treatment, and (d) the disorder is not treated; rather, the component parts of the disorder are treated (J. S. Beck, 2011). The therapeutic process is based on the principles of empirical investigation, reality testing, and problem-solving in a collaborative process between the therapist and the client. Distortions in perception and thinking create and reinforce learned errors in logic and reason. Figure 8.1 provides a visual representation of the flow of thoughts, behaviors, and emotions that demonstrate the development of emotional or behavioral reactions to events.

■ DEFINITION OF MENTAL HEALTH AND PSYCHOPATHOLOGY IN CBT

CBT is based on a cognitive theory of mental health and psychopathology. When perceptions of situations are accurate and functional, clients will have appropriate emotional reactions and behaviors. When perceptions of situations are inaccurate and distorted, emotional and behavioral reactions will be dysfunctional. Clients' perceptions are often distorted and dysfunctional when they are distressed.

■ THERAPEUTIC GOALS IN CBT

CBT is the treatment of choice for clients with dysfunctional automatic thoughts and core beliefs. The goal is to assist clients in changing their dysfunctional thoughts and core beliefs to ones that are functional. CBT aids in developing skills and tools that will enhance internal resources and coping skills. CBT is collaborative; thus, the therapist and client together structure each session and set reasonable, measurable, and specific goals. Goal setting allows both participants to assess if, when, and how progress has been made. Goals include both problems to overcome as well as positive changes that need to be made (S. M. Freeman, 2008). Each session ends with assigned homework, which is then reviewed at the beginning of the next session. CBT is based on treatment plans that are clearly conceptualized and incorporated from empirically validated approaches that guide the clinician through each session and overall plan of care (J. S. Beck, 2011). Clients learn to identify

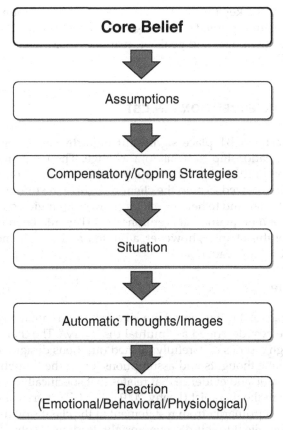

FIGURE 8.1. Diagram representing the flow of thoughts, behaviors, and emotions that generate emotional or behavioral reactions to events.

and evaluate their automatic thoughts and to correct their thinking so that it more closely resembles reality. When clients do so, their emotional distress usually decreases, their physiological arousal abates, and they are able to behave more functionally.

■ PERSPECTIVE ON ASSESSMENT IN CBT

Assessment in CBT includes a comprehensive intake evaluation that assesses the client's chief complaint, history of the current problem, psychiatric history, developmental history, family history, physical health history, current and previous medications, prior experience with therapy, and collateral information. As the client discusses these aspects, the therapist notices any CDs. If the client tells a story about a difficult situation, it is common for the therapist to ask him or her what he or she was thinking as the situation took place. The therapist is interested in the client's interpretation of events. For example, if a client states that he or she felt depressed after the death of his or her dog, the therapist should inquire as to the interpretation of the loss. For example, if the client states, "I will never be happy again," this interpretation by the client is key, for it will become one of the initial targets for therapy. The therapist identifies core beliefs that underlie the automatic thought such as, "I am a miserable person that never has any luck in this world." The therapist also assesses any concomitant behaviors that are dysfunctional.

Beck believed that the key for positive outcomes is the development of a solid plan for treatment. Treatment is guided by the cognitive conceptualization, which is, in turn, guided by the assessment data and goals of treatment (S. M. Freeman Clevenger et al., 2015)

■ THERAPEUTIC INTERVENTIONS IN CBT

Therapists who practice CBT place significant importance on cognitive information processing and its relationship to behavioral change. The resultant theoretical model combines features of traditional psychotherapy within a unique conceptual framework. Clinical strategies are utilized to help the client recognize the thinking patterns that are illogical or dysfunctional, and to help the client changes their views and/or conclusions. A complete review of therapeutic interventions in CBT would be massive and therefore beyond the scope of this chapter; however, a limited review of some of the basic techniques are outlined for the reader.

Socratic Dialogue

The Socratic Dialogue (SD) is the central model of communication employed by the CBT therapist. SD can be best described as "mutual discovery." The therapist guides the client using SD through a series of carefully posited questions designed to elicit responses that uncover automatic thoughts and assumptions. Once the thought is uncovered, the client examines the logic and evidence that relates to it specifically, with or without additional prompting from the therapist (Leahy, 2001). The CBT therapist uses SD to ask specific questions derived primarily from restatement of the client's own words as the major technique, leading the client to self-discover insight, leading to subsequent changes. Self-discovery increases the probability that the client will incorporate and modify automatic thoughts based on his or her own observations (S. M. Freeman & Freeman, 2005).

There are seven types of questions involved in the SD: memory, translation, interpretation, application, analysis, synthesis, and evaluation. These purposeful questions skillfully guide the client to an insightful response, rather than didactically providing the answer. It is a powerful technique to have the client obtain the answers through self-discovery. Box 8.1 describes the types of questions used in the SD method of therapeutic interactions (A. Freeman & Freeman, 2005b; S. M. Freeman, 2008).

BOX 8.1 SD: Types of Questions

1. History questions: *"How many children did you have in your first marriage?"* (non-SD)
2. Memory questions: (remembering that the client's recall is influenced temporally, with interference and "facts" being considered inconsequential) *"When did you first notice that your sleep patterns had changed?"*
3. Translation questions: (asks the client how the data refers to the individual) *"When you say you become anxious, explain to me what it feels like to feel anxious to you."*
4. Interpretation: (helps the client identify relationships between facts and experiences) *"How does your sensitivity to criticism play out with your husband?"*

(continued)

BOX 8.1 SD: Types of Questions (*continued*)

5. Application: (asks the individual to apply previously mastered skills to a new situation) "*How can you use what you learned with your boss in your discussion with your son?*"
6. Analysis: (requires breaking a problem into a number of parts) "*What evidence do you have to support this conclusion?*"
7. Evaluation: (asks the individual to make decisions/judgments based on data) "*On a scale of 0-10, where would you rate your level of anxiety today?*" "*And how does that compare to 4 months ago?*"

SD, Socratic Dialogue.

Source: Data from Freeman, A., & Freeman, S. (2005b). Socratic Dialogue. In A. Freeman, S. H. Felgoise, A. M. Nezu, C. M. Nezu, & M. A. Reinecke (Eds.), *Encyclopedia of cognitive behavior therapy* (pp. 380–384). New York, NY: Springer.

Box 8.2 illustrates the basic rules for SD adapted from Freeman and Freeman and is used in conjunction with the question types in Box 8.1 (2005b).

BOX 8.2 SD: Basic Rules

1. The techniques are embedded in the collaborative dialogue and are goal-directed and specific.
2. The therapist has a problem list that generates the plan of direction that begins the SD process. SD is not a series of drifting questions that "follow the client." Each question must be strategically placed in order to reach the predefined goal. This is where the concept of "guided discovery" comes from for the therapeutic interaction.
3. The questions must be short, focused, and targeted. For example, "Do you experience difficulty agreeing with your husband?" "Is this similar to interactions with others?" "How does this play itself out in this situation?" "Can you think of another way to respond that may result in a less defensive response from him?"
4. The questions must progress in a manner that keeps anxiety at a minimum for the client.
5. The SD questions should be framed in a way to elicit an affirmative response. For example, in a reluctant client: "There are probably a lot of places you would rather be than here, right?"
6. The additional point to the previously mentioned is that negative responses to questions mean that the therapist must reframe the question to gain an affirmative response. "Is it your idea to come to therapy today?" "No! I don't want to be here!" "There are probably a lot of things you would rather be doing today than sitting here." "Yeah! That's for sure!"

(*continued*)

BOX 8.2 SD: Basic Rules (*continued*)

7. The therapist must monitor the client's reactions and moods on an ongoing basis. If a question increases a reaction, the therapist needs to address it immediately. "What just happened—I noticed a reaction—what was that?"
8. The therapist must pace the questions to suit the individual's mood, style, and content of information.
9. The questions must be planned and in logical sequence. The therapist must have an internal map for the session and move the session in a planned direction toward the desired goal.
10. The therapist must be careful to self-monitor and not "jump in" to offer interpretations or solve the client's problems. This is not only more respectful to the client, but it allows for greater clarity.
11. Self-disclosure should be extremely limited and only used with extreme caution and great care as to the motive for the disclosure. Comparing what the therapists did or does with what the client did or does moves away from SD into discussion and possibly misjudgment.
12. The therapist may use everyday experiences as therapeutic metaphors. For example, this author uses Aesop's Fables and other well-known story characters to make a point such as "sour grapes" that can elicit both content and affect.

SD, Socratic Dialogue.

Source: Data from Freeman, A., & Freeman, S. (2005b). Socratic Dialogue. In A. Freeman, S. H. Felgoise, A. M. Nezu, C. M. Nezu, & M. A. Reinecke (Eds.), *Encyclopedia of cognitive behavior therapy* (pp. 380–384). New York, NY: Springer.

Downward Arrow

First used by Beck in 1979, downward arrow refers to elicitation of sequential reasoning. Assumptions in logic are elicited through careful SD questioning by the therapist asking, "If this is true, then what happens?" For example, Mrs. Delany, a successful business owner, was concerned that Martha, a staff member she was having problems with, would undermine her business if she terminated her. Martha and Ms. Delany had not been able to work out their differences for months. The therapist asked her what specifically would happen if she fired Martha.

Mrs. Delany:	She would bad mouth me to her friends and everyone in town and that would give me a bad name!
APPN:	And how would that affect your business?
Mrs. Delany:	Everyone would believe her, and I have a lot of customers that she knows!
APPN:	How many customers do you have currently that she knows?
Mrs. Delany:	(*Thinking*) Gosh. I've never thought about it (*pauses*). I guess about 15.
APPN:	How many customers do you have in total, or perhaps just in any given week?
Mrs. Delany:	About 250.

APPN: How many of the 15 customers that Martha knows would believe Martha and drop you?

Mrs. Delany: (*Laughing*) OK, about two or three, maybe.

APPN: So, if you fired Martha, two or three customers out of 250 would possibly drop you.

Mrs. Delany: (*Laughs*) That's true. I do this to myself all the time! I've been making a mountain out of a molehill over nothing!

Idiosyncratic Meaning

Idiosyncratic meaning is the clarification of statements and terms used so that both the therapist and the client have a clear understanding of meaning. For example, Mr. Smith says, "When she makes those little faces it just puts me out! You know what I mean." Therapist: "No, I don't know what you mean. Please explain what you mean by 'puts you out'."

Daughter Technique

A distancing technique (analogical comparison) presents a hypothetical situation to externalize the conversation with someone near and dear to the client. The person "talks" to an important person in his or her life in session. This technique is more powerful when the person's dilemma is placed on the other person and the client is asked to give that person advice (hypothetically his or her "daughter" but you can use sister, son, niece, nephew, etc.).

Labeling of Distortions

Individuals are helped to identify automatic thoughts that are "dysfunctional or irrational" as a type of self-monitoring for more accurate descriptive terminology. Table 8.1 contains examples of CDs. The therapist provides a list of CDs to the client, then asks the client to choose four or five of his or her "favorite" CDs as homework and to bring this information to the next session. This information is then integrated into future sessions as educational material as it is noticed in the client's verbalizations and/or written information. The client is stopped and asked to "notice" what he or she has said (thought) and encouraged to reframe the information. Other spontaneously elicited examples of distorted automatic thoughts are also "caught" and similarly restructured as needed.

TABLE 8.1 EXAMPLES OF COGNITIVE DISTORTIONS	
Distorted Thought	**Example**
All-or-nothing	*"No one will ever like me!"*
Mind reading	*"They probably think that I'm weird."*
Emotional reasoning	*"I feel lazy today so I might as well just lie in bed."*
Personalization	*"I know she meant me when she said that."*
Global labeling	*"Everything I do turns out wrong."*
Catastrophizing	*"If I start to cry everyone will hate me!"*
Should statements	*"I really should exercise, I shouldn't be so lazy."*

(*continued*)

TABLE 8.1 EXAMPLES OF COGNITIVE DISTORTIONS (*CONTINUED*)	
Distorted Thought	**Example**
Overgeneralization	*"Everything always goes wrong for me."*
Control fallacies	*"If I'm not in complete control all the time, I will go out of control."*
Comparing	*"I'm the only one who isn't on a sports team!"*
Heaven's reward	*"If I do everything perfectly, they will see how valuable I am, and I will be rewarded."*
Disqualifying the positive	*"She doesn't really like me. She was just being polite."*
Perfectionism	*"When I don't get 100% correct it means I'm stupid."*
Time tripping	*"I screwed up my past and now I must be vigilant to secure my future."*
Objectifying the subjective	*"I have to be funny to be liked."*
Selective abstraction	*"All of the good men are taken or gay."*
Externalization of self-worth	*"My worth is dependent upon what others think of me."*
Fallacy of the change of others	*"If you do exactly as I say and change your behavior, I won't yell at you anymore."*
Fallacy of worrying	*"If I worry about it enough, it will be resolved."*
Ostrich technique	*"If I ignore it, maybe it will go away."*
Unrealistic expectations	*"I must be the best absolutely all of the time."*
Filtering	*"I must focus on the negative details while I ignore and filter out all the positive aspects of a situation."*
Being right	*"I must prove that I am right as being wrong is unthinkable."*
Fallacy of attachment	*"I can't live without a partner." "If I was in a relationship, all of my problems would be solved."*

Table 8.2 contains examples of CBT techniques, and Box 8.3 contains steps for cognitive restructuring.

TABLE 8.2 COGNITIVE BEHAVIORAL THERAPY TECHNIQUES		
Technique	**Example**	**Intervention**
Questioning the Evidence	"I know my wife is not satisfied with our love making"	How do you know? What did she tell you? Did she lie to you when she said she enjoyed it?

TABLE 8.2 COGNITIVE BEHAVIORAL THERAPY TECHNIQUES (*CONTINUED*)		
Technique	**Example**	**Intervention**
Examining Options and Alternatives	"There is no way I can tolerate being with my son-in-law for an entire week!"	What are your options? Do you have to spend all 7 days with your son-in-law? What else have you considered doing during your vacation?
Reattribution	"I am such a loser!"	You were married for 22 years and knew of at least five affairs that your husband had; how does that make you a loser?
Decatastrophizing	"I can't stand not to sleep! I can't live like this anymore!"	How much sleep are you getting? Is 4–5 hours the same as not getting any sleep? What is the worst thing that could happen if you continue to get 4–5 hours sleep instead of 7 hours of sleep? What have you tried to help you get more sleep?
Advantages and Disadvantages	The client is "stuck" between two options	What are the pros and cons of option A? B? What are the advantages of A? of B? Disadvantages?
Turning Adversity to Advantage	"I didn't get the job," again.	Review the job requirements, using SD to highlight the places where the job didn't fit the client. Brainstorm possibilities for jobs that fit the client better. "Now you are available to go for the kind of job you really want!"
Paradox or Exaggeration (be careful with this one or it could be seen as sarcasm)	The wife of a client who has obsessive compulsive neatness is upset because they cannot agree on how to organize a new garden they were putting in their yard.	"Oh my goodness! He wants the plants in rows and to be neat and orderly! Where on earth would he get an idea like that?"
Cognitive Rehearsal	"I can't imagine what I will say if they ask me about . . . ."	"Let's practice that out loud and see what happens.".

(continued)

TABLE 8.2 COGNITIVE BEHAVIORAL THERAPY TECHNIQUES (*CONTINUED*)		
Technique	**Example**	**Intervention**
Thought-Stopping	The client begins obsessing and is spiraling.	(Makes a loud noise) Ask the client to report his or her thought pattern after the loud noise. Reinforce how interruption is effective at stopping negative thought patterns.
Cognitive Restructuring	The client identifies negative thought patterns using an automatic thought record.	Brainstorm alternative explanations to what the client has concluded, then evaluate the mood before and after restructuring (see Box 8.3 for Cognitive Restructuring).

SD, Socratic Dialogue.

BOX 8.3 Steps in Cognitive Restructuring

1. Tune in . . . keep a thought diary.
2. Focus on the words that are unhealthy.
3. Stop the messages.
4. Change the negative to positive.

Automatic Thought Records

The automatic thought record (ATR) is the backbone of the cognitive component of CBT. The thought record was first introduced by Beck in 1979 to capture and analyze automatic thoughts both during and between sessions (A. T. Beck et al., 1979; Gilson, Freeman, Yates, & Freeman, 2009). The ATR is used as homework after introducing the process within the therapy session. The client completes the columns identifying a troubling situation, resulting in emotion and thoughts associated with both. The therapist and client work on clarification and development of "rational" responses in order to debate or challenge the original reaction. When practiced and repeated, the process of clarification and debate becomes internalized in the individual (Gilson et al., 2009). An ATR is included in Appendix A.

■ BEHAVIOR THERAPY IN CBT

Behavioral techniques are utilized along with cognitive techniques. Most clients will be treated with a combination of cognitive and behavioral techniques with the predominate type of intervention depending upon the sophistication, ability, and interest of the client.

Assertiveness Training

Assertiveness training involves a combination of cognitive and behavioral practice. Prior to beginning an assertiveness training program, the therapist needs to define the terms *assertive, aggressive,* and *passive.* The therapist may model assertive or passive behaviors, then assist the client within the session with role-play, then eventually develop *in vivo* experiments that increase in complexity over time until the new behavior is internalized.

Behavioral Rehearsal

Use of behavioral experiments helps clients gather more evidence, or to develop more effective responses and styles. Rehearsal is usually practiced first in the therapy session itself, often with role-playing and then as often as possible outside of the session. Modification of behavior practice is conducted using direct observation, or self-report by the client. Behavioral rehearsals are repeated until the client reports comfort, or even excitement: "Okay, I can do that—that's cool." It is important to evaluate for safety as well as understanding of behavioral boundaries when using out of session behavioral assignments.

Contingency Management

Contingency management is based on generally accepted principles of human behavior in that an undesirable behavior is more likely to recur if it is immediately followed by a reinforcer that is pleasurable (positive reinforcement). Positive reinforcers or rewards are more effective at changing behaviors than punishment (aversive reinforcement). A recommended component of contingency management is a contingency contract, which is a written agreement developed in a collaborative manner. The contract should explicitly state the positive and negative reinforcers for performing the desired behavior, as well as aversive reinforcers for failure to perform the behavior. Suitable targets are those behaviors that are observable, and sequential. See Box 8.4 for a checklist to assist the therapist in developing a contingency contract.

BOX 8.4 Checklist of Client Outcomes for Contingency Contract

	1. Identify target behavior
	2. Explore reasons for behavior
	3. Verbalize knowledge of consequences of behavior
	4. Identify secondary gains from behavior (i.e., attention)
	5. Keep diary of when problem behavior occurs
	6. Keep log of sequence and pattern of behavior (who, what, when, how, and why)
	7. Identify feelings that precede and follow behavior
	8. Keep a diary of behavior and feelings
	9. Identify alternatives to behavior
	10. Write conditions under which desired behavior will occur and how behavior will be observed and measured
	11. Select positive reinforcers (i.e., weight loss, rewards)

(continued)

BOX 8.4 Checklist of Client Outcomes for Contingency Contract (*continued*)

	12. Select aversive consequences for failure of desired behavior (i.e., chores)
	13. Carry out plan for 1 week
	14. Practice desired behavior, step-by-step
	15. Keep diary of practice
	16. Involve family/friends in feedback/encouragement
	17. Identify other positive aspects associated with changed behavior
	18. Monitor ongoing weekly progress

Source: Data from Dykes, P., Wheeler, K., & Boulton, M. (1998). Psychiatric copathways. In P. Dykes (Ed), *Psychiatric clinical pathways: An interdisciplinary approach* (pp. 265–275). Gaithersburg, MD: Aspen.

Bibliotherapy

Assignment of specific readings related to the individual's difficulties. Readings and references can be given to the client of the many CBT-based self-help books as an adjunct to in-session work.

Guided Relaxation, Mindfulness Training, and Meditation

This grouping includes techniques aimed at reduction of autonomic nervous system responses to anxiety. Examples might include deep breathing, relaxation training, meditation, mindful meditation, walking a labyrinth, and other exercises. These techniques help the client train himself or herself to refocus away from upsetting thoughts and to increase awareness of conscious control over breathing, heart rate, and other anxiety symptoms and thoughts.

Social Skills Training

This includes various behavioral interactions that many people may take for granted. It is helpful to practice in-session, then in-office (maybe interacting with the receptionist when he or she leaves the office). An example might be teaching an adolescent with Asperger's disorder who wants to interview for jobs to look at a person in the eyes and shake his or her hand firmly (but not too firmly!) at the beginning and end of an interview.

Shame-Attacking Exercises

This technique, first introduced by Albert Ellis, the father of Rational Emotive Therapy (RET), includes engaging the individual in exercises that emphasize their concern for what others think of them. For example, a person who is afraid of drinking soup in public may be assigned the task of going to a restaurant with a friend, ordering soup, and drinking it loudly while the friend makes note of how many people are really interested in what they are doing.

Homework

Homework is a critical component of CBT. Homework reinforces what was learned in the therapy session with specific assignments intended to reinforce or practice skills. This results in a truly collaborative process between client and therapist. Some homework assignments might include deep-breathing practice, role-play, and assertiveness exercises. Homework also allows clients to "try on" and experiment with new skills in order to give feedback to the therapist on which techniques work and which do not work. Techniques that do not work can then be modified or discarded as needed.

Psychoeducation

In CBT the educational component is skillfully interwoven within the specific therapeutic techniques that the therapist is choosing, and then supplemented with bibliotherapy if that is appropriate.

Exposure Therapy

The most powerful, and most well-known, behavioral therapies are developed for phobias, panic attacks, posttraumatic stress disorder (PTSD), obsessive compulsive disorder, and habit reversal for tics, skin-picking, and hair pulling. There are now numerous types of exposure therapy, but the common theme is to expose the person in a structured way to the feared thoughts or situation in order to extinguish the fear response. Some examples of exposure therapies include Exposure and Response Prevention (ERP; Lindsay, Crino, & Andrews, 1997; McLean et al., 2015; Steinglass et al., 2014), Eye Movement Desensitization and Reprocessing therapy (EMDR; Novo et al., 2014), Prolonged Exposure (PE; Foa, McLean, Capaldi, & Rosenfield, 2013; Granato, Wilks, Miga, Korslund, & Linehan, 2015; Lee, Gavriel, Drummond, Richards, & Greenwald, 2002), Cognitive Processing Therapy (CPT; Resick et al., 2015), Systematic Desensitization (Triscari, Faraci, Catalisano, D'Angelo, & Urso, 2015), and Trauma-Focused CBT (TF-CBT; Bisson & Andrew, 2007). Exposure can be in vivo, in-session, through virtual reality, or imaginal in nature. A systematic review of therapies for trauma found that of the treatments evaluated (TF-CBT, stress management, supportive therapy, nondirective counseling, psychodynamic therapy, hypnotherapy, group CBT, and EMDR), TF-CBT and EMDR administered by trained clinicians were the most effective (Bisson & Andrews, 2007).

An excellent resource for clinicians and clients on using CBT for anxiety is *Stopping the Noise in Your Head* (Wilson, 2016), with an accompanying free video series (noiseinyourhead.com/free-video-series) by Reid Wilson, PhD.

■ CASE STUDY

Background

Wendy is a 35-year-old married female who was referred to me for psychotherapy by her primary care practitioner (PCP) following the sudden death of her only sister, who died at the age of 32, 6 months prior. The sister had been seen by her family doctor for a routine physical, had been pronounced healthy, and then shockingly dropped dead of a sudden heart attack 4 days later. Wendy reported an inability to sleep more than 3 hours per night for almost a month. Her PCP prescribed an antidepressant, a benzodiazepine, and sleeping medications to try to help her. Wendy followed her prescribed treatment plan; however, she reported that she was getting worse. Worsening of her symptoms was interpreted by her PCP as "attention seeking," and she was referred for psychother-apy. Wendy was still in shock, horribly grief stricken, and extremely tearful when she arrived for her first appointment. I conceptualized her care based on knowledge inte-grated from REBT, CBT, normal grieving processes, stress models, sleep models, and an understanding of the effects of some of her prescribed medications. This case is intended to demonstrate how creatively following rational, practical, evidence-based standards of practice may help to guide treatment. Prior to beginning psychotherapy, Wendy com-pleted a comprehensive intake that included personal history, family history, physical health history, medications current and previous, prior experience with therapy, and collateral information from her PCP and spouse. I saw Wendy for 24 sessions over a 5-month period of time.

Transcript of Cognitive Behavioral Psychotherapy Sessions

The transcripts were selected from segments of the beginning, middle, and final phase of therapy.

Beginning Phase

The following session is a beginning brief therapy session following the initial intake:

Wendy:	(*Tearful, agitated, wringing her hands, apologizing for crying*) I'm so very sorry! I am never like this! I just can't seem to stop crying!
APPN:	You said that your crying and insomnia have been getting worse. What do you mean by that? (*seeks to understand her experiences*)
Wendy:	After Linda died, I was in a fog for about 2 or 3 weeks. I couldn't eat, but I didn't cry . . . well, at least like this! My husband took me to my family doctor, and he gave me something to help me sleep and to calm me down. At first it worked great! I was sleeping for almost 12 hours at first, but I couldn't go to work, or take care of the house.
APPN:	How long did that last?
Wendy:	That lasted about a month, I guess, and then I started getting worked up for no reason! I was crying if the mail came, if it rained, if I couldn't find my toothpaste—stupid things! And now I can't stop crying, it's almost constant—like this!
APPN:	You said you were prescribed a nerve pill (*alprazolam*) and sleeping medication (*zolpidem*)? How are they working? (*understands that chronic use of benzodiazepines and benzodiazepine receptor agonists such as zolpidem can cause memory issues and exacerbate symptoms due to tolerance and with-drawal effects*)
Wendy:	I still can't sleep! I can't fall asleep and if I do, I'm awake after an hour. I'm just exhausted! And I can't remember the stupidest things! (*Wendy may be experiencing negative effects from her anxiety medications. I make a note to continue to evaluate her symptoms and response.*)
APPN:	You also said you can't stop thinking about your sister. Is that right? (*clarification of ineffective process*)
Wendy:	(*Another burst of crying*) Yes! She was my best friend! We talked every day! She would help me deal with this if she was here. That's what she

	always did. I try to move on like everyone tells me, but no matter how hard I try not to think about her, I just do!
APPN:	Your PCP also prescribed an antidepressant (*sertraline*). Are you taking it every day? (*interruption of ineffective rumination*)
Wendy:	Yes, just like he said, but it's not working at all! Nothing works! I'm going to be like this forever!
APPN:	Your sister was very important to you. Her loss so suddenly just pulled the rug out from under you and now you don't have her to help you get through this. (*Summarizes important points from Wendy's statements—a Socratic technique. I am going to use their relationship to help Wendy cope by helping her connect with her sister's advice.*)
Wendy:	That's true! I am so lost!
APPN:	If you could reverse things, and your sister was sitting here with me, what would you say to her right now? (*Daughter technique, Socratic question*).
Wendy:	(*Pauses looking startled*) I would tell her to knock it off! And then tell her that she should remember our fun times! (*smiles, then becomes tearful but not sobbing*)
APPN:	You look like that conversation with your sister calmed you down a little (*continuation of SD to set the stage for Wendy to "channel" her sister's advice and to discontinue her double standard for grief*).
Wendy:	It did help. I even smiled a little! I haven't done that in forever . . . .
APPN:	Maybe you keep crying about her because you are trying too hard NOT to think about her. (*Begin process of reinforcing using her sister to cope. Interrupt her cyclical thinking—avoidance techniques that are unstructured often increase symptoms.*)
Wendy:	What?
APPN:	Your sister was your best friend. You talked every day. You did things together every day. She was one of the most important people in your life (*demonstrates empathy and understanding regarding the loss*).
Wendy:	I know! I miss her so much!
APPN:	So, maybe you should stop avoiding her (*smiles*). I wonder if you might want to learn how to do this more often, and to use what you know your sister would say to help you feel better (*reinforces the plan to develop the Daughter technique with her and to get her to commit to therapy*).
Wendy:	If you think that might help, I'm game—it did seem to settle me down for a few minutes! (*Wendy is now sad but not sobbing.*)
APPN:	Can you summarize what you learned today, and then decide what you might want to practice before our next meeting?
Wendy:	I learned that it helps to talk with Linda. Maybe I should try that at home?
APPN:	What do you think about that?
Wendy:	I think it might help!

Commentary: I complete the assignment by asking Wendy how often she wants to practice, what days of the week she is going to practice, how long she will practice each time, and so on. Then, I summarize "her" plan back to her.

Middle Phase

APPN: Last time we met, you thought about what you would say to your sister if things were reversed and that was helpful. Did you practice that this week? (*Review of last session homework, use of Daughter technique*)

Wendy: Yes. I did that like we planned, and even added a few extra times. It helped, but it seemed to work better when I was here.

APPN: Would you like to practice something like that again today? (*set goals for this session*)

Wendy: OK, but I'm a little nervous because I can't stop crying if I think about Linda! (*begins to sob*)

APPN: Grieving is healthy. It's normal. We are the only animal that weeps, cries with tears. Since we have tear ducts, we must be meant to use them. And the most reasonable time to use them is when we are grieving someone who we have lost who was very important to us (*normalizes her experience*).

Wendy: (*Smiles weakly*) But all I do is cry.

APPN: Is that ALL you do? (*challenges irrational all-or-nothing thinking*)

Wendy: Of course not, it just seems any time I stop working or doing something, I remember Linda and start to cry again. It's endless!

APPN: What do you mean it is endless? (*clarification of another irrational expectation to prompt automatic revision of catastrophic thought*)

Wendy: It seems like it will never end, it just gets worse and worse. It *seems* endless. The worst is when I try to sleep! As soon as I lay down, I start to sob because I miss her so much.

APPN: You caught yourself and changed things from it *is* endless to it *seems* endless (*scaling technique to break all-or-nothing thinking into a range of intensities*).

Wendy: (*Smiles*) That does *seem* different! (*smiles at her use of "seem" as a modifier*)

APPN: (*Smiles*) Little differences *seem* to make things more reasonable and not so catastrophic, don't they?

Wendy: Yes. It does *seem* like such a small thing, but it does *seem* different! (*laughs*)

APPN: Let's focus on something else you said earlier. You said you try to avoid thinking about Linda, so you don't cry all day, but as soon as you let your guard down you start thinking about her again and start to sob again. Is that accurate?

Wendy: Yes. I really try hard to not think about her!

APPN:	Are you sure you have given yourself time to grieve her, or are you mostly trying to avoid grieving her? (*observes dichotomy that she has created*)
Wendy:	I thought I was grieving her all the time, and that is why I can't stop crying. But I'm not grieving, am I? I am mostly avoiding it.
APPN:	Is avoiding it working? (*reality-based REBT technique*)
Wendy:	Apparently not! So, what you are saying is that I should cry about her on purpose? That sounds scary!
APPN:	What is scary? (REBT *observation of automatic negative expectation*)
Wendy:	I'm afraid I won't be able to stop crying.
APPN:	Do you know anyone who was never able to stop crying? (*REBT technique to help her observe irrational fear*)
Wendy:	(*Laughs*) No. It sounded silly as soon as I said it (*observation of irrational belief*).
APPN:	Okay then, how can you cry about her on purpose? (CBT *technique: using her own words to begin to form a plan*)
Wendy:	I don't have any idea!
APPN:	What places have you been where it is normal, or expected, to cry on purpose? (*Notice that I do not solve the problem for her. Instead, I use Socratic questioning to have her solve her problem.*)
Wendy:	People cry at cemeteries. I guess I could go to her gravesite and talk to her. (*Eyes open widely*) That sounds really scary! But, if it helps, I'll try anything! (*calmed herself*)

Commentary: The remaining part of the session develops the experiment of going to the graveside (when, how often, how long to stay there) and set up additional opportunities to "cry on purpose" in controlled ways.

Final Phase

Wendy:	I am doing so much better! I have now visited with Linda three times by going to her grave and talking with her. It is funny to say this out loud, but I almost heard what she would say to me!
APPN:	What did she say to you?
Wendy:	She loves me and that I should live my life, and be happy, and that would make her happy.
APPN:	Did that change how you felt?
Wendy:	Yes! I have so much more peace now. I mean, I am really sad, and I miss her so much; but I don't feel like I am falling apart anymore. And, I stopped taking all those medications and now I have a cup of chamomile tea in the evening and I really like the lavender. I noticed I'm sleeping better too.

(*She remained on the sertraline but discontinued the benzodiazepines.*)

Commentary

This case example illustrates three components:

- The importance of recognizing normal, rational grief
- An understanding of creatively combining evidence from multiple models
- An illustration of some of the specific techniques used in CBT to guide treatment practices and outcomes

The reader should note that I do not interpret, direct, or solve Wendy's problems. The client should perceive active listening and restating by the therapist and the techniques used should sound conversational and invite her to use her own logic. The case conceptualization begins with knowing that grieving, like many uncomfortable emotions, is not necessarily bad, or abnormal (Ellis, 1985). When emotions are normal, rational responses to life events, it is healthier to acknowledge them and honor them instead of seeking ways to avoid experiencing them (Ellis, 1994). Also, given that the longer someone is taking sedatives, the more likely he or she is to experience anxiety, agitation, and insomnia, I chose not to address this directly by exploring ways to soothe herself that she has used in the past. I observed to Wendy the changes that occurred as she gradually discontinued sedatives and began to choose more natural, soothing options (chamomile tea, lavender essential oil). I used basic CBT and RET techniques to help her to notice irrational negative expectations, CDs, and ineffective responses. When negative or irrational thoughts were voiced, I guided her toward experiments using rational, normal grieving cognitions and behaviors.

DISCUSSION QUESTIONS

1. Can you identify a situation with a client or family member where the "Daughter technique" might be useful?
2. Grieving is a normal, but uncomfortable process. What other normal, uncomfortable life processes have you or someone else tried to avoid?
3. In this case, I indicate that it is not therapeutic to solve a client's problem. Do you agree or disagree? Why, or why not?
4. Were there other CBT techniques that you would have used with Wendy? If so, which ones and why would you have used them?
5. Do you live life from the front row, or the third row?

REFERENCES

Adler, A. (1917). *Study of organ inferiority and its physical compensation: A contribution to clinical medicine*. New York, NY: Nervous Mental Disorders.

Beck, A. T. (1976). *Cognitive therapy and the emotional disorders*. New York, NY: Meridian.

Beck, A. T. (1989). Psychiatry: Cognitive therapy for depression and panic disorder. *Western Journal of Medicine*, 151(3), 311. Retrieved from https://www.ncbi.nlm.nih.gov/pmc/articles/PMC1026864

Beck, A. T., Rush, A. J., Shaw, B. F., & Emery, G. (1979). *Cognitive therapy of depression*. New York, NY: Guilford.

Beck, A. T., & Weishaar, M. E. (1986). *Cognitive therapy*. Philadelphia, PA: Center for Cognitive Therapy.

Beck, J. S. (2011). *Cognitive behavior therapy: Basics and beyond* (2nd ed.). New York, NY: Guilford Press.

Bisson, J., & Andrew, M. (2007). Psychological treatment of post-traumatic stress disorder (PTSD). *Cochrane Database of Systematic Reviews* (3), CD003388. doi:10.1002/14651858. CD003388.pub3

Clark, D. A., Beck, A. T., & Alford, B. A. (1999). *Scientific foundations of cognitive theory and therapy of depression*. New York, NY: Wiley.

Dreikurs, R. (1949). *Fundamentals of Adlerian psychology*. Chicago, IL: Alfred Adler Institute.

Dykes, P., Wheeler, K., & Boulton, M. (1998). Psychiatric copathways. In P. Dykes (Ed), *Psychiatric clinical pathways: An interdisciplinary approach* (pp. 265–275). Gaithersburg, MD: Aspen.

Ellis, A. (1957). *How to live with a neurotic*. Oxford, England: Crown Publishers.

Ellis, A. (1985). Expanding the *ABC's* of rational-emotive therapy. In M. Mahoney & A. Freeman (Eds.), *Cognition and psychotherapy* (pp. 313–324). New York, NY: Plenum Press. doi:10.1007/978-1-4684-7562-3_13

Ellis, A. (1994). *Reason and emotion in psychotherapy* (2nd ed.). Secaucus, NJ: Citadel Press.

Ellis, A., & Grieger, R. (1977). *Handbook of rational-emotive therapy*. New York, NY: Springer Publishing Company.

Foa, E. B., McLean, C. P., Capaldi, S., & Rosenfield, D. (2013). Prolonged exposure vs supportive counseling for sexual abuse-related PTSD in adolescent girls: A randomized clinical trial. *Journal of the American Medical Association, 310*(24), 2650–2557. doi:10.1001/jama.2013.282829

Freeman, A., & Freeman, S. (2005a). Understanding schemas. In A. Freeman, S. H. Felgoise, A. M. Nezu, C. M. Nezu, & M. A. Reinecke (Eds.), *Encyclopedia of cognitive behavior therapy* (pp. 421–426). New York, NY: Springer.

Freeman, A., & Freeman, S. (2005b). Socratic dialogue. In A. Freeman, S. H. Felgoise, A. M. Nezu, C. M. Nezu, & M. A. Reinecke (Eds.), *Encyclopedia of cognitive behavior therapy* (pp. 380–384). New York, NY: Springer.

Freeman, S. M. (2008). Cognitive-behavioral psychotherapy. In K. Wheeler (Ed.), *Psychotherapy for the advanced practice psychiatric nurse* (pp. 177–202). St. Louis, MO: Mosby/Elsevier.

Freeman, S. M., & Freeman, A. (2005). *Cognitive Behavior Therapy in nursing practice*. New York, NY: Springer Publishing Company.

Freeman Clevenger, S. M., Miller, L., Moore, B. A., & Freeman, A. (2015). *Behind the badge: A psychological treatment handbook for law enforcement officers* (p. 296). New York, NY: Routledge, Taylor & Francis.

Gilson, M., Freeman, A., Yates, M. J., & Freeman, S. M. (2009). *Overcoming depression: A cognitive therapy approach: Therapist guide*. New York, NY: Oxford University.

Granato, H. F., Wilks, C. R., Miga, E. M., Korslund, K. E., & Linehan, M. M. (2015). The use of dialectical behavior therapy and prolonged exposure to treat comorbid dissociation and self-harm: The case of a client with borderline personality disorder and posttraumatic stress disorder. *Journal of Clinical Psychology, 71*(8), 805–815. doi:10.1002/jclp.22207

Leahy, R. L. (2001). *Overcoming resistance in cognitive therapy*. New York, NY: Guilford Press.

Lee, C., Gavriel, H., Drummond, P., Richards, J., & Greenwald, R. (2002). Treatment of PTSD: Stress inoculation training with prolonged exposure compared to EMDR. *Journal of Clinical Psychology, 58*(9), 1071–1089. doi:10.1002/jclp.10039

Lewinsohn, P. M., Hoberman, H. M., & Teri, L. (1985). An integrative theory of depression. In S. Reiss & R. R. Bootzin (Eds.), *Theoretical issues in behavior therapy* (pp. 331–359). New York, NY: Academic Press.

Lindsay, M., Crino, R., & Andrews, G. (1997). Controlled trial of exposure and response prevention in obsessive-compulsive disorder. *The British Journal of Psychiatry: The Journal of Mental Science, 171*, 135–139. doi:10.1192/bjp.171.2.135

McLean, C. P., Zandberg, L. J., Van Meter, P. E., Carpenter, J. K., Simpson, H. B., & Foa, E. B. (2015). Exposure and response prevention helps adults with obsessive compulsive disorder who do not respond to pharmacological augmentation strategies. *Journal of Clinical Psychiatry, 76*(12), 1653–1657. doi:10.4088/JCP.14m09513

Meichenbaum, D. H. (1977). *Cognitive-behavioral modifications: An integrative approach*. New York, NY: Springer.

Novo, P., Landin-Romero, R., Radua, J., Vicens, V., Fernandez, I., Garcia, F., . . . Amann, B. L. (2014). Eye movement desensitization and reprocessing therapy in subsyndromal bipolar clients with a history of traumatic events: A randomized, controlled pilot-study. *Psychiatry Research*, *219*(1), 122–128. doi:10.1016/j.psychres.2014.05.012

Resick, P. A., Wachen, J. S., Mintz, J., Young-McCaughan, S., Roache, J. D., Borah, A. M., . . . Peterson, A. L. (2015). A randomized clinical trial of group cognitive processing therapy compared with group present-centered therapy for PTSD among active duty military personnel. *Journal of Consulting and Clinical Psychology*, *83*(6), 1058–1068. doi:10.1037/ccp0000016

Steinglass, J. E., Albano, A. M., Simpson, H. B., Wang, Y., Zou, J., Attia, E., & Walsh, B. T. (2014). Confronting fear using exposure and response prevention for anorexia nervosa: A randomized controlled pilot study. *The International Journal of Eating Disorders*, *47*(2), 174–180. doi:10.1002/eat.22214

Triscari, M. T., Faraci, P., Catalisano, D., D'Angelo, V., & Urso, V. (2015). Effectiveness of cognitive behavioral therapy integrated with systematic desensitization, cognitive behavioral therapy combined with eye movement desensitization and reprocessing therapy, and cognitive behavioral therapy combined with virtual reality exposure therapy methods in the treatment of flight anxiety: A randomized trial. *Neuropsychiatric Disease and Treatment*, *11*, 2591–2598. doi:10.2147/NDT.S93401

Wilson, R. (2016). *Stopping the noise in your head*. Deerfield Beach, FL: Health Communications.

Manualized Cognitive Behavioral Therapy: An Adolescent With Anxiety and Depression

Pamela Lusk

■ PERSONAL EXPERIENCE WITH COGNITIVE BEHAVIORAL THERAPY

I had an exceptional psychiatric nursing rotation on a small adolescent unit at a private psychiatric hospital in the late 1970s during my bachelor of nursing degree program. My psychiatric nursing instructor and the psychiatric inpatient treatment team, which included a psychiatric clinical nurse specialist, were inspiring. I found working with this population to be the most interesting rotation of my nursing education, and I knew when I graduated that my goal was to practice psychiatric nursing with older children and adolescents. Soon after graduation, I was hired as the adolescent team nurse at a psychiatric hospital for children and adolescents. I loved my work there and became increasingly interested in learning more and expanding my role in this specialty area of psychiatric nursing.

A few years later when exploring options for graduate school, I found a master's degree program in psychiatric nursing that prepared students to conduct psychotherapy with adults during the first year and, with faculty approval, to specialize in conducting psychotherapy with children and adolescents during the second year of the program. After starting the program, I was approved for the second year in the child and adolescent specialty and was able to register for courses in child psychotherapy and developmental psychology in the university's clinical psychology graduate program. During my second year of specializing in children and adolescents, half of my time was spent working on an inpatient children's unit where I was supervised by a psychiatrist with a psychoanalytic play therapy background and the other half of my time was spent working in the community with adolescents where I was supervised by a clinical psychologist, who was an expert in developmental psychopathology and the author of our developmental psychopathology textbook. After graduation with my master's degree in psychiatric nursing, I became certified as a child and adolescent psychiatric clinical nurse specialist. Since then, I received a post-master's degree in a psychiatric-mental health nurse practitioner program and became certified as a psychiatric mental health nurse practitioner (PMHNP). For the past 15 years, I have practiced as a PMHNP at a variety of primary care settings where I have integrated behavioral health into primary care. Currently, I am the PMHNP at a large pediatric medical practice and see children and adolescents from our practice as well as those who are referred from other community agencies and practices for behavioral healthcare.

Ten years ago, I decided to go back to graduate school for a doctorate in nursing practice (DNP) degree. While reviewing the literature on evidence-based psychotherapy for adolescents with depression, my topic for my clinical scholarly project, it became very clear to me that cognitive behavioral therapy (CBT) had the strongest evidence of support for the first-line treatment of adolescents with anxiety and depression. At that time, I only had a rudimentary understanding of this therapeutic approach. Consequently, I attended an introductory training in CBT and began to use the approach with teens I was working with at a community mental health center. Experiencing great outcomes with the teens I saw for depression, I decided to obtain further training. I completed the Beck Institute training in CBT with children and adolescents in 2011. I have attended additional trainings at the Beck Institute since that initial training and continue to learn more with each course. In a primary care setting, most of my referrals are for teens experiencing anxiety and depressive symptoms that are significantly impairing their functioning at school, home, or in social situations. CBT is an evidence-based approach indicated for this population with these types of problems.

▪ FOUNDER OF COGNITIVE BEHAVIORAL PSYCHOTHERAPY

Aaron Beck (1921–) and Albert Ellis (1913–2007) are recognized as the fathers of CBT. Aaron Beck, an American psychiatrist and professor emeritus in the department of psychiatry at the University of Pennsylvania, found in his work as a psychoanalyst in the 1960s that his clients with depression had automatic negative thoughts about certain situations they encountered. He discovered that the content of these thoughts fell into three categories that he eventually called the cognitive triad of depression: negative ideas about oneself, negative ideas about the world, and negative ideas about the future (Beck, 2011). Beck found that he could lessen the depressive symptoms of his clients by helping them identify and evaluate these negative thoughts and develop alternative, more probable thoughts. By doing so, clients were able to think more realistically, feel better emotionally, and behave more functionally. CBT soon after became a model of psychotherapy with principles and strategies for implementation and eventually many outcome studies to support the approach (Beck, 2011). Since that time, Beck and his colleagues have found CBT to be efficacious in treating a wide variety of disorders in addition to depression including anxiety disorders, bipolar disorders, personality disorders, psychotic disorders, and substance use disorders, among others. In addition, CBT has been shown to be very effective in working with children and adolescents (Beidas & Kendall, 2014).

Albert Ellis, an American clinical psychologist, was first trained as a psychoanalyst like Aaron Beck. Ellis became dissatisfied with aspects of the psychoanalytic method and developed Rational Therapy in the 1950s. His approach focused on helping clients understand their self-defeating irrational beliefs (rational analysis) that led to upsetting emotional consequences and behaviors and then develop more rational constructs (cognitive reconstruction) and functional behaviors. His well-recognized ABCD model specified that it is not the activating event that causes the upsetting emotions, but the irrational beliefs (self-talk) about the event.

- A is the Activating Event
- B is the Self-Talk or Irrational Beliefs about the event
- C are the Upsetting Emotional Consequences
- D is the Disputing of the Irrational Idea

During his life, Ellis authored over 75 books for professionals as well as the lay public. He founded The Institute for Rational Living in 1959 to train other therapists and to provide therapy for clients in the community. In 1993, he changed the name of his therapy to Rational Emotive Behavior Therapy (REBT). His institute continues to thrive in New York City and is now known as The Albert Ellis Institute: The Home and Headquarters of Rational Emotive Behavior Therapy.

■ PHILOSOPHY AND KEY CONCEPTS OF CBT

CBT is a structured, short-term, present-oriented psychotherapy, which is well received by adolescents and their parents. Adolescents are, according to Piaget's theory of cognitive development, in the formal operations stage—the stage in which the young person gains the ability to think abstractly and draw conclusions about information. Using one's cognitive abilities to problem-solve and identify coping strategies in therapy fits well with this cognitive developmental level described by Piaget. Erikson's psychosocial theory of development emphasizes mastery of developmental tasks. For the adolescent, the task is identity versus role confusion, which is the ability to understand oneself and others, the ability to see oneself as a unique and integrated individual, and the ability to have success in relationships with others (Adler-Tapia, 2012). Adolescents are very interested in exploring where they fit in the world; thus, the self-exploration required in CBT is appealing to them.

In CBT, the therapist works with clients on cognitive restructuring, problem-solving, and behavioral activation. Cognitive restructuring refers to identifying, evaluating, and modifying faulty thoughts and beliefs that are responsible for negative mood states. Adolescents are curious about their thinking and beliefs of others. They develop skills in challenging beliefs and coming up with creative ways to solve problems. When they apply CBT skills to their own cognitions, clients learn to solve their own problems. Behavioral activation is the identification of activities that are pleasurable and then increasing these activities in their life. This allows teens to express their individual preferences and choices for activities, develop skills in those activities, and increase time in those activities that are fun and interesting for them. They often learn to experience these activities as "being in the zone"—a time where usual worries don't intrude (Adler-Tapia, 2012).

■ DEFINITION OF MENTAL HEALTH AND PSYCHOPATHOLOGY IN CBT

CBT is based on a cognitive theory of mental health and psychopathology. CBT believes that mental health is the result of sound information processing that manifests itself in realistic and accurate thinking, which leads directly to appropriate emotions and adaptive behaviors. In contrast, psychopathology is the result of faulty information processing that reveals itself in distorted and dysfunctional thinking, which leads directly to negative emotions and maladaptive behaviors (Beck, 2011).

■ THERAPEUTIC GOALS IN CBT

CBT is an evidence-based short-term psychotherapy. Typically, clients attend weekly sessions over a period of several months and will then be able to independently use the strategies learned in the therapy sessions. The goal of CBT is for clients to develop thought patterns that allow them to live a more functional and satisfying life. As each session is tailored to meet the needs of individual clients, the goals vary. For example, teens may have a need to develop more friendships, speak in front of class without performance anxiety, or overcome symptoms of depression. Goals are examined to determine the thought patterns, emotions, physical reactions, and behaviors that are associated with specific problems and to then develop new thought patterns that result in more functional behaviors (Beck, 2011).

■ PERSPECTIVE ON ASSESSMENT IN CBT

In CBT, assessment is a collaborative process of joint discovery between the client and the therapist. The client identifies the problem believed to be important and the therapist helps the client determine the thoughts, emotions, physiological reactions, and behavior relevant to the identified problem. The therapist also seeks additional information about the problem such as when and where it occurs; the frequency, intensity, and duration of symptoms; and the specific triggers for the problem.

■ THERAPEUTIC INTERVENTIONS IN CBT

According to Beck, there are 10 CBT principles to guide the therapists' interventions (Beck, 2011). These are as follows:

- CBT is based on an ever-evolving formulation and conceptualization of the client's problems in cognitive terms.
- CBT requires a sound therapeutic alliance.
- CBT emphasizes collaboration and active participation by the client as well as the therapist.
- CBT is goal oriented and problem focused. The client is viewed as a detective finding the solutions to the problems.
- CBT emphasizes the present and is a here-and-now approach to therapy. Parents and teens find that exploring issues that are part of the teen's life now are less intimidating and more relevant.
- CBT is educative and aims to teach clients the skills to be their own therapist, which is important in relapse prevention.
- CBT aims to be time-limited (four to 14 sessions). For teens, I use the COPE (Creating Opportunities for Personal Empowerment) for Teens program, which is a seven-session, manualized approach to treatment.
- CBT sessions are structured and include a check in, agenda setting, homework review, session work, summary, feedback, and assigning homework. Knowing how each session will be organized decreases anxiety for teens. It is predictable and they know what will be asked of them.
- CBT teaches clients to identify their automatic self-critical or negative thoughts, evaluate the truth of the thought (is it entirely true or partially true and is there an

alternate explanation), and change the dysfunctional thought to a more accurate, useful thought.
• CBT uses a variety of techniques and teaches a variety of skills to change thinking, mood, and behavior. Some of these include relaxation strategies, mindfulness, and thought stopping.

Strong research evidence exists to support the effectiveness of CBT treatment manuals with depressed and anxious teens. The use of manuals assures that each client receives the same intervention. Treatment manuals have sometimes been criticized as an impersonal, cookbook approach to therapy; however, a study of manual-based treatments found that they are not inflexible, impersonal, or uncreative; rather, they continue to require clinical skill in their flexible implementation (Beidas & Kendall, 2014). Training is also available to orient therapists to specific treatment manuals.

In my practice, I use the teen manual COPE when working with adolescents. COPE, developed by Bernadette Melnyk in 2003, is a Seven-Session Cognitive Behavioral Skills Building Program, presented in a colorful, developmentally appropriate manual (Melnyk, 2003). It is a highly structured manual that I have been trained in to use. Each teen is evaluated for the ability to think abstractly in order to use the COPE manual for teens. Using the COPE manual allows me to provide a workbook to the teen at the beginning of therapy. The teen then takes ownership of the workbook and uses it for reference during our sessions, as well as after our sessions have been completed. Meta-analysis research of effective psychotherapy for adolescents with depression has identified 12 necessary components of therapy, which are included in the COPE CBT manual for teens. These are as follows:

• Achieving measurable goals and competency
• Adolescent psychoeducation
• Self-monitoring
• Relationship skills and social interaction
• Communication training
• Cognitive restructuring
• Problem-solving
• Behavior activation
• Relaxation
• Emotion regulation
• Parent psychoeducation
• Improving the parent–child relationship (McCarty & Weisz, 2007).

There have been 17 intervention studies using the COPE treatment manual, which are listed on the COPE training website at www.Cope2thrive.com. Other CBT manuals are available for teens. One that is especially valuable is the Adolescent Coping With Depression Course (CWD-A) (Clarke & Lewinsol, 1989), which is useful in treating adolescents with depression (Rohde, Lewinsohn, Clarke, Hops, & Seeley, 2005).

■ CASE STUDY

Background

Stephanie, a 16-year-old high school junior with dark, free-flowing, shoulder length curly hair, came to our pediatric practice with her mother. She was dressed in a loose, flowing cotton top and pants that were consistent with her description of herself as an artist. She was referred from an urgent care practice where she was recently seen for gastrointestinal (GI) distress, depression, and anxiety. Her Patient Health Questionnaire-9 (PHQ-9) for adolescents revealed a score of 22, indicating severe depression. Stephanie, seen individually and together with her mother, stated very clearly that she wanted help for her depression and anxiety. Stephanie lived with her mother, stepfather, and younger brother in a home in a nearby small town in Arizona. Her parents divorced 10 years ago. Her mother, a junior high school teacher, is very supportive of Stephanie, especially of her interests in art and yoga. Although Stephanie believes her depression and anxiety began a few years ago, she did experience two recent losses, which may have increased the intensity of her symptoms. These losses were the death of her biological father from an alcohol-related illness and the estrangement from her best friend Angie who left her behind for a new boyfriend and new friends. Stephanie views herself as an artist and hopes to continue studying art in college. She achieves good grades (A's and B's) and is in advanced art classes. She has a new boyfriend and a group of friends, but misses her closest long-term friend Angie. Stephanie's GI symptoms, for which she has had numerous workups, revealed no definitive cause for the symptoms. Her mother was very concerned about Stephanie's symptoms of depression followed by anxiety, especially a recent panic attack. I shared with Stephanie and her mother that adolescent treatment studies indicate that CBT has the strongest evidence as a psychotherapy for adolescent depression and anxiety, while for the most severe depression and anxiety disorders, the combination of CBT and antidepressant medication provide the most robust treatment. Both Stephanie and her mother were interested in starting CBT without medication as soon as possible. Both felt she would benefit greatly from talk therapy. Stephanie is very interested in psychology and enjoys discussions of self-improvement and self-help topics. I showed Stephanie and her mother the CBT COPE manual for teens (Melnyk, 2003) and provided an overview of this approach to treatment. They agreed for Stephanie to be seen individually by me with her mother reviewing the sessions and homework pages between sessions. In the CBT approach with teens, it is very helpful for parents to follow along with the skills being taught in order for the cognitive restructuring, behavioral activation, and problem-solving approach to be reinforced at home.

I have used the CBT COPE manualized program teens for 10 years and I present each of the topics in the manual in 30-minute visits (Lusk & Melnyk, 2011). I present the material to the client word for word in order to ensure fidelity to the interventions and flexibility in individualizing the examples. The Teen COPE 7 Session CBT manual has the following session topics:

- Session 1: Thinking, Feeling, and Behaving: What Is the Connection?
- Session 2: Self-Esteem and Positive Thinking/Self-Talk
- Session 3: Stress and Coping
- Session 4: Problem-Solving and Setting Goals
- Session 5: Dealing With Your Emotions in Healthy Ways/Effective Communications
- Session 6: Coping With Stressful Situations
- Session 7: Putting It All Together for a Healthy You!

Because the manual presents the content in clear, concise, well-illustrated lessons with the subsequent homework assignment in a "fill in the blank" format, the session can easily be completed in 30-minute visits, which is the recommended session time for teens. This time period is age appropriate for the teens I see and still allows time for the teen or parent to bring up pressing concerns. The fast pace of the 30-minute session keeps the interest level high and is long enough for the attention span of most teens. The structure of the session provides a continuity that reduces anxiety for the client. It progresses in the following order:

1. Check in—the teen brings up any pressing concern and a PHQ-9 for adolescents is administered. The PHQ-9 assesses for suicidal ideation and other symptoms of depression.
2. Homework—a review of the homework from the last session takes place.
3. Lesson content—the content for the weekly lesson is reviewed.
4. Summary of content—the content for the weekly lesson is summarized.
5. Feedback—feedback is provided by the client and the therapist.
6. Homework—a plan for the next session is made by reviewing the required homework pages. Homework (also called an action plan) extends the session and gives the client an opportunity to reinforce what was covered in the session and to continue working on self during the week.

Transcript of Therapy Sessions

Each of the seven sessions will be presented with an overview of the skill and a brief transcript of the dialogue between Stephanie and me.

COPE Session 1: Thinking, Feeling, and Behaving: What Is the Connection?

I gave Stephanie her COPE manual and she was eager to get started.

APPN:	I'd like to start by having you fill out the PHQ-9.
Stephanie:	OK.
APPN:	Your score decreased to a 14, which indicates moderate depression. So, let's do a check-in about your past week.
Stephanie:	I met a guy at school named Mick and we have been spending time together. I feel better about myself since this happened.
APPN:	That may be the reason why your test number decreased.
Stephanie:	Yes.
APPN:	The content for this week is an overview of the Thinking, Feeling, Behaving Triangle. Often in our lives something happens that is an anticipatory event or trigger. The trigger event happens, and we may have an automatic negative or not helpful thought. These thoughts happen reflexively, quickly, before we even have time to think things through. For example (*reads from COPE manual*), Sarah, a student in art class, has a classmate walk by her table and say, "Your art project is weird." Sarah's automatic thought is "I can't do anything right." Following her thought is a feeling of sadness and discouragement and a behavior of not putting any more effort into that art project or in fact any schoolwork for the rest of the day. She walks down the school hallway changing classes with her head down, not interacting with anyone. So, how you think affects how you feel and how you behave. (*I show her the following visual*)

How you think

affects how you feel

and how you behave.

APPN:	Do you understand this, Stephanie?
Stephanie:	Yes.
APPN:	Then, let's go to the next example in the workbook of the teen named Darcy. Darcy gets good grades, but the teacher has just handed the test papers back and Darcy got a D. Darcy thinks, "I really blew the test this time, but I will study hard for the next test and do well and bring the grade up." How do you think Darcy feels? Fill in the feeling Stephanie.
Stephanie:	I guess Darcy feels just fine.
APPN:	What do you think about Darcy's subsequent behavior?
Stephanie:	I think she probably just goes on with her day—no problems.

There is a brief discussion in the manual about how we can reprogram our brain from negative thoughts to more realistic, positive thoughts, resulting in feeling better and behaving more positively. Then, the teen is asked to identify a trigger with automatic thoughts and then subsequent feelings and behaviors.

APPN:	So, can you identify a situation that happened for you this week that was difficult?
Stephanie:	It's still hard for me to see my best friend Allie being with her new boyfriend and new group of friends at lunch.
APPN:	What thought do you have when you see this?
Stephanie:	"I'm not good enough to be in that group of kids. Allie is spending her time with people that are cooler than me. I'm not good enough to be in that group."
APPN:	What feelings do you have after having these thoughts?
Stephanie:	Sadness and disappointment in myself.
APPN:	What do you do?
Stephanie:	I guess I walk around with my head down, go to the other side of the cafeteria, and sit by myself and read.
APPN:	Although you can't change how other people think or what they say, you can choose how you react to them.

I review the Thinking, Feeling, Behaving Triangle and the next session skill, which is positive self-talk.

APPN:	Positive self-talk is one way to begin to change your negative thinking. Here are some examples in the manual:

- I am a good friend.
- I did that well.
- I'm not going to give up.

- I'm going to stay calm.
- This won't last forever.
- I am in control of my feelings.
- I'm going to try harder next time.

APPN:	Which of these positive self-statements resonate with you?
Stephanie:	"This won't last forever" and "I have some other good friends."
APPN:	That's very good. So, if you use these self-talk messages, your feelings and your behavior will change.

Another CBT skill taught in this first session is "staying in the moment." An activity of clapping and following the cadence of the APPN who claps first provides an experience of concentrating totally on what one is doing, and thereby not regretting the past or worrying about the future. With this activity, both the teen and APPN are trying so hard to keep the clapping cadence followed, there isn't time for problematic thoughts or worries.

APPN:	OK Stephanie. Let's review all of the content covered—triggers, automatic negative thoughts, the Thinking, Feeling, Behaving Triangle, positive self-talk, and staying in the moment.
Stephanie:	*(Reviews and summarizes the content)*
APPN:	I'd like to review the situation you provided earlier in the session when you saw Allie with her new boyfriend and new group of friends and thought, "I'm not good enough to be part of that group and felt sad and disappointed, and isolated yourself at lunch." What positive statements might you tell yourself?
Stephanie:	"I have other friends that I fit in with, that have been friends for a long time. I fit in well with them and they are my cool artistic friends. We have a good time."
APPN:	Let's spend a few minutes on you and I giving each other feedback.
Stephanie:	I like the CBT model and think I understand it.
APPN:	You have picked up the CBT model very quickly and are very forthright and self-aware. It's going to be fun to work through the manual with you and with all your cognitive strengths.
Stephanie:	This makes sense and will be helpful for me. I like psychology.
APPN:	Terrific. Let's review the homework pages for you to fill out in the manual before our next meeting. First, I want you to write on an index card two positive self-statements and say those statements out loud 10 times a day.
Stephanie:	*(she writes)* I am good at art.

In the waiting room, I check in with her mother and suggest they review the homework pages together so Stephanie can explain the CBT approach we are using. It is a positive part of CBT when parents also learn the process and can provide their own examples of triggers, automatic negative thoughts, and their learned strategies for coping.

COPE Session 2: Self-Esteem and Positive Thinking/Self-Talk

Stephanie arrived for Session 2 with her manual in hand. First, I administer a PHQ-9, which is done at each session, and her score was 7, much lower than before and indicating her symptoms are now in the mild range of depression. I also asked about suicidal thoughts, which she did not have.

APPN: Let's review your homework.

Stephanie: *(Shows the APPN her homework. In the manual, Stephanie had identified examples from her week where she had autonomic negative thoughts and subsequent feelings and behaviors. She was also able to identify times she was able to catch the negative thoughts, question if the situation was all negative, and identify a more realistic, useful interpretation.)*

APPN: Tell me about a negative thought you had this week.

Stephanie: My brother and I were fighting and I said to myself, "We never can just have a peaceful evening." I realized quickly that is not true and caught myself by saying, "Sometimes we fight, but many times we have a good time together."

The content of Session 2 begins with the explanation of self-esteem—how the teen views and feels about self. The manual focuses on the fact that self-esteem comes from within and that positive self-talk can change the way we see ourselves.

APPN: The manual here lists signs of poor self-esteem. Can you relate to any of these examples for yourself?

Stephanie: Yes. Two of them sound like me—not trying things for fear of failure and being worried too much about what others think of me.

APPN: Now, there is a list of signs of positive self-esteem. Can you identify with any of these?

Stephanie: Yes. I have no trouble standing up for what I believe in with peers.

APPN: Practicing positive self-talk is a very effective way to build self-esteem. Can you list five people or things you are thankful for?

Stephanie: I am thankful for my family, especially my supportive mother and my new boyfriend who just introduced me to his family. I am enjoying my art projects this semester. They are going to be part of an art exhibit at the local college.

APPN: That is terrific.

Stephanie: Sometimes, when I feel pressure about the art show, I find myself saying things like, "I'll never get my projects finished in time" or "My project will be lame compared to my classmates." Then, I feel hopeless and don't want to do anything. I have been catching myself though and substituting, "I will get my projects finished in time and they will be good."

Further content for Session 2 focused on identifying habits and learning how to change unhealthy habits focusing on stages of change: (a) make a decision to change; (b) set the goal; (c) believe you can do it, because anything is possible when you believe;

and (d) take action one step at a time. Stephanie told me that she smoked cigarettes in the past, but stopped smoking completely. Stephanie then summarized the session by reviewing the Thinking, Feeling, Behaving Triangle and I reiterated the point: "Although you can't change how other people think or what they say, you can choose how you think and how you react to them." Stephanie fully understands the concept of cognitive restructuring and is enjoying catching automatic negative or catastrophic, hopeless thoughts. We ended the session with giving mutual feedback and reviewing the homework pages for the week, which focused on identifying positive and negative habits and plans for change. She also added to her index card: "I am a good friend."

COPE Session 3: Stress and Coping

This session is one of the most helpful for most teens. It focuses on teaching teens to recognize symptoms of anxiety—how anxiety is experienced physically, emotionally, and behaviorally. It is noted that during the initial psychiatric evaluation, Stephanie spoke of having panic attacks as well as a history of GI symptoms with negative diagnostic tests. These presenting symptoms indicated to me that Session 3 would be particularly helpful in providing strategies for Stephanie when experiencing high levels of anxiety. In week 3, I did a quick check-in and administered the PHQ-9, which remained at a score of 7. I then reviewed Stephanie's homework.

APPN:	Can you describe an event that happened this past week where you changed your thinking from negative to positive?
Stephanie:	My parents and I were having a major conflict. Mom thinks my grades are dropping. I responded angrily that I have so many obligations, school, babysitting, needing to spend time with my friends and my new boyfriend, and that I am so overwhelmed. I said, "I never can get everything done." I realized I was so exhausted and irritable that I told Mom that I needed to take time in my room to regroup and then I would make a workable plan to get caught up with my two classes in which I received lower grades.
APPN:	Let's review the Thinking, Feeling, and Behaving Triangle with your thought, "I will never get everything done, feeling exasperated, and stomping around, but then quickly catching the thought, and modifying that to "I'm exhausted right now. I will think straight after some time in my room." (*Reviews the situation and subsequent thoughts, feelings, and behavior*)
Stephanie:	When I went to my room and regrouped, I came up with a plan to get my grades up in the two courses telling myself to take one step at a time and then I felt hopeful.

Following this, the manual introduces the topic of stress with the following COPE definition: "Stress is when you do not have the ability or skills to deal with things that you see as frightening or unpleasant (like taking a test that you didn't study for or missing your curfew). Stress can also be helpful; for instance, when it helps you finish an assignment before the deadline, but too much stress, not handled in healthy ways, can contribute to bad health in both your body and mind" (Melnyk, 2003, p. 21). There is a list of the 13 most common causes of stress and worry for teens. These include whether you are liked by your peers, pressure from parents, school and grades, feelings of anxiety or depression, and what you will do when finished with school.

APPN: What are your common stressors?

Stephanie: School and grades, feelings of anxiety and depression, and pressure from my parents are my greatest causes of stress.

APPN: In all my years of delivering this session, nearly every teen—about 99%—has chosen "pressure from parents" as a top cause of their stress. This seems to be universal—young teens, older teens, rural, from urban areas, all feel the expectations of their parents as stressful, so you are not alone.

The next section of content is a list of 11 physical responses to stress. The list includes fast or pounding heart rate, breathing fast, anger, restlessness, headaches, stomach aches, and feeling tired all the time.

APPN: What are your physical responses to stress?

Stephanie: Stomach aches, fast heart rate, and breathing fast.

The next section identifies emotional signs of stress, like feeling irritable, feeling anxious, feeling hopeless, feeling burned out, and so on.

APPN: What happens to you emotionally when you feel stressed?

Stephanie: I feel anxious, hopeless, irritable, and at times burned out.

The next section is a list of behaviors associated with stress and includes examples such as arguing with parents, bad grades, smoking, overeating, and drugs/alcohol.

APPN: What behaviors associated with stress do you have?

Stephanie: Oh definitely, arguing with my parents, especially my mother.

The emphasis in the session then moves to identifying healthy coping with the stresses of life including a list of possible healthy coping strategies. The list includes these suggestions:

- Talking about how you feel
- Exercising
- Seeking out family and friends for support and help
- Writing thoughts and feelings in a journal
- Turning a negative thought in response to a stressor into a positive one
- Using positive self-talk (I can do anything that I set out to do, I can remain calm)
- Doing relaxation techniques like deep breathing or guided imagery
- Taking small steps when working toward a goal or starting something new

The teen identifies how he or she currently copes and then identifies ones from the list that might work well in the current life situation. These behavioral strategies are then reinforced. In CBT, the B stands for behavioral activation, which focuses on increasing one's participation in the activities he or she enjoys and works for him or her as a coping strategy. Behavioral activation is critical for improving depressive symptoms and improving anxiety symptoms.

APPN:	Is there anything from the list that would work for you? You can identify any healthy strategy that works for you and that does not cause harm to you or others.
Stephanie:	I love yoga, but since I have been so overwhelmed with school assignments, family obligations, and my boyfriend and friends wanting to spend time together, I have not been going to my yoga studio. I will think about putting yoga back into my week and figure out how often I can go.
APPN:	Is there anything else?
Stephanie:	Well, I prefer doing my artwork and using self-talk, deep breathing, and of course yoga.

The rest of the session includes a list of clinical symptoms from the *Diagnostic and Statistical Manual of Mental Disorders* (5th ed.; *DSM-5*; American Psychiatric Association, 2013) of depressive disorders and anxiety disorders. Reviewing these symptoms provides an opportunity for anxiety and depression psychoeducation and to teach the teen that they are treatable medical conditions. Thoughts of death and suicide are also explored with a list of resources for the teen as well as any friend in need. Session 3 content ends with practice of abdominal breathing.

APPN:	OK. Let's summarize and give some mutual feedback.
Stephanie:	OK. But I want you to know that I am having some bad dreams and have awakened with worries about not meeting my deadlines.
APPN:	I would like for you to track how often you have these bad dreams with increased anxiety in the morning.
Stephanie:	I can do that. (*She summarizes the session and gives feedback.*)
APPN:	The homework for the week is to identify a most stressful situation and then identify how you thought, felt, and behaved. Then, identify the coping strategies that worked and those coping practices that you would like to add to your list of strategies for coping with stress.
Stephanie:	OK. I will do that.
APPN:	Also, for homework, I would like you to make a chart of how often you are able to repeat your positive self-statements on your index card and also a chart of how many days you utilize your coping strategies.
Stephanie:	OK. I am also going to add to my index card: "I am capable of doing what I need to do once I make up my mind to do it."

Session 4: Problem-Solving and Setting Goals

Stephanie arrived for Session 4 with her homework pages filled out. She had been feeling a high level of stress during the past week related to school deadlines, especially because several of her advanced art projects for the art show were taking longer than expected to complete. Her thoughts were: "I can't possibly get this done like I planned and wanted." Her PHQ-9 score was more elevated to 13, which is a moderate level of depression. She was feeling conflicting pressure from parents and her boyfriend. Her parents wanted her to keep her grades up and so did she, but she also wanted to spend time with her boyfriend. During the check, she spoke about the difficulty of getting her art work done.

Stephanie:	I was having a hard time getting my art work done this week realizing that I could not possibly get them done as I had planned.
APPN:	I wonder what happened when this was realized?
Stephanie:	Well, I realized that I needed to modify my multistage project to a simpler plan.
	I used my self-talk and also met with my art teacher and explained that I would have to do a simpler plan.
APPN:	And . . . .
Stephanie:	I told myself that the simpler art project is fine. It is still beautiful and still shows my idea and artistic creativity, even if not the grand design. It is good art and it is doable in my time frame. But, sometimes, I am unable to say these positive thoughts.
APPN:	What happened then?
Stephanie:	I admit I sometimes say that I messed up and didn't complete the awesome project. Then, I feel sad about not doing the larger, awesome project. But it doesn't last long. I am able to go back to the positive thoughts and not have the sad feelings.

We then continue with the focus of Session 4, which is problem-solving and setting goals. This topic is of great interest for Stephanie for she is in her last few months as a high school junior and post high school plans were weighing heavily on her mind. The lesson asks if the teen dreams about what he or she wants to do as an adult and what kind of things are needed to do to achieve those dreams? This helps the teen identify things to do now in order to move toward reaching the goals and dreams. The manual has an example of a 13-year-old boy who has a goal of becoming a teacher and the client is asked to identify what he can do now to prepare to become a teacher. Stephanie easily comes up with ideas for the 13-year-old.

APPN:	Now. Can you write down a long-term dream for yourself?
Stephanie:	OK. I would like to go to college to study forestry as my major and also participate in all of the art clubs and take art courses so I can keep up with my art work. I have decided that art is not the best day job career plan, but forestry would allow me greater employment opportunities. We live in a state with several National Parks and forests surround us. Forestry is a difficult major, but a field of study with much promise. I love being outdoors and providing education to people about the natural resources in the area.
APPN:	What can you do in the next 1 to 2 years? Can you write down weekly tasks and goals to achieve your dream?
Stephanie:	Yes. I know I need to continue to make good grades in my junior and senior years of high school.
APPN:	Are there any barriers such as people, events, or situations that you might encounter that might prevent you from reaching your dreams and goals?

Stephanie:	The cost of college. I don't know how I will afford college. I don't even have a car yet, so I can't get a good job to start saving money.
APPN:	And what could you do to overcome these barriers?
Stephanie:	Apply for scholarships. My mom knows how to apply for them. I can meet with her and begin to realistically plan to overcome the cost barrier. I don't want to burden my family with my financial needs, so I have not brought up my worries.

The last part of the session includes four steps of problem-solving and addresses the following questions:

- What is the problem?
- What is the cause?
- What are all the possible solutions and the pros and cons?
- What is the best solution?

Some example situations from teens are presented in the manual and the client is asked to go through the four steps of problem-solving to help the teen in the manual examples figure out the best solutions. Stephanie is exceptional at problem-solving, so solving the situations were fun for her.

APPN:	But how about problem-solving your conflict?
Stephanie:	Yes. I am feeling conflicting pressure from my parents and my boyfriend. My parents want me to keep my grades up and so do I, but I also want to spend time with him.
APPN:	This is a good problem to work on during the week using the four steps of problem-solving for your homework.
Stephanie:	Will do.

Stephanie is very capable of solving this for herself, and when we review the homework pages, she smiles confidently stating that this is the type of challenge she enjoys. As with other teens, the challenge of using their cognitive skills to figure out problems leads to a feeling of accomplishment and pride.

The session ends with a summary and feedback and the words: Success happens when:

- You start achieving your goal by taking small steps
- You overcome barriers to your goal by problem-solving
- You build on your strengths and BELIEVE in yourself

Session 5: Dealing With Your Emotions in Healthy Ways/Effective Communications

By this time in the CBT program, the effort on the part of the therapist has been teaching the principles of CBT, walking the client through the areas where he or she expresses struggle, and choosing the coping strategies that fit best. In the last two sessions, the teen assumes the major part of coming up with his or her own strategies for dealing with common and possible future problematic situations. The teen practices the skills and becomes very good at identifying targets and the associated automatic negative thoughts. The teen has learned how to challenge the automatic thoughts with Socratic questions such as, Is this entirely correct? Or is it only partially true? Are there other explanations? Once the teen learns the basic concepts of catching his or her unhelpful automatic negative or self-critical thoughts, the teen is able to evaluate the thoughts with the CBT lens, and modify them to be more realistic. The teen then becomes more in charge and gains mastery of his or her thoughts and well-being. The teen strengthens the skills of self-talk and uses strategies to cope with stress and anxiety. The teen uses problem-solving skills and goal setting skills. Stephanie is at the point where she identifies her usual negative thoughts such as, "I will never finish the art project" or "If I don't do my original project plan, this isn't worthy of entry into the exhibition." She is able to catch these thoughts quickly and often laughs as soon as the all or nothing statements are spoken and modifies these thoughts to more realistic, accurate statements such as "I will get the modified art project done for the exhibit" or "I am totally capable of quality work." She now has an appreciation of how the process takes a great deal of practice during the week. With the next three sessions teens are honing the skills they learned and giving thought to future challenging situations.

Session 5 begins with a check-in; administration of the PHQ-9, which was back down to 7 indicating mild depression; and a review of her homework.

APPN: So, let's take a look at your homework.

Stephanie: You remember my conflict last week of wanting to both spend time with my boyfriend and also keep up my grades.

APPN: Yes. Go on.

Stephanie: Well, I had a heart-to-heart talk with my boyfriend and came up with some solutions. We decided that during the school week, our time together will be study dates. We are both happy with this plan to be able to keep up with our assignments while also enjoying being with each other. My mom was impressed that I came up with this plan, and for the first day or two the study dates worked out well.

APPN: I too am impressed with the plan you came up with to solve your problem.

The next part of the homework page asks the teen what she is thankful for today and to write down two or three good things about herself. The homework reminds her to add to the positive self-statements on the index cards. The content in this session relates to additional ways of dealing with stress and introduces the technique of mental imagery.

APPN: Mental imagery is a healthy way to cope that involves imagining that you are in one of your most favorite places or doing one of your favorite things. Close your eyes and think of a place that is pleasant for you, a peaceful place, a place of no worries. Be in this place—take in the smells, the sights, the temperature of being. This is the time to simply enjoy being at your peaceful pleasant place.

After the experience, the point is made that she can close her eyes and return to her peaceful place at any time. This is a favorite skill for teens. They realize that when anxiety increases, a trip to this peaceful place can be made and it results in relaxation. The importance of practicing going to the special place is emphasized. As with all the skills, practice is critical and makes the skill become part of the teen and available when needed.

The next part of Session 5 focuses on regulation of emotions. Emotional regulation is a positive way to gain control over sadness, anxiety, fear, jealousy, and anger—healthy, normal emotions that everyone has, but that need to be regulated when they are too strong. The subsequent behaviors of what the teen does with the emotions is most important. A list of self-control strategies is presented, so that the teen can choose the strategy that best fits. The manual includes the following:

- Positive thinking
- Positive self-talk
- Counting to 100 or reciting the ABCs
- Deep breathing
- Walking away and finding a quiet place to practice a relaxation technique (e.g., breathing, imagery)
- Talking with a friend or adult who will listen and support you
- Going for a walk or run or bike ride.

APPN: Talking about what you will do next time you experience a stressful situation will help you use the self-control strategies you choose. Healthy choices are under your control, and as you practice them, they will become easier and easier. So, from this list of healthy coping strategies, which ones do you choose Stephanie?

Stephanie: Spending time with a friend and quiet time in my room with my art supplies.

APPN: Other strategies in the manual include listening to your favorite music, exercise, taking time with a friend, relaxation techniques, writing in a journal, reading a positive book, watching a funny movie, singing, having quiet time, and doing hobbies. Do any of these fit?

Stephanie: Yes. Listening to music and writing in my journal.

APPN: Terrific. You have a number of strategies. It is important to practice and rehearse your self-control strategies when you are calm—so when something happens that annoys you or makes you feel angry or anxious, you will be ready to deal with it in a healthy way.

There is also a section in Session 5 that describes effective communication (tone of voice, word choice, active listening, body language). Even though Stephanie is an excellent communicator and is very good at these skills, we still go over them for the CBT program as presented in the manual needs to be fully completed for fidelity; thus, all the portions of the program are read, even those that aren't needed as much by an individual client. I always read the manual word for word, then reinforce the individualized examples the teen has provided. Thus, that is what I did with Stephanie. We ended the session with a summary, feedback, and a review of the weekly homework.

APPN: The homework for the week is to identify a situation during the week when you feel anxious and/or angry and discuss how you coped with the situation. You are then to reflect on how you might have coped in other healthy ways in the particular situation. (*Stephanie will also record how many times she practices going to her peaceful place.*)

Session 6: Coping With Stressful Situations

Stephanie's homework was reviewed.

APPN: I am always so impressed with the time you put into filling out the homework pages. Can I make a copy of some of your homework pages to use as an exemplar to share with my students?

Stephanie: Of course. I am proud of my work and pleased that you will show it to students. (*She gave permission for this example—as did her mother.*)

Exhibit 9.1 is an example of one of Stephanie's homework pages, which she gave permission to use for this chapter.

The content for Session 6 begins with a review of a trigger followed by the Thinking, Feeling, Behaving Triangle.

APPN: What event occurred this week that led you to use the strategies that we have talked about in this program?

Stephanie: I had a stressful time with my art work that wasn't turning out the way I had hoped.

APPN: What did you do?

Stephanie: I first did my positive self-talk and then went to my peaceful place. That worked and I was able to get back to my art.

EXHIBIT 9.1

Completed homework assignment.

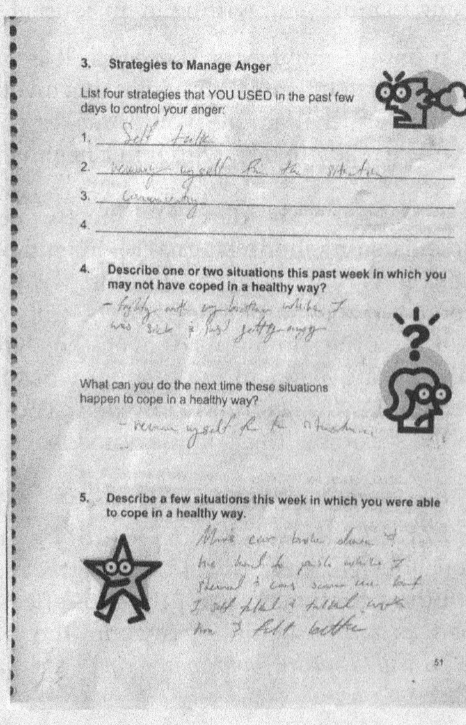

The rest of Session 6 consists of questions about how the teen can apply the COPE lessons. Some examples are the following:

- How do you express your feelings when you are hurt or disagree with another person? (*Use "I" statements instead of accusing the other person or calling him or her a name.*)
- How do you ask for help or for what you need? (*Asking for help is not a sign of weakness for everyone needs help at times in his or her life.*)
- How to say "no" to others (*When you don't give into peer pressure you are less likely to get into trouble, less likely to get into a dangerous situation, be seen as a positive leader rather than a follower, and serve as a role model for other teens.*)

We end the session by summarizing the content, giving mutual feedback, and reviewing the weekly homework, which is to give examples of the questions provided and to specific situations in his or her life. And, they are also asked to add another positive statement to the index card.

Stephanie: (*smiles and adds to her card*) I do a great job on my COPE homework!

Session 7: Putting It All Together for a Healthy You!

This final session is a review of the COPE program. After a check-in, administering the PHQ-9, which was now down to 4 (minimal or no signs of depression), we began the session:

APPN: Over the past few weeks you have learned how to handle some difficult situations by thinking more positively and coping in healthy ways. Can you describe a situation that occurred this past week that you think you handled differently because of the things you learned through the COPE program?

Stephanie: I've learned that when I am faced with something stressful and start to think negatively, I can turn the negative thought into a positive one to feel better and act in a positive way.

APPN: Can you describe a situation where you "turned around" your negative thinking to a positive thought?

Stephanie: Well, my situation with my art. When I start saying negative things about it, I just turn it around to a positive message.

APPN: Terrific. I would like to go over the important review points:

- Positive thinking is up to YOU!
- When you think and talk positively, you will feel happier—remember to say your positive self-statements every day!
- Stay in the present moment to lessen your worries.
- Focus on what you have, not what you don't have.
- You cannot change other people. You can only change how you react to them.
- You can change a habit or reach a new goal through practice.
- You can make a decision to change.
- Set a goal and picture yourself reaching it.
- Believe you can do it.
- Take action one step at a time.
- Ask yourself what is the best solution?
- Act on the best solution.

Stephanie:	Those are really good points to remember.
APPN:	To deal with stress, practice the things that help you, like relaxation techniques, write in a journal, talk to someone, or exercise. When you are angry, practice your self-control strategies, like counting to 10, blowing your anger away, listening to music, or exercising. Communicate effectively and ask for help when you need it. Remember, anything the mind can conceive and believe, it can achieve. You can continue to think positively for a healthier you! Congratulations! You did it! Stephanie, you did it! You completed the manual!

Commentary

Stephanie felt great about completing the COPE CBT program. As I reviewed our therapy process, I initially provided psychoeducation and taught the CBT process of cognitive restructuring. In each session, new skills were taught and practiced. The theme of positive self-talk and recognizing individual strengths via the index card of positive self-statements was a focus during all seven sessions. In the fourth session, the responsibility for the session moved from my teaching to encouraging Stephanie to do the work. She identified her dysfunctional thoughts, and caught the thoughts, evaluated the thoughts, and modified and changed the thoughts to more accurate, positive, helpful thoughts. Stephanie would quietly laugh when she caught herself stating negative thoughts such as, "I will never finish my art project" or "That isn't good enough—my high goals have to be met or it is nothing." She was very quick at catching the automatic negative thought and this was quite impressive. She informed me about the strategies and skills that worked best for her in coping with anxiety, dealing with stressful situations, and self-regulating her strong emotions. She shared her dreams and set short- and long-term goals to achieve these dreams. She now knows strategies to address barriers she might encounter on her way. Stephanie has excellent cognitive abilities and enjoys using her mind to solve problems.

It took Stephanie approximately 16 weeks to complete the seven sessions. This is usual, for many teens and families have many competing obligations (e.g., school breaks, illnesses, activities) and cannot come in weekly. A 16-week course of therapy is great to both finish a time-limited therapy and allow for the practice of new ways of thinking, feeling, and behaving as well as new skills and strategies. This time frame was perfect for Stephanie.

By the end of our work together, Stephanie's GI symptoms and panic attacks had not reoccurred. Her grades were good and her PHQ-9 was low (was 4). She felt positive and hopeful and confident that she had done the hard work of CBT and mastered this form of cognitive restructuring and problem-solving. She still struggles with getting back to yoga on a regular basis. We agree to meet periodically for "booster" follow-up sessions. Stephanie became very engaged in therapy and would always bounce into the sessions with her homework carefully done. She related warmly and showed me photos of her art projects. She has been a joy to watch as she met the challenges of each session and grown in self-confidence. She is hopeful about her future and aware of her strong capabilities.

ADDENDUM from a follow-up booster visit: Stephanie is now a high school senior. She talked with a guidance counselor and found out that if she attends the local community college for her first 2 years, she will be able to attend her last 2 years at the State University with their exceptional forestry program on full scholarship. It is a special scholarship program put together by the two colleges in order to encourage students to stay in the state and contribute to the state. This is a great relief for Stephanie and it has decreased her senior stress level. Stephanie is working part time after school. Her grades are good. Over the summer, she and her boyfriend had some difficult times and spent some time apart, but now are back together and doing fine. Her mother is supportive of her busy schedule with work and school and tries to ensure she gets some down time. Stephanie's efforts are recognized by her family. She remains hopeful about her future. She continues to use her coping strategies. We continue to meet every 3 months for booster sessions and any time she requests an appointment. I am always so happy to see Stephanie bounce into the office and share her great art projects.

DISCUSSION QUESTIONS

1. What are the pros and cons of using a CBT treatment manual with adolescents? Discuss fidelity with flexibility.
2. What is an automatic negative thought that you "catch" yourself saying to yourself in times of stress?
3. CBT requires collaboration and active participation from the teen. If you are working with a naturally quiet teen or an angry, resistant teen, what strategies might you use to increasehis or her participation in the sessions?
4. With the content of the sessions just described, and skills taught, what do you think adolescents might take from their therapy into their young adult/adult years?

REFERENCES

Adler-Tapia, R. (2012). *Child psychotherapy: Integrating developmental theory into clinical practice.* New York, NY: Springer Publishing Company.

Beck, J. (2011). *Cognitive therapy: Basics and beyond* (2nd ed.). New York, NY: Guilford Press.

Beidas, R., & Kendall, P. (Eds.). (2014). *Dissemination and implementation of evidence-based practices in child and adolescent mental health.* New York, NY: Oxford Press.

Clarke, G., & Lewinsohn, P. M. (1989). The coping with depression course: A group psychoeducational intervention for unipolar depression. *Behaviour Change,* 6(2), 54–69. Retrieved from https://psycnet.apa.org/record/1990-05300-001

Lusk, P., & Melnyk, B. M. (2011). The brief cognitive-behavioral COPE intervention for depressed adolescents: Outcomes and feasibility of delivery in 30-minute outpatient v isits.*Journal of the American Psychiatric Nurses Association,* 17(3), 226–236. doi:10.1177/1078390311404067

McCarty, C., & Weisz, J. (2007). Effects of psychotherapy for depression in children and adolescents: What we can (and can't) learn from meta-analysis and component profiling. *Journal of the American Academy of Child & Adolescent Psychiatry,* 46(7), 879–886. doi:10.1097/chi.0b013e31805467b3

Melnyk, B. (2003). *COPE (Creating opportunities for personal empowerment) for teens: A 7-session cognitive behavioral skills building program.* Columbus, OH: COPE2THRIVE, LLC. Retrieved from https://www.COPE2Thrive.com

Rohde, P., Lewinsohn, P. M., Clarke, G. N., Hops, H., & Seeley, J. R. (2005). The adolescent coping with depression course: A cognitive-behavioral approach to the treatment of adolescent depression. In E. D. Hibbs & P. S. Jensen (Eds.). *Psychosocial treatments for child and adolescent disorders. Empirically based strategies for clinical practice* (pp. 219–237). Washington, DC: American Psychological Association. Retrieved from https://psycnet.apa.org/record/2005-00278-010

10

Dialectical Behavior Therapy: A Client With Complex Trauma

Danielle Conklin

■ PERSONAL EXPERIENCE WITH DIALECTICAL BEHAVIOR THERAPY

I first encountered Dialectical Behavior Therapy (DBT) during my graduate studies at New York University. DBT was presented as an approach well suited to treating the needs of the young adult population, especially those with severe emotional dysregulation. I remember sitting in that first lecture and thinking to myself, "outside of being a psychotherapy, DBT seems to be a pretty comprehensive life skills program." I was struck by how the skills taught within DBT seemed to be valuable tools for anyone to learn and apply to navigate difficult personal and relational experiences.

My first practicum rotation was at the Manhattan Veterans Administration Hospital where I co-led a weekly DBT skills group with a senior psychiatric clinical nurse specialist (CNS). These clients presented with the range of psychiatric illness including major depressive disorder, posttraumatic stress disorder (PTSD), bipolar disorder, schizophrenia, and personality disorders. Despite the clinical heterogeneity of the group, learning of DBT skills was valuable to all who attended in order to help support their learning and integration of techniques to manage symptoms of emotional dysregulation which were ubiquitous across their varying complex clinical presentations. I experienced DBT as a very effective treatment model; however, due to my naiveté at the time, I did not seriously consider developing an advanced skillset in DBT because I wanted to do the "deep and meaningful" trauma work with clients.

Early in my advanced practice career, I knew I wanted to work with a population of individuals who had experienced psychological trauma. I first received training in the trauma-focused psychotherapy Eye Movement Desensitization and Reprocessing (EMDR) and embraced the approach for its value in working directly with the traumatic memories underlying most mental disorders: trauma and stressor-related disorders to major depression, obsessive compulsive disorder, phobias, and personality disorders. I then completed training in emotion-focused therapy for complex trauma, which is an evidence-based, short-term treatment for complex trauma that focuses on the therapeutic relationship and emotional processing of trauma material as the key mechanism of healing and change (Paivio & Pascual-Leone, 2010).

When I entered private practice, I specialized as a "trauma-focused" psychotherapist. I began to see clients with a variable range of trauma exposure from single-incident traumas, repeated trauma, to complex developmental and attachment-related trauma. Upon completing an initial evaluation, it became increasingly clear to me that many of my clients were survivors of repeated early childhood abuse and neglect. Their clinical presentations differed significantly from the "single-incident" adult-onset trauma clients in that these clients, who were clearly struggling with unresolved traumatic memories, were also needing support in building their affect regulation capacity and in learning strategies to manage emotional distress that were not ultimately self-destructive. Many of the clients I saw with complex trauma presentations required a comprehensive treatment approach which first and foremost required addressing the immediate issues of suicidality and self-harm prior to engaging in any traumatic memory reprocessing. I thus attended training in DBT at the New Jersey Institute for Psychotherapy Training and Supervision. More recently, I was on a national panel that developed trauma competencies for nursing education and completed my Doctor of Nursing Practice (DNP) project, which focused on integrating trauma-focused psychotherapy training in graduate Psychiatric-Mental Health Nurse Practitioner (PMHNP) programs.

■ FOUNDERS OF DBT AND COMPLEX TRAUMA

Judith Herman, an American psychiatrist, professor of clinical psychiatry at Harvard University, and director of training at the Victims of Violence Program at the Cambridge Health Alliance, first introduced the term *complex trauma* in her seminal book, *Trauma and Recovery* (Herman, 1992). In this book, she developed the concept of "complex posttraumatic stress disorder" to define the symptom constellations present in those who had suffered repeated instances of trauma, especially those originating from childhood adversity. This more comprehensive definition of complex PTSD included domains of alterations in: affect regulation, consciousness, self-perception, perception of the perpetrator, relations with others, and systems of meaning. The importance of this cannot be understated as it provided a language for researchers, academicians, and clinicians to use to capture the experiences of individuals with a history of repeated and prolonged exploitation and therefore allowed for the research and application of evidence-based treatment approaches.

Herman also developed a three-stage sequence of trauma treatment and recovery that entailed: (a) regaining a sense of safety through a therapeutic relationship, medication, or relaxation exercises; (b) actively working on the trauma, fostered by that secure base, and employing a range of psychological techniques; and (c) advancing to a new posttraumatic life recognizing the experience of surviving the trauma and moving on to live a successful life (Courtois, 2014; Herman, 1992).

The field of traumatology has bourgeoned over the past few decades. Contemporary scholars in traumatology define complex trauma as resulting from exposure to severe stressors that (a) are repetitive or prolonged, (b) involve harm or abandonment by caregivers or other ostensibly responsible adults, and (c) occur at developmentally vulnerable times in the victim's life, such as early childhood or adolescence (Courtois, 2014) with the subsequent posttraumatic sequelae, which includes problems with dissociation, emotion dysregulation, somatic distress, or relational or spiritual alienation.

DBT was developed by Marsha Linehan, an American psychologist, professor of psychology and psychiatry and behavioral sciences at the University of Washington, and director of the Behavioral Research and Therapy Clinics, in the late 1980s to treat clients diagnosed with borderline personality disorder (BPD). The existing psychotherapeutic approaches, at the time, proved limited in their ability to assist clients with reducing symptoms of chronic suicidality, impulsivity, and self-injury.

As a teenager, Linehan was admitted to an inpatient psychiatric unit, diagnosed with schizophrenia, and treated with electroconvulsive therapy and antipsychotic medication. She believes that she was misdiagnosed and actually had borderline personality disorder. After this experience, she went on to receive a PhD in psychology from Loyola University and completed a postdoctoral internship at the Suicide Prevention and Crisis Service in Buffalo. After a number of university positions, she took a position at the University of Washington where she developed DBT. Linehan has published extensively in scientific journals and has authored and coauthored many books, including her two seminal treatment manuals: *Cognitive-Behavioral Treatment of Borderline Personality Disorder* (1993a) and *Skills Training Manual for Treating Borderline Personality Disorder* (1993b).

DBT emerged as an evidence-based, hybrid approach, focused on assisting clients, not only with managing their dysfunctional thinking patterns and changing dysfunctional behavior, but as a comprehensive treatment package consisting of individual therapy and group skills building to address severe emotional dysregulation and entrenched self-destructive behavioral patterns.

■ PHILOSOPHY AND KEY CONCEPTS OF DBT

Dialectical Theory

In DBT, dialectics reflect the relative nature of truth, which is subject to change according to the frame of reference. Reality is considered within a systems perspective in which a part of an experience cannot be held separately from the whole of that experience as each invariably shifts in relation to the other. Reality is comprised of opposing forces ("thesis" and "antithesis"), and the integration ("synthesis") of such forces results in a new set of opposing forces (Linehan, 1993a). According to this philosophy, opposing forces do not cancel each other out, but rather exist in a shared and dynamic system. Essentially "the self" is both individual and social, existing within a matrix of relational exchanges and obligations. In DBT, both the therapist and client are tasked with holding multiple yet often disparate truths as in the dialectics of acceptance and change, flexibility and stability, nurturing and challenging, and capabilities and deficits. DBT reinforces the client's ability to hold multiple, sometimes opposite and ambiguous truths at the same time, therefore fostering a synthesis of a wise middle ground—that space in which the client's experience is validated AND the client is held accountable to his or her commitment to change. The "wise-mind" perspective assumes that each client has within himself or herself the potential that is necessary for change (Linehan, 1993a).

Client and Therapist Assumptions

Inherent to DBT are specific assumptions pertinent to the client and therapist. Such assumptions facilitate the function of motivating clients, teaching skills, generalizing skills to natural environments, motivating and improving the skills of therapists, and structuring the treatment environment (Linehan, 1993a).

1. Clients are doing their best in the moment and need to do better.
2. Clients cannot fail in therapy.
3. Clients want to improve yet need skills to do so.

4. Skills need to be generalized to all relevant areas of life.
5. Therapists assume a nonjudgmental approach to clients.
6. Therapists require consultation to stay motivated and effective.
7. Therapists, like clients, need to practice skills.

These core assumptions of DBT apply to clients who struggle with emotional sensitivity, interpersonal crises, behavioral instability, and heightened vulnerability. One of the key considerations is that the client and therapist are thought to be doing the best they can at any given point in time and, at the same time, are able to "do better" in the future. In DBT the client is directed toward changing behavior after he or she has achieved a relative acceptance of the need to change. Additionally, while clients may not be responsible for causing their difficulties, they are still responsible for how they react or respond to those challenges.

■ DEFINITION OF MENTAL HEALTH AND PSYCHOPATHOLOGY IN DBT

In DBT, a mentally healthy individual can regulate his or her emotions without relying upon maladaptive behaviors to manage distress. According to Gottman, Katz, and Hooven (2013), affect or emotion regulation requires the ability to (a) change physiological arousal induced by the affect; (b) refocus attention away from the affective stimuli; (c) inhibit mood-dependent behavior; and (d) organize one's actions to achieve a non-mood-dependent goal.

In the biosocial theory of DBT, the client's struggles are thought to originate from a combination of biological vulnerability and an invalidating early environment leading to difficulty with emotional vulnerability and emotion regulation. Invalidating early environments contribute to emotion dysregulation as they fail to teach the child how to label and regulate arousal, how to tolerate emotional distress, and when to trust his or her emotional responses as reflective of valid interpretations of events.

The combination of emotional vulnerability and impaired capacity for emotion regulation results in repeated behaviorally conditioned problematic patterns. Through operant conditioning, a client's problematic behaviors may have been reinforced over time by a positive internal or external response to the behavioral stimulus. Posttraumatic symptomatology is also understood within a learning theory framework. For example, a client who experiences a flashback in response to reminders of a previous trauma experiences a classically conditioned response of anxiety, fear, and helplessness to benign yet conditioned stimuli (Linehan, 1993a). Thus, the combination of biological vulnerability, an invalidating early environment, and repeated conditioned problematic patterns lead to emotion dysregulation and psychopathology.

■ THERAPEUTIC GOALS IN DBT

The overarching goal of DBT is for the client to change behavioral patterns toward building a life worth living. That process is facilitated through increasing emotional experiencing and modulation, self-validation, realistic decision-making, and good judgment and problem-solving to support improving the client's engagement in life (e.g., going to school, seeing friends, going to work). Throughout the treatment, emphasis is placed on enhancing emotional regulation and behavioral self-management through validation and teaching of the skills of mindfulness, emotion identification, distress tolerance, and interpersonal effectiveness. In treating complex trauma, after an initial focus on developing basic skills, the focus then shifts toward applying skills specifically on symptoms associated with PTSD.

■ PERSPECTIVE ON ASSESSMENT IN DBT

DBT emphasizes initial and ongoing behavioral assessment as fundamental to successful treatment. Clinicians utilize formal and informal assessment strategies to guide treatment decisions (Swales & Dunkley, 2020). While therapists may conduct a distinct initial biopsychosocial assessment at the outset of treatment, behavioral assessment continues within each subsequent client encounter. Problematic behaviors are identified and organized within a behavior hierarchy, which identifies the priority treatment target(s) of each session (Figure 10.1).

Often, survivors of complex trauma, especially when they first come to treatment, struggle with a range of potentially life-threatening and self-harming behaviors including nonsuicidal self-injury, suicidal attempts, impulsivity, excessive alcohol and/or substance use, and other risk-taking behaviors. The initial target of therapy is on helping the client to reduce self-destructive behaviors through a process of developing strategies to support emotion regulation, self-soothing, and learn more adaptive behaviors to use in response to emotional activation.

■ THERAPEUTIC INTERVENTIONS IN DBT

Traditional DBT is considered a comprehensive treatment model and in its truest form includes the client attending (a) weekly individual therapy sessions and group skills training, (b) skills coaching via telephone or other means of communication to support the client's application of skills to real-life situations, and (c) a team consultation to assist the therapist with maintaining fidelity to the treatment frame. However, DBT can be adapted and integrated into other therapeutic modalities as a contextualized approach.

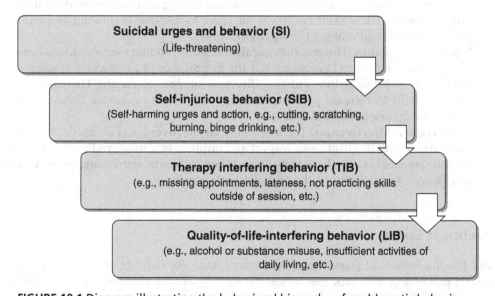

FIGURE 10.1 Diagram illustrating the behavioral hierarchy of problematic behavior

Individual Therapy

Individual therapy has a recommended structure for each session (Linehan, 1993a), whether the therapy is a component of a comprehensive DBT program or if it occurs as a standalone individual treatment. The session begins with a mindfulness exercise for the first several minutes. The therapist guides the client in this practice and checks in with the client after the exercise to get a sense of how the experience was for him or her and builds upon positive internal shifts with validation and positive reinforcement. Next, the therapist checks in with the client about other aspects of the client's treatment including asking about what was focused on in the skills group, updates on meetings with other providers, and any pressing issues to be included in the agenda. The focus is then shifted to the diary card review and the client and therapist collaborate in prioritizing the target behaviors according to the treatment hierarchy. The remaining 30 to 40 minutes of the session are organized according to the agenda and techniques such as behavioral analysis, which may be focused on to gain clarity around previous difficulties with refraining from problematic behaviors or anticipated future difficulty. The last several minutes of the session include assigning homework to be completed prior to the next session, followed by a closing mindfulness exercise.

Skills Training

Linehan (1993b) identified four distinct skills modules: *mindfulness, distress tolerance, emotional regulation,* and *interpersonal effectiveness.* The modules are comprised of didactic psychoeducation on the specific skills, with experiential application exercises to facilitate the client's mastery of the skills.

Mindfulness. Mindfulness is the first skills module taught with the goal of helping the client to practice being present, with a nonjudgmental attitude toward inner and outer experience. The dialectic of emotion and reason is synthesized in the creation of a "wise mind" perspective to support decision-making that is grounded, responsive, and effective.

Distress Tolerance. The distress tolerance skills module teaches the client healthy coping behaviors to use in place of maladaptive coping in situations that are impossible to change. These skills empower the client to respond to difficult and painful experiences without making the situation worse.

Emotion Regulation. The emotion regulation skills module teaches clients how to identify and understand emotions and the importance of proactively engaging in self-care in order to reduce vulnerability and support resiliency. The focus is on learning skills to increase positive emotions and how to decrease behaviors that maintain negative emotional reactions.

Interpersonal Effectiveness. The interpersonal effectiveness skills module outlines skills to increase the client's self-respect and improve relationships through increasing interpersonal skills. These skills include setting limits; expressing needs, wants, and desires; and building and negotiating relationships.

Treatment Stages

DBT has five treatment stages: (a) pretreatment stage, (b) stability and behavioral control, (c) processing traumatic memories, (d) solving routine problems, and (e) finding freedom, joy and spirituality.

Pretreatment Stage. The pretreatment stage creates the foundation for successful psychotherapy. The focus is on establishing a secure, mutually agreed upon, treatment frame for the therapy to follow. While an initial focus is on building the therapeutic relationship, the therapists' job is also to elicit the client's motivation and commitment to participate in treatment. The structure of treatment should be clearly defined including a detailed orientation including an informed consent and clarity around frequency of sessions, extra-session contact, the role of homework, client and therapist responsibilities, and protocol in case of emergency in addition to clear expectations regarding session fees, attendance, cancellation, and early discharge from treatment.

Stage One: Stability and Behavioral Control. This stage is an especially important and necessary stage of treatment with a complex trauma survivor. The initial focus in this stage is the development of a safe and trusting relationship between the client and the clinician. As many of these clients have experienced insufferable abuse and neglect by primary caregivers including attachment-related trauma and subsequent attachment difficulties, establishing a "good-enough" and "safe-enough" therapeutic relationship is paramount to creating safety in the treatment and begins the process of repairing attachment-related difficulties. This relational foundation may be the client's first exposure to a secure attachment and provides a meaningful opportunity for the client to experience a secure attachment. With a strong therapeutic alliance in place, the therapy can then focus on skills training to assist the client with refraining from engaging in ineffective and destructive target behaviors. Symptom control and safety is essential for successful treatment. Stage one lasts until clients reach a place of personal and environmental safety and adequate stabilization prior to continuing in more trauma-focused therapy.

Stage Two: Processing Traumatic Memories. In this stage, attention is placed on treating PTSD and significant stress reactions. The treatment is focused on the processing of traumatic memories while maintaining dual awareness through mindfulness and containment techniques.

Stage Three: Solving Routine Problems of Living. In this stage, clients have typically achieved successful trauma resolution. The focus of treatment shifts to navigating the more "routine" challenges of being a human and creating a values-based life.

Stage Four: Finding Freedom, Joy, and Spirituality. During this stage of treatment, clients experience low levels of functional impairment. They are ready to address any existential concerns in their work toward actualizing and maintaining a life of peace and fulfillment.

Specific Techniques

Commitment Strategies. Therapists utilize "foot in the door" concepts to enhance clients' commitment to treatment by emphasizing aspects of DBT most appealing to them. The goal is to increase clients' willingness to engage in treatment. With clients who may be overly eager to change problematic behavior, a "door-in-the-face" devil's advocate approach may be the best route for increasing commitment. For example, if a client was to commit to refraining from all self-harm behavior, the therapist might respond with: "Self-harm can be an effective solution for managing overwhelming emotions. Why change now?" Through this questioning, the client builds commitment through articulating counterarguments to the clinician's statements and questioning.

Validation. Therapists use validation to support the change process by creating a relationship in which clients feel valued and understood. Through validation, the therapist seeks to create a trusting experience and connect deeply with the experiences of the client with presence and authenticity. The experience of validation, while not directly eliciting behavioral change, provides an opportunity for relational healing. DBT therapists use six levels of validation: (a) mindfully attentive and alert, (b) acknowledgment of what the client says, (c) acknowledgment of what is communicated nonverbally, (d) articulate how the client's experience makes sense given history or biology, (e) articulate how the client's experience makes sense in the present, and (f) being in genuine human contact with clients (Linehan, 1993a).

Self-Monitoring. Self-monitoring in DBT is achieved through use of the diary card (Exhibit 10.1). Clients are responsible for recording their day-to-day experiences to

EXHIBIT 10.1

Diary Card

Dialectical Behavior Therapy	Instructions: Circle the days you worked on each skill	Filled out in session? Y N	How often did you fill out this side? ____Daily___ Two to Three Times____Once				
1. Wise mind	Mon	Tues	Wed	Thurs	Fri	Sat	Sun
2. Observe: just notice (urge surfing)	Mon	Tues	Wed	Thurs	Fri	Sat	Sun
3. Describe: put words on	Mon	Tues	Wed	Thurs	Fri	Sat	Sun
4. Participate: enter into the experience	Mon	Tues	Wed	Thurs	Fri	Sat	Sun
5. Nonjudgmental stance	Mon	Tues	Wed	Thurs	Fri	Sat	Sun
6. One-mindfully: in-the-moment	Mon	Tues	Wed	Thurs	Fri	Sat	Sun
7. Effectiveness: focus on what works	Mon	Tues	Wed	Thurs	Fri	Sat	Sun
8. Objective effectiveness: DEARMAN	Mon	Tues	Wed	Thurs	Fri	Sat	Sun
9. Relationship effectiveness: GIVE	Mon	Tues	Wed	Thurs	Fri	Sat	Sun
10. Self-respect effectiveness: FAST	Mon	Tues	Wed	Thurs	Fri	Sat	Sun

(continued)

EXHIBIT 10.1

Diary Card *(continued)*

Dialectical Behavior Therapy	**Instructions: Circle the days you worked on each skill**	**Filled out in session? Y N**		**How often did you fill out this side? ____Daily___ Two to Three Times____Once**			
11. Reduce vulnerability: PLEASE	Mon	Tues	Wed	Thurs	Fri	Sat	Sun
12. Build MASTERY	Mon	Tues	Wed	Thurs	Fri	Sat	Sun
13. Build positive experiences	Mon	Tues	Wed	Thurs	Fri	Sat	Sun
14. Opposite-to-emotion action (Alt. Rebellion)	Mon	Tues	Wed	Thurs	Fri	Sat	Sun
15. Distract (Adaptive denial)	Mon	Tues	Wed	Thurs	Fri	Sat	Sun
16. Self-soothe	Mon	Tues	Wed	Thurs	Fri	Sat	Sun
17. Improve the moment	Mon	Tues	Wed	Thurs	Fri	Sat	Sun
18. Pros and cons	Mon	Tues	Wed	Thurs	Fri	Sat	Sun
19. Radical Acceptance	Mon	Tues	Wed	Thurs	Fri	Sat	Sun
20. Building Structure/Work	Mon	Tues	Wed	Thurs	Fri	Sat	Sun
21. Building Structure/Love	Mon	Tues	Wed	Thurs	Fri	Sat	Sun
22. Building Structure/Time	Mon	Tues	Wed	Thurs	Fri	Sat	Sun
23. Building Structure/Place	Mon	Tues	Wed	Thurs	Fri	Sat	Sun
Urge to use (0–5): Before therapy session: ______After therapy session: ______						BRTC Diary Card Copyright 1999 Marsha M. Linehan	
Urge to quit therapy (0–5): Before therapy session: ______ After therapy session: ______							

(continued)

Diary Card (continued)

Dialectical Behavior Therapy Diary Card															Initials	ID No.	Filled out in session? Y N	How often did you fill out this side?			Date Started
																		Daily	Two to Three Times	Once	
Day and Date	Use	Suicide	SH	Pain	Sad	Shame	Anger	Fear	Illicit	ETOH	Prescrip	OTC	S-H	Lying	Joy	Skills	R				
	0–5	0–5	0–5	0–5	0–5	0–5	0–5	0–5	No. Specify	No. Specify	No. Specify	No.	Y/N	No.	0–5	0–7	✓				
Mon																					
Tues																					
Wed																					
Thur																					
Fri																					
Sat																					
Sun																					

*USED SKILLS
0 = Not thought about or used
1 = Thought about, not used, did not want to
2 = Thought about, not used, wanted to
3 = Tried but could not use them
4 = Tried, could do them but they did not help
5 = Tried, could use them, helped
6 = Did not try, used them, did not help
7 = Did not try, used them, helped

Belief in control of . . .	Before	After
Emotions:		
Behaviors:		
Thoughts:		

	Before	After
Urge to use (0–5):		
Urge to quit therapy (0–5):		
Urge to harm (0–5):		

BRTC Diary Card
Copyright 1999 Marsha M. Linehan

track their emotional experience, behavioral responses, distress tolerance skill use, and daily emotion regulation practices. The diary card helps guide the agenda for each session with priority assigned according to the behavior hierarchy. Reviewing the diary card in session provides an opportunity for the therapist to validate the client's emotional struggles in between sessions as well.

Functional Behavioral Analysis. Behavioral analysis allows the client and therapist to explore the antecedents and consequences of a behavior and work together to identify moments in which skills could have been applied to emotions, cognitions, physiological reactions, or other contributors to target behaviors. A chain analysis is often conducted in response to use of target behaviors (see Figure 10.2); however, it is important for the therapist to make sure that it is not used for or perceived as punishment.

Communication Techniques. DBT therapists utilize both reciprocal and irreverent communication in a balanced dialectic to facilitate the therapy process. Reciprocal communication builds the therapeutic relationship through warm engagement, validation, and support. Therapist self-disclosure of personal information may be judiciously used to facilitate the process of the client's therapy. The therapist may use examples of his or her own application of a skill to teach or reinforce the skill, role model the skill, or affirm the client's use of the skill. Self-disclosure may also express the therapist's experience of the client in that moment. Irreverent communication, on the other hand, is a paradoxical technique that is used to shift emotions, thoughts, or behaviors. It encourages the client to consider the multiple meanings of the therapist's response, thereby fostering greater cognitive flexibility in the client. The therapist may respond in an unexpected way using humor to encourage dialectical thinking.

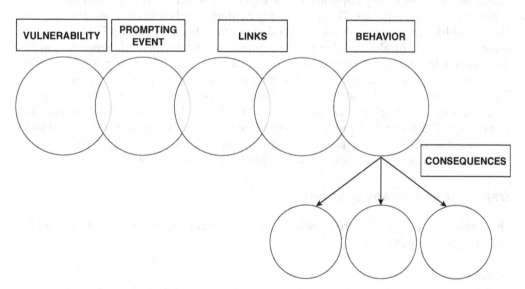

FIGURE 10.2 Chain analysis template diagram.

■ CASE STUDY

Background

I chose to include my work with a 22-year-old female client whom I saw for outpatient psychotherapy for approximately 3 years. She was referred to me by a colleague who had been seeing her for the past 6 months for psychiatric medication management and recommended she begin trauma-focused psychotherapy.

Emma presented with significant emotion dysregulation including symptoms of depressed mood, generalized anxiety, insomnia, recurrent flashbacks and nightmares, and repeated self-injurious behavior, all of which were present since her childhood. Her chaotic household, experiences of childhood sexual abuse, and parental neglect likely resulted in a reliance on defensive dissociation to distance herself from experiencing overwhelm in the presence of ongoing threat to her physical and emotional integrity. Her emotional landscape vacillated between extreme anxious hyperarousal and shutdown depressive hypoarousal. She maintained a core schema that she is "bad and evil" which likely developed to help her maintain her attachment bonds to her parents, who were both perpetrators of the abuse she experienced. Additionally, Emma did not learn how to regulate her emotions or self-soothe as the trusted adults in her life did not effectively role model such behavior, and she frequently relied upon the use of alcohol and restricting caloric intake. As a result of her profound shame and low self-esteem, Emma struggled with maintaining interpersonal relationships. On one hand, she desires closeness and intimacy, and on the other, she maintains emotional distance, fearing criticism or rejection.

My treatment targets for Emma included her life-threatening behaviors, her therapy-interfering behaviors, her quality-of-life-interfering behaviors, and her emotional vulnerability. Emma had been hospitalized one time, approximately 3 years ago, after expressing suicidal intent to her roommate in college. She was voluntarily admitted to an inpatient psychiatric unit and was discharged after 1 week. She occasionally experiences passive suicidal ideation;, however, she denies any intent to act on those thoughts. Nevertheless, these life-threatening behaviors were a treatment target. Emma would often miss or forget therapy appointments, especially when she experienced an increase in posttraumatic symptoms. Thus, her therapy-interfering behaviors were also a target. Quality-of-life-interfering behaviors included the targets of decreasing Emma's cutting behavior, overuse of alcohol, depressive symptoms, and financial dependence on her parents and increasing social contact and self-care with respect to her regular undernourishment. By addressing these behaviors, Emma could improve the quality of her life by improving her relationships, increasing positive experiences, and addressing her health concerns. Emma's emotional vulnerability included her emotional dysregulation based upon her biological predisposition to be highly sensitive to emotional stimuli in addition to her early experiences of growing up in an invalidating environment in which her emotional expressions were minimized and/or dismissed.

Transcript of Therapy Sessions

The transcripts presented here were selected from segments of the beginning, middle, and final phase of therapy.

Beginning Phase

APPN: One of your goals for our work together is to decrease your alcohol use. Can you tell me more about that?

Emma: Well, my previous therapist Lauren was concerned that maybe I was drinking too much.

APPN: Do you agree with her assessment?

Emma: Yes and no. I have been drinking more than usual these days, maybe five nights a week, but it's always social. I never drink by myself or anything and I don't get out of control.

APPN: Part of you feels that your drinking is just fine, it's social, it's never out of control, so, what's the problem with that?

Emma: *(Taken aback)* I guess Lauren is worried that I may be using alcohol to self-medicate when I'm stressed. And the truth is, she's not wrong. After a long day at work, I really enjoy grabbing a few drinks with friends to relax and decompress.

APPN: Alcohol seems to help you feel better at the end of your day. You mentioned a "long day" at work contributes to your feeling stressed. Are there any other factors contributing?

Emma: I'm not sure.

APPN: *(silence)* Hmm, can we imagine for a moment a day that you ended work feeling stress free, having worked just the right amount of time with exerting just enough effort to leave work feeling neutral or positive? Might you feel compelled to drink?

Emma: Probably. I think too that I tend to feel more anxious in the evening, especially after daylight savings when it gets dark so early . . . I would prefer to not have to be commuting home when it's dark out, but it is what it is, kinda. I've always been this way, even when I was a kid. That's when I can feel very triggered into a very bad memory.

APPN: *(Observing dissociated affect; slightly allowing my saddened affect to show)* It must be so challenging to feel anxious and vulnerable most nights of the week, Emma.

Emma: *(tears filling her eyes, nods)*

APPN: *(silence)* Emma, I can understand your wanting to feel relief from those painful feelings. Anyone would. And, if you'd like, I can help you learn and apply skills to help you manage your anxiety and stress in the evenings. How does that sound?

Emma: It sounds good. I know I am drinking more than I should, and I do need to figure out how to take better care of myself. I just want to feel better, which is what I'm striving for.

Commentary: After collaborating on identifying treatment targets, the early sessions focused on reviewing the diary cards.

APPN: In our last session, we went over how to use the diary cards and their role in our treatment together. I am wondering if you were able to try it out.

Emma: Umm, kinda. I did it for 5 days and then I think I forgot about it.

APPN: Emma, it's great that you were able to complete it for those 5 days!

Emma: *(Looking down, appearing sad; significant silence)*

APPN: *(After a pause)* You're quiet.

Emma: Yea, it's just . . . I appreciate you saying that but I'm angry at myself for failing and not doing it like I was supposed to. It's more evidence that I am a lazy piece of crap and therapy will never work for me.

APPN:	You're angry at yourself for not meeting your goal.
Emma:	Yea, it's like, I want more than anything to get better and to feel better, but this is what I always do. I always say I'm going to do something and then I don't. I know therapy is only going to work if I do the work.
APPN:	Do you have a sense of what may have gotten in the way of your completing the diary card?
Emma:	Well, I remember that on Friday night I was having a lot of flashbacks and I just couldn't fall asleep. So, then I overslept and was late for work on Saturday and didn't have time to complete my 24-hour recall before having to leave.
APPN:	It sounds like it was really challenging for you to fall asleep on Friday evening because you were experiencing flashbacks. I can understand how that could make it difficult to wake up in time for work the following day.
Emma:	Yea, it IS really hard. I hate that I have to deal with all of this.
APPN:	Your PTSD symptoms?
Emma:	Yes.
APPN:	You're angry and it feels unfair that you re-experience the trauma you've been through.
Emma:	Yea. It's infuriating and I hate that I'm too lazy to get to work on time and too lazy to complete my diary card.
APPN:	Is it possible that some of the anger you feel toward yourself around not completing your diary card has more to do with your anger at having recurrent flashbacks?
Emma:	Yes.
APPN:	Perhaps it's less about your being a "lazy piece of crap" and more about your feeling helpless and frustrated that despite being committed to therapy you continue to re-experience the terrible and traumatic things you've been through?
Emma:	Yes . . . .. It seems really unfair (*begins to cry*).
APPN:	It is unfair . . . and yet, despite tremendous struggle, you continue to show up for yourself and for your healing.
Emma:	(*Looks up, smiles slightly*)

Middle Phase

The middle sessions focused on Emma and I completing a behavioral chain analysis and reviewing distress tolerance skills in order to explore the factors contributing to her use of cutting behaviors in between sessions.

APPN:	Emma, it looks like you were really struggling on Tuesday.
Emma:	Yea, I guess (*looks down*).

APPN:	Can you say a little more about what was going on that you decided to cut yourself?
Emma:	I don't know. I don't really want to talk about it, but I know I need to.
APPN:	(*After a pause*) What are you noticing right now?
Emma:	I don't know. I feel a lot of shame right now and I just want to hide.
APPN:	It seems a part of you is wanting to go away right now and there is a part of you that is present and willing to share openly. I wonder if a chain analysis might help us to look at what happened objectively—might that be an okay way to approach talking about this?
Emma:	Yes, so when I got home from my date with Joe on Tuesday, I was feeling really overwhelmed—so much that I'm not sure that I was even in my body. I sat down at my desk in my bedroom and I took out my razor blade and cut myself on my thighs.
APPN:	Tuesday night sounds incredibly difficult. Before we continue talking about it, I want to make sure that you are physically okay, okay?
Emma:	(*nods*)
APPN:	How many times do you think you cut yourself and did you draw blood?
Emma:	Like four times and it was bleeding a little, but it stopped pretty quickly and then I cleaned it up in the bathroom after and now it's just scabbed over.
APPN:	Okay, so it seems like it's in the healing process.
Emma:	Yup.
APPN:	Shifting gears, let's go back to the chain analysis. I'm going to draw it out on the whiteboard and let's fill in the bubbles together. (*We develop chain analysis; see Figure 10.3.*)

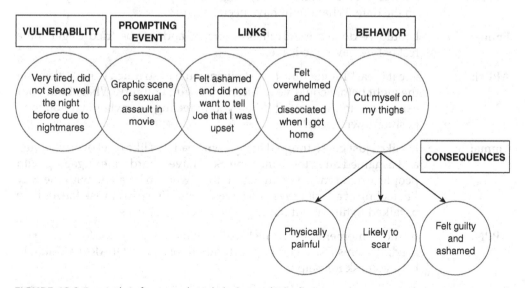

FIGURE 10.3 Example of a completed chain analysis diagram.

APPN:	Let's zoom-out for a moment. What stands out to you?
Emma:	That it was a stupid thing to do.
APPN:	Cutting yourself?
Emma:	Yea, it's so clear that it made the situation worse and my thigh is still hurting.
APPN:	The cutting behavior resulted in some pretty negative consequences. I imagine the cutting behavior may have also served a purpose. How do you understand that?
Emma:	What do you mean?
APPN:	Well, let's look at what led up to it.
Emma:	I think maybe it helped me to feel less overwhelmed and in a way it felt like it brought me back to earth—like I was less dissociated.
APPN:	At the time it seems like you were desperate for relief and cutting provided that, albeit, temporarily.
Emma:	Umm hmm. I think the movie was really triggering for me and I had already felt so on edge earlier in the day, so it was like a double whammy. I felt bad for Joe because I didn't want him to think that I wasn't having a nice time, but I also felt too embarrassed to say anything about what was going on with me.
APPN:	What you just said is super important in putting together and understanding how you arrived at the cutting behavior. It seems you were already in a vulnerable place before the date, felt triggered by the content of the movie, and then you had to hide the way you were feeling because you felt embarrassed. No wonder you felt overwhelmed and dissociated when you got home! (*smiling*)
Emma:	(*Slightly giggles*) Yea, I guess it makes sense.
APPN:	Let's look at the vulnerability you were experiencing before you went on the date. What might have been helpful?
Emma:	I could've done a mindfulness exercise, and maybe tried to get some rest before having to leave.
APPN:	Great ideas! Taking time to rest given you had so much trouble sleeping the night before could've reduced some vulnerability. What about your experience in the movie? When you're feeling overwhelmed you tend to shut down, right?
Emma:	It's like I just get so trapped in my own head. It's like I feel overwhelmed and ashamed all at the same time. So, I have a hard time engaging with people around me, even though I don't want to be alone with the way I'm feeling at all. (*after a pause*) I guess I could've tried to ask Joe for help or talked to him about the way I was feeling, I guess.
APPN:	In those moments it can feel really challenging to ask for what you need. It seems like a good opportunity to use your DEARMAN skill to help you ask for help.
Emma:	That would've been helpful. It would've made me feel less pressured to figure out how to explain what was going on with me.

APPN:	How might you have asked for what you need using the DEARMAN skill? Let's start with the D for describe.
Emma:	(*Describe*) "Joe, the scene in the movie triggered a traumatic memory."
APPN:	Next—the E for express.
Emma:	(*Express*) "I am feeling really afraid."
APPN:	Next, the A for assert.
Emma:	(*Assert*) "I would like if you could remind me that I am okay and that I am safe."
APPN:	And the R for reinforce.
Emma:	(*Reinforce*) "It would really help me to feel less overwhelmed."
APPN:	Excellent! How do you think he would've responded?
Emma:	I think he would've been happy to help me when I needed him to. He's been super supportive in the past and I think he would've appreciated knowing what I was feeling and being there for me in that way.
APPN:	Let's say for whatever reason you are not able to elicit the support of someone around you when you are feeling triggered. Looking at the other night as an example, was there another point in time that you could've done something differently?
Emma:	Well, when I got home, I could've used my distress tolerance skills.
APPN:	What skills would you have used?
Emma:	It really helps me to hold an icepack or an ice cube while I do deep breathing. That usually helps me to come back to the present.
APPN:	What a great idea! I want to acknowledge how awesome it is that just now you were able to identify three choice-points in which skills could have helped you to manage your flashbacks and intense feelings without feeling so overwhelmed that cutting seemed like the only option.
Emma:	(*Smiling*) It's a good feeling when I think about having a choice, having options, like I'm not just helpless, that I can do things differently.
APPN:	(*Smiling*) Can we sit with and enjoy the positive feelings you are experiencing right now?
Emma:	(*smiling, nods*)

Final Phase

The final sessions focused on reviewing progress made in the course of therapy, identifying areas for continued growth, and processing the experience of ending treatment. This is an excerpt from our last session.

APPN:	So, here we are, it's our last session.
Emma:	Oh my gosh, you're going to make me cry. I can't believe this is the last time we'll be meeting.

APPN:	In our usual fashion, let's take a moment to do some grounding (*smiling*).
Emma:	Of course! (*chuckles*)
APPN:	Go inside and take a moment, and when you're ready let me know what you notice.
Emma:	I notice that I am feeling really pretty sad right now.
APPN:	How do you experience that sadness?
Emma:	Well, I'm noticing that my eyes are becoming teary, and it feels like I have a pit in my stomach. I'm also aware that I'm having a hard time looking you in the eyes right now.
APPN:	What do you think is contributing to your difficulty of making eye contact with me right now?
Emma:	(*Still looking down*) I don't know, I guess in a weird way, I am afraid that if I look up at you, that I might break down into tears.
APPN:	And if you did, what would your tears be communicating?
Emma:	Just how grateful I am for the work we've done together these past years, and how grateful I am for our relationship and how I'm really going to miss you (*crying*).
APPN:	The feelings are mutual.
Emma:	Well, since I've already opened the floodgates, I can look at you now (*chuckles*).
APPN:	(*Smiling*) Well, there you go!
Emma:	(*smiling*)
APPN:	The last time we met, we were talking about the ups and downs of our journey together, the challenges and the successes. I would like for us to spend some time reflecting upon the progress you've made from day 1 to now. What comes to mind for you?
Emma:	A lot of things. I guess what stands out the most, in this moment, is that I have not engaged in cutting behaviors at all in almost 2 years.
APPN:	That is quite the accomplishment.
Emma:	Totally. Although, at this point I feel so far removed from that behavior that I almost can't believe that there was a long time where I was certain that cutting would always be my security blanket, and one of my go-to strategies to deal.
APPN:	When you first began treatment, you used quite a few maladaptive behaviors—cutting, excessive drinking, restricting calories—all of which helped you to manage the intensity of the way you were feeling. Then, you learned and worked really hard to practice other more effective ways to tolerate and regulate your emotions.
Emma:	Yea, it's like these new behaviors have become more like second nature for me. In fact, I remember, maybe after a year of treatment, I noticed this shift in which I found myself wanting to proactively take good care

of myself. It was like self-soothing began to feel more natural. I also got a lot better at asking and letting others in when I needed help.

APPN: It seems like you were able to develop a more intuitive compassion for yourself and in that process were better able to let others support and nurture you.

Emma: Yes, self-compassion was definitely not in my vocabulary 3 years ago (*chuckles*). Don't get me wrong. I still have a ways to go, but remember that time when in a session, you said to me, "You are stronger than you feel right now," and I snapped back in a very snarky way something like, "What, do you have that on a mug at home or something?"

APPN: (*Smiling*) Oh yes, I do remember that time.

Emma: (*Chuckling*) I'm sorry about that. It was a pretty mean thing to say. Honestly, I am so surprised that you didn't fire me as a patient in the beginning of treatment. I was truly a terror at times (*smiling*).

APPN: (*Smiling*) Hmm, how do you think I was able to hold on for so long?

Emma: Well, I think it was because you saw me as a whole person. It's like no matter what was going on, what had happened in between sessions, you were always genuinely interested in knowing what was going on with me. I remember feeling like I really mattered and that my feelings were important. Thank you (*smiling*).

APPN: It has been an honor and a pleasure to be on this journey with you. I am also holding a strong sense of gratitude right now and appreciation for your courage and resilience throughout this process.

Commentary: Emma and I continued to reflect upon the progress she made toward achieving her therapeutic goals and then we switched our focus to areas for future continued growth.

APPN: You've heard me say quite a few times, but as you know, I feel strongly that one's work on him- or herself is never done. While holding what you have been able to accomplish in our work together, let's also spend some time thinking about worthwhile targets for future continued self-growth.

Emma: Okay, I need to think about that . . . .

APPN: Take your time.

Emma: I think another area I would like to work on is improving my relationship with my parents. I think I am solid enough in myself to begin to work through some of those issues.

APPN: What could that look like?

Emma: Well, like with my relationship with my mom, for instance, I know she is not all bad and she too has been through a lot in her life. I guess I feel ready to work on having a better relationship with her. In a way I want to redefine our relationship where we have healthier boundaries than in the past.

APPN: You have done a lot of great work on setting and maintaining good boundaries with quite a few important people in your life, which will serve you well when you are ready to work on negotiating limits with your parents.

Emma: I also want to continue to develop different hobbies and interests, and engage in more activities outside of work that I find enjoyable. It's strange that for so long, I just didn't have the bandwidth to add anything additional to my plate. No pun intended. I feel like I have achieved a greater balance in my life and have opened a lot of space for me to live in a more meaningful way.

Commentary

Emma presented for treatment wanting to decrease her use of self-destructive behaviors to manage her complex trauma-related symptoms of hyper- and hypoarousal. We met for 120 sessions over a 32-month time period. In our early sessions, I helped Emma to identify the problematic behavioral targets which, on the one hand, provided temporary relief; however,, on the other hand, they contributed to her distress and interfered with her ability to "lead a life worth living." I helped her to contextualize her experiences of emotional distress as understandable traumatic responses to experiences of childhood trauma. She self-monitored the treatment-related aspects of her life in-between sessions and presented her diary card in each session. We prioritized the treatment targets using a behavioral hierarchy to better understand the factors contributing to her use of dissociation, avoidance, cutting behavior, excessive alcohol use, and food restriction to modulate her emotional arousal. The use of a chain analysis helped Emma to be more reflective and curious about her experiences; she was then able to identify choice points in which to apply distress tolerance and self-regulatory skills. As Emma learned and mastered skills to assist her with managing distress and supporting emotion regulation, she exhibited greater emotional resilience and capacity for affect modulation.

DISCUSSION QUESTIONS

1. What is meant by the term *complex trauma* and how does the symptomatology differ from single-incident trauma presentations?
2. Describe the overarching goals of DBT and the approach for prioritizing treatment targets.
3. What is the purpose of the diary card in DBT and how does this facilitate the change process?
4. What techniques might you use in session to address a client's use of nonsuicidal self-injurious behavior in-between therapy sessions?

REFERENCES

Courtois, C. A. (2014). *It's not you, it's what happened to you: Complex trauma and treatment*. Dublin, OH: Telemachus Press.

Gottman, J. M., Katz, L. F., & Hooven, C. (2013). *Meta-emotion: How families communicate emotionally*. Abingdon, England: Routledge.

Herman, J. (1992). *Trauma and recovery: The aftermath of violence--from domestic abuse to political terror*. New York, NY: Basic Books.

Linehan, M. M. (1993a). *Cognitive-behavioral treatment of borderline personality disorder*. New York, NY: Guilford Press.

Linehan, M. M. (1993b). *Skills training manual for treating borderline personality disorder: Diagnosis and treatment of mental disorders*. New York, NY: Guilford Press.

Paivio, S., & Pascual-Leone, A. (2010). *Emotion-focused therapy for complex trauma: An integrative approach*. Washington, DC: American Psychological Association.

Swales, M., & Dunkley, C. (2020). Principles of skills assessment in dialectical behavior therapy. *Cognitive and Behavioral Practice*, 27(1), 18–29. doi:10.1016/j.cbpra.2019.05.001

11

Interpersonal Psychotherapy: A Client With Complicated Bereavement

Candice Knight

■ **PERSONAL EXPERIENCE WITH INTERPERSONAL PSYCHOTHERAPY**

Approximately 20 years ago, significant changes in the mental health insurance payer system initiated industry-wide policies that limited psychotherapy for many clients to 12 to 16 sessions. As a clinician practicing long-term Gestalt, person-centered, and existential psychotherapy, I was motivated to consider training in a short-term, problem-focused approach that had the potential to meet the needs of clients who were precluded the luxury of long-term therapy due to the limitations of their insurance. As many of my clients had mood disorders and initiated psychotherapy for interpersonal problems, I decided to train in Interpersonal Psychotherapy (IPT), a time-limited, structured approach based on the belief that interpersonal problems are frequently the cause of mood disorders and other psychological disorders.

I was further intrigued by IPT based on its integration of concepts from John Bowlby's attachment theory, Adolf Meyer's biopsychosocial theory, and Harry Stack Sullivan's interpersonal psychoanalysis, three seminal theories of personality and psychotherapy that I greatly admire and in which I was extensively trained during my graduate school education in psychiatric nursing and clinical psychology. IPT frames psychotherapy around a central interpersonal problem in the client's life. By mobilizing and working collaboratively with the client to resolve the interpersonal problem, IPT seeks to improve interpersonal skills, decrease interpersonal stress, enhance social support, and facilitate emotional processing. IPT accomplishes these tasks in a very focused, short-term context; thus, it beckoned as an appealing solution to my dilemma of limited sessions. Accordingly, I attended a number of workshops in this approach and completed beginning and advanced level training as well as supervision at the Institute for Interpersonal Psychotherapy. I have found this approach to be of great utility for clients with interpersonal problems whose only option is short-term psychotherapy.

■ FOUNDERS AND LEADERS OF IPT

IPT emerged as a psychotherapeutic treatment modality in the 1970s when Gerald Klerman, Myrna Weissman, and Eugene Paykel participated in a comprehensive research project at Yale University that investigated the efficacy of an antidepressant medication, alone or in combination with psychotherapy, for the maintenance treatment of clients diagnosed with major depressive disorder (MDD). Occurring concurrently, there was a groundswell movement to develop standardized and manualized psychotherapy treatment that could be tested and reliably replicated. Consequently, the psychotherapy developed for this project was standardized and manualized and named "high contact therapy." As the study revealed the efficacy of the combination approach, the psychotherapy was further developed, became more comprehensive, and was aptly renamed IPT (Klerman, Dimascio, Weissman, Prusoff, & Paykel, 1974; Weissman et al., 1979).

Soon after, a three-way comparison acute treatment trial was conducted using antidepressants and IPT to treat MDD. Results revealed that the combination of medication and IPT was the most efficacious treatment for acute treatment rather than medication or psychotherapy alone. The original IPT manual, *Interpersonal Psychotherapy of Depression*, was published in 1984 for this research project (Klerman, Weissman, Rounsaville, & Chevron, 1984). These studies led to the inclusion of IPT in the 1989 National Institute of Mental Health Treatment of Depression Collaborative Research Program, which compared IPT to imipramine, placebo, and cognitive behavioral therapy (CBT) for acute treatment of MDD. Results of that extensive study revealed that IPT and CBT were both effective psychotherapies in treating clients with MDD (Elkin et al., 1989).

From that time forward to the present, IPT has been adapted for other disorders such as dysthymia, bipolar disorder, eating disorders, substance use disorders, postpartum depression, cyclothymia, and borderline personality disorder. IPT has effectively been applied to children, adolescents, and older adults as well as with different delivery methods such as in groups, community settings, and by telepsychiatry (Weissman & Markowitz, 1998). IPT is recognized as an efficacious, evidence-based, short-term psychotherapy by the American Psychiatric Association, the American Psychological Association, the United States Department of Veterans Affairs, and the National Institute for Health and Clinical Excellence in the United Kingdom. Today, there are thousands of empirical studies supporting the efficacy and effectiveness of IPT (Cuijpers, Donker, Weissman, Ravitz, & Cristea, 2016; Markowitz & Weissman, 2012; Mufson, 1999).

■ PHILOSOPHY AND KEY CONCEPTS OF IPT

IPT is a brief, evidence-based, manualized psychotherapy that focuses on resolving a client's interpersonal issues. Those interpersonal issues are identified as major factors in the development and maintenance of depression and other psychiatric disorders (Frank et al., 1990). IPT is provided in an individual psychotherapy format that is highly structured, time-limited, and delivered within a 12- to 16-week time period (Cornes & Frank, 1994). Some key concepts of IPT are as follows.

A Medical Illness

In IPT, depression is viewed as a medical illness, rather than the client's fault or personal shortcoming. Although IPT posits that depression is the result of interpersonal problems, clients are specifically informed at therapy's initiation that they have a medical illness. As a medical illness, the psychiatric problem is considered a treatable condition, which has the effect of removing self-blame from the client (Markowitz & Weissman, 2004; Weissman, Markowitz, & Klerman, 2007).

Linkage Between Mood and Interpersonal Situation

IPT establishes strong linkage between the mood disorder and the problematic interpersonal situation of the client. The interpersonal situation is viewed as either a trigger for the mood disorder or emerges as a result of the mood disorder. Simply expressed, an interpersonal situation is inevitably paired with a mood disorder (Markowitz & Weissman, 2004; Weissman et al., 2007).

Types of Interpersonal Issues

IPT identifies four types of issues in which a client may have interpersonal difficulties. They are as follows:

1. **Grief or Complicated Bereavement.** Grief or complicated bereavement exists when the onset or maintenance of the depressive episode is associated with the death of a loved one. In this type, there may be an obstacle to mourning as well as blocks to developing new relationships. The goal is to help the client comprehend their experience isn't entirely the natural consequence of their loss, but rather indicative of a mood disorder.
2. **Interpersonal Disputes.** Interpersonal disputes exist when the onset or maintenance of the depressive episode is associated with an unsatisfying, conflictual interpersonal relationship characterized by nonreciprocal role expectations between two parties. It is common for an interpersonal dispute to emerge in problematic focus when there is an increase in responsibilities, as with the birth of a child or the purchase of a new home.
3. **Interpersonal Role Transitions.** Interpersonal role transitions exist when the onset or maintenance of the depressive episode is associated with a situational or developmental role transition that is characterized by difficulty adapting to the change in that new role. Role transitions involve a change from one role to another such as moving from a state of health to physical illness or moving from a secure family home to an unfamiliar college dormitory. Many role changes reflect normal developmental stages; nonetheless, when depression is experienced, the client is likely to view the role transition as a loss.
4. **Interpersonal Deficits.** Interpersonal deficits exist when there is a long-standing history of interpersonal difficulties or social isolation prior to the onset of the depressive episode. In this type, given the prolonged nature of the interpersonal difficulties, the goals are more limited and aim to establish a greater sense of connection with existing interpersonal relationships or establish new interpersonal relationships (Lipsitz & Markowitz, 2013).

■ DEFINITION OF MENTAL HEALTH AND PSYCHOPATHOLOGY IN IPT

In IPT, mental health exists when a client is free from depression and other psychiatric disorders. This goal is achieved by solving interpersonal problems, which are identified as the cause of the depression or other psychiatric disorder. Psychopathology exists when clients have psychiatric symptoms. For example, once a client becomes depressed, symptoms of the illness compromise their interpersonal functioning further. Many depressed clients withdraw by turning inward, blame themselves, and become disengaged from their interpersonal environment. Whether life events follow or precede mood changes, the client's task in therapy is to resolve the disturbing life event, build social skills, and decrease symptoms. If the client is able to solve the life problem, it follows that depressive symptoms should resolve as well. This coupled effect has been borne out in clinical trials demonstrating the efficacy of IPT for major depression (Lipsitz & Markowitz, 2013; Markowitz & Weissman, 2012).

■ THERAPEUTIC GOALS IN IPT

The goals of IPT are symptom reduction and improved functioning in one of four problematic interpersonal areas: grief or complicated bereavement, interpersonal dispute, interpersonal role transition, or interpersonal deficits. The client learns to link changes in their mood to events occurring in their identified problematic interpersonal relationships. During the course of therapy, communication skills are improved and social support networks developed. Problem-solving solutions in regard to the problematic interpersonal area are learned and are then employed in future interpersonal difficulties (Lipsitz & Markowitz, 2013; Markowitz & Weissman, 2012).

■ PERSPECTIVE ON ASSESSMENT IN IPT

IPT has three phases: beginning, middle, and end. The beginning phase is simply another name for the assessment phase and it usually takes two to three sessions. There are specific tasks in the beginning phase. These are to obtain a psychiatric history, to develop a therapeutic relationship, to complete an interpersonal inventory, and to offer a case formulation.

Beginning Phase: Assessment

Psychiatric History. In obtaining a psychiatric history, standard areas are addressed such as the chief complaint, history of the current illness, past psychiatric history, physical history, substance use history, family history, personal history, psychosocial history, and mental status exam. Assessment instruments may be employed such as the Beck Depression Inventory or the Hamilton Depression Rating Scale in order to reify the problem as a medical illness rather than a personal defect.

Therapeutic Relationship. A therapeutic relationship is established based on warmth, empathy, authenticity, affective attunement, and positive regard. This results in a positive relationship with a low level of resistance. The therapeutic relationship also serves as a significant transitional source of support, providing a reassuring, safe connection during a problematic interpersonal situation. The therapeutic relationship bridges the gap created by a lost relationship, reduces tension in an interpersonal dispute, provides support in an interpersonal role transition, and creates connection with social isolation (Lipsitz & Markowitz, 2013; Markowitz & Weissman, 2012).

Interpersonal Inventory. An interpersonal inventory is completed. This serves as a careful review of the client's patterns in relationships and their capacity for intimacy as well as an evaluation of the important people in the client's life and the quality of those relationships. The therapist seeks to understand the client's sources of social support, interpersonal communication style, and relationship difficulties that may be a cause or consequence of the depressive episode. The information garnered from the interpersonal inventory is employed to select the interpersonal problem area (e.g., grief or complicated bereavement, interpersonal dispute, interpersonal role transition, or interpersonal deficits), which then becomes the focus for treatment. At times the client may have more than one interpersonal problem, and a decision has to be made as to which one is the most salient (Lipsitz & Markowitz, 2013; Markowitz & Weissman, 2012).

Linking Diagnosis to the Interpersonal Focus (Case Formulation). A *Diagnostic and Statistical Manual of Mental Disorders*, (5th ed.; *DSM-5*; American Psychiatric Association, 2013) diagnosis such as MDD is determined and linked to an interpersonal problem identified in the interpersonal inventory. The combination of diagnosis and linked interpersonal problem is considered the case formulation and is explained to the client as a treatable illness that is not their fault. This imparts for the client a temporary status of being in a "sick role" and recognizes for them that it is the MDD that keeps the client from functioning at peak capacity. The connection between the MDD and the interpersonal problem is correlational, not etiological; thus, there is no pretense that this is what causes depression. Treatment parameters, such as time limits and the expectation that therapy will focus on recent interpersonal interactions, are established. The case formulation defines the remainder of the therapy. With the client's collaborative agreement on this focus, treatment moves into the middle phase (Markowitz & Weissman, 2004, 2012).

■ THERAPEUTIC INTERVENTIONS IN IPT

The middle phase is the active treatment phase, when the therapeutic work takes place. The final phase is the termination phase and the end of treatment.

Middle Phase: Active Treatment Phase

The middle phase usually takes three to 13 sessions and is focused on resolving the interpersonal problem chosen in the beginning phase of assessment. Treatment focuses on the client's outside environment, not on what is occurring within the therapy. During sessions, the therapist and client review the past week's events. Specific interventions are employed for each of the four interpersonal problem areas. Two overarching interventions used for all four of the interpersonal problem areas are improving communication and exploring options and decision-making. In the service of improving communication, detailed information about interpersonal exchanges is analyzed followed by role-plays, with the therapist coaching the client in order to improve communication. In order to explore options and decision-making, clients are queried about what they desire to occur in any given interpersonal situation. This is followed by decision-making, taking into consideration all the options and resources necessary to achieve the desired outcome. Then, a specific plan is developed. When the client succeeds in an interpersonal situation, the therapist gives abundant support, reinforcing healthy interpersonal skills. When the outcome is adverse, the therapist offers sympathy, helps the client to analyze what went wrong in the situation, brainstorms new interpersonal options, and role-plays them with the client in rehearsal for real life. The client then tests these interventions in the course of their life during the week. The following interventions are used for the four interpersonal problems:

Grief or Complicated Bereavement. In grief or complicated bereavement, clients are encouraged to describe their relationship with the deceased including current and past memories. A comprehensive review of the entire interpersonal relationship is secured including both positive and negative memories as well as the expression of feelings associated with the memories. Attention is paid to the time period surrounding the death and the ways in which grieving may have been hampered, such as with a traumatic loss. Attention is also paid to the implementation of social support and how social support could be developed.

Interpersonal Disputes. With interpersonal disputes, clients are helped to understand how the dispute is prolonged by identifying and resolving problematic communication patterns and expectations. Difficulty expressing feelings or communicating needs would be an example. Detailed reconstructions of unsatisfactory communication exchanges are reviewed in terms of what was said, how it was said, how it was received, what was left unsaid, and the achievement of the desired outcome. Improved communication patterns are explored through role-play where more empathic and direct responses are enacted and practiced.

Interpersonal Role Transitions. In interpersonal role transitions, three interrelated steps are taken: (a) mourning and moving away from the old role, (b) reevaluating the opportunities in the transition, and (c) clarifying and becoming proficient and self-efficacious in regard to the demands of the new role. The intervention first explores the context of the change, how it came about, and the resulting emotions. For example, the context and resulting emotions will be very different when losing a job because the company closed versus being fired from the job. The intervention also identifies obstacles that have blocked successful completion of the transition, such as lack of support. Attention is given to all of the opportunities available in the new role, which may not have been considered, as well as to reengage with social support in the new role.

Interpersonal Deficits. Relationships are expected to be inadequate by scarcity as a result of clients' interpersonal deficits. Thus, previous relationships are reassembled to understand how these relationships functioned, to identify the successes achieved, and to explore the manner in which these relationships may have faltered. Direct attention is given to the therapeutic relationship, an aspect of treatment which is infrequent in the other interpersonal problem areas (e.g., grief and uncomplicated bereavement, interpersonal disputes, interpersonal role transitions). In this case, the therapeutic relationship may be the best example for the difficulties the client encounters in their interpersonal relationships. Giving direct attention to the therapeutic relationship provides an opportunity to work collaboratively, to understand the emerging difficulties, and to provide constructive feedback to the client, which may otherwise be unavailable. It also provides repeated opportunities for the therapist to model alternative ways of dealing with the problems that the client repeatedly may face in interpersonal relationships, problems which have frequently led to the termination or poor quality of the client's previous interpersonal relationships.

Final Phase: Termination

The final phase, which usually takes two to three sessions, focuses on termination. The client is informed that termination is imminent. The therapist helps the client to feel more capable and independent by reviewing the course of treatment, the client's accomplishments, and the client's future treatment needs. IPT looks at termination as similar to a graduation where the client recognizes the achievement of meaningful gains, feels better, and is ready for something different such as a new treatment, maintenance treatment, or no treatment. The therapist notes that ending therapy is itself a role transition, with inevitable good and painful aspects. If the depression has not fully remitted, the therapist blames the treatment rather than the client and suggests alternative or adjunctive treatments that might address remaining symptoms. The therapist may also identify interpersonal issues that have not been adequately addressed in IPT, such as ongoing marital discord or job dissatisfaction, and perhaps recommends follow-up care for those areas. As IPT has also demonstrated efficacy as a maintenance treatment for recurrent MDD, and as clients who have had multiple episodes are very likely to have more, the therapist and client may decide to end acute treatment as scheduled and then to recontract for ongoing treatment, perhaps of less intensive dosage, for example, monthly rather than weekly sessions.

▪ CASE STUDY

Background

In this case, I will be using IPT to treat Zoe, a 23-year-old, single woman who recently graduated from college with a bachelor's degree in animal science. The therapy consisted of 16 weekly individual sessions lasting 45 minutes each. Zoe sought therapy for symptoms of depression that commenced 6 weeks ago, soon after Lucky, her three-legged, 12-year-old dog, died. Lucky had become incapacitated, and with a great deal of personal resistance, Zoe had made the difficult decision to have him euthanized. Approximately 1 year prior to the death of Lucky, her mother had died of pancreatic cancer. Zoe was a junior in college when her mother was first diagnosed, and she returned home as much as possible during that academic year and summer. Her mother insisted she go back to college for her senior year, which she did. Sadly, her mother died the day before Thanksgiving when Zoe was at home. Her mother was cremated and a memorial service was held the Saturday after Thanksgiving. Zoe returned to college the following week. She finished her senior year, graduated, and returned home. Upon arriving home, Zoe discovered that her stepfather, who married her mother when Zoe was only 2 years old and whom Zoe considered to be a loving, doting father, had remarried several weeks prior (only 6 months after the death of her mother), and his new wife had moved into the house with her three teenage daughters. Knowing nothing of the marriage, Zoe was thoroughly shocked. Although everyone was pleasant, she soon observed that all pictures of her mother had been removed from the common areas and relegated to Zoe's bedroom, the only area of the house that she felt was still home to her. She felt that she no longer belonged there and made plans to leave. Her stepfather was loving and pleasant and apologized that he kept Zoe in the dark about the marriage, but said he felt she might be upset and wanted her to be able to finish college and graduate. She and Lucky left the house a few weeks later and she went to live in a cottage on a large farm 60 miles away owned by her biological father, with whom she had a distant but amicable relationship. She chose to move there because she was able to take Lucky and her horse Lacey. She had been living on her biological father's farm for several months when her dog died. I met with her 6 weeks after Lucky's death.

Transcript of Therapy Sessions

The transcripts presented here were selected from segments of the beginning, middle, and final phase of therapy.

Beginning Phase

This is a segment from the first psychotherapy session and focuses on obtaining a psychiatric history, developing a therapeutic relationship, completing an interpersonal inventory, and deciding on times to meet. Zoe had more than one interpersonal problem, and thus it required the selection of the most salient problem, and linking it to her symptoms of depression.

APPN: You told me on the phone that your dog Lucky died 6 weeks ago and since his death you have been feeling depressed. Is that correct?

Zoe: Yes.

APPN: Tell me about Lucky.

Zoe: He was a golden retriever.

APPN: What was he like?

Zoe: He was wonderful—intelligent, friendly, gentle, trustworthy, and devoted to me. He was light golden in color and loved to swim and run. In college, I lived off campus, so I was able to have him with me. He was with me almost all the time, except when I went to class.

APPN: He sounds wonderful and your loss of him has to be very hard for you.

Zoe: (*Cries*) Yes. Plus, he was given to me by my mother when I was only 11 years old—he was a birthday present.

APPN: And you lost your mother as well not too long ago.

Zoe: I think that as long as I had Lucky, my mother in some way was still with me—it was like she didn't die.

APPN: Tell me a little about your mom.

Zoe: She was a wonderful person—a fantastic mother. She loved horses and had two of her own that she trained and rode daily. She had them my whole life. We had a barn on our property and the space to board six more horses, so we always had eight horses. When I was a young girl, I would help out in the barn and of course ride with her. I loved it. When I was about 8, she bought me my own horse – Lacey—who I still have and who lives with me on my father's farm.

APPN: What was it like for you when she got sick?

Zoe: Well, she was diagnosed with pancreatic cancer during my junior year of college. In the beginning, she was fine and had few symptoms. I came home as much as possible, which was mainly for holidays—I was in school in Kentucky. I came home that following summer. Mom was tired from the chemotherapy and had lost some weight, but had a positive spirit. We actually had a great time that summer and I spent a lot of time with her. She had stopped riding, but would come with me to the barn and watch me ride Lacey. After I went back to Kentucky for my senior year, she went downhill fast. She died the day before Thanksgiving. I got home to say goodbye, but hospice was already there and she was in-and-out of consciousness and heavily sedated with opioids for her pain. I went back to college the following week and didn't come home again until after graduation. I didn't even go to graduation—it didn't seem right without my mother.

APPN: So, when you went back home that was the first time you were back in the house without your mother.

Zoe: Yes. And, it didn't really feel like home with my stepfather's new wife and her three teenage daughters (*laughs*).

APPN: What's the laughter about?

Zoe: Well, I know it sounds crazy, but I don't blame my stepfather. He's moved on and found someone who's very nice. I wish him well.

APPN: What makes you think it sounds crazy?

Zoe: Well, you know, you might think I should hate him for getting married so soon.

APPN: Do you think that?

Zoe: Actually, I don't. My mother would have wanted him to move on. That's how she was. Plus, they knew each other before—from work. They were friends and she was very supportive to my stepfather during my mother's illness.

APPN: I see. Do you see him?

Zoe: Yes. I don't like going back to the house, but we have dinner once a month. He usually comes down here and picks me up and we go out to a restaurant. He is interested in my life and loves to see Lacey and Lucky. He's a good guy.

APPN: What's he like?

Zoe: He married my mother when I was only 2. He was a father to me. He was very smart, nice, loving, and taught me a lot of things. He was in finance and made a lot of money and was very good to me. He and my mother had a very good relationship—a good life. He supported her in her love of horses and my mother didn't have to work, so she was always around. I had a nice upper-middle class life with tennis lessons, nice vacations, private schools, and horses. And, he fully paid for my college.

APPN: You told me on the phone that you were shocked when you returned from college and found your stepfather had remarried and his new wife and three daughters took over the house and relegated you and your mother—in terms of pictures—to your bedroom.

Zoe: I know it might sound strange to you, but my stepfather is a very kind man. I think he did that to make his new wife feel comfortable in the new home. As I said, they knew each other from work and were friends. Her husband was killed in a car crash a few years back. During my mother's illness and then after she died, she was there for him.

APPN: As you're telling me this, what are you experiencing?

Zoe: I actually feel happy for him—that he moved on. I wish he told me about it, but he didn't. With his new wife, I don't have to worry about him and can go on with my life. I would have moved out anyway, even if my mother was alive. I'm not the type to be dependent.

APPN: It sounds as if you did move on—moving into the cottage on your father's farm. How's that?

Zoe:	It's a small four room cottage—a bedroom, living room, kitchen, dining area, bathroom. It's very cute actually. And, there's a small barn right next to it where I keep my horse Lacey. My mother left me some money that I've been living on since I moved to the farm. I know I need to get a job, but I don't feel like doing anything.
APPN:	Tell me a little about your father.
Zoe:	My parents divorced when I was very young—I think I was about 1-year-old. My father bought the farm soon after the divorce and then my mother remarried and we moved about 2 hours away. It was hard for my father to make ends meet on the farm—it's a working farm—he grows livestock crops—mainly soybeans and corn and he has lots of farm animals. I rarely saw him though. He remarried a woman who was also a farmer and they built a life together. They had a son named Chad—my half brother, who works on the farm and will probably inherit it when my father and his wife eventually pass away.
APPN:	What's your father like?
Zoe:	He's a quiet man—doesn't talk much—very stoic—never expresses his feelings. He's not the type to show affection easily. Sometimes, I'll go to the farmhouse and have dinner with them. There's not much conversation. But I know he loves me and will be there for me if I need him.
APPN:	Did you see him much growing up?
Zoe:	No. I spent a week there in the summer and would see him for major holidays. He was always so busy. My mother would take me there and I would play with my half brother and run around the farm. I didn't see much of him, but he and his wife were always nice to me. He seemed more like an absent uncle than a Dad, but that was just the way it was. I was always glad to go back home though.
APPN:	I see. You told me that you are depressed. I'm wondering what that looks like in terms of your symptoms and your functioning?
Zoe:	Well, my mood is depressed. It's like everything is tinged with the color gray. I cry at the drop of a hat. I don't feel like doing anything. I've lost weight.
APPN:	How many pounds?
Zoe:	About 6.
APPN:	What else?
Zoe:	I isolate myself in my cottage and with my horse. I do feed and ride Lacey, but even riding doesn't make me feel happy. And, I have a hard time falling asleep. I think about Lucky and my mother. Sometimes, I wake up in the middle of the night and can't go back to sleep.
APPN:	I see. It sounds like it is very difficult for you right now.
Zoe:	Yes (*cries*).
APPN:	(*After a period of time*) Would you be willing to fill out this depression scale (Beck Depression Inventory), so I can get a sense of all your symptoms and how severe they are?

Zoe: Sure. (*She fills it out.*)

APPN: Well, you received a score of 42, which according to the instrument evaluates you as severely depressed. What are your thoughts about that?

Zoe: It's true. So, what's next?

APPN: We've spent a lot of time looking at what might be linked to your depression. You spoke about your grief over the loss of Lucky and your mother, the relationship with your stepfather and the fact that you were not prepared for his new marriage, the loss of your old life where you were raised, and the transition of moving on to a new life in a cottage on your father's farm.

Zoe: Yes. As you lay all these things out, I think what's bothering me most is the death of Lucky and my mother—they are somehow linked together.

APPN: As we've discussed, you're suffering from major depression, which is a treatable medical illness and certainly not your fault. From what you've told me, your depression seems related to the loss of Lucky and your mother. You went right back to college after your mother died and got right back into the swing of things there. You never really grieved her death. Then, when you returned home and saw the changes made, you moved out with Lucky and Lacey. But, soon after the move, Lucky died. You soon began to feel depressed. You had difficulty sleeping and awakened during the night. Your appetite decreased and you were tearful and sad much of the time. You isolated yourself and stayed in your cottage, only leaving to ride your horse. We call your type of depression *complicated bereavement*, which is a common and treatable form of depression.

Zoe: I never heard that term before, but it sounds right.

APPN: I suggest that we spend the next 14 weeks working on the loss of Lucky and your mother. If you can work through these losses, I believe your mood will improve and the depressive symptoms will decrease.

Zoe: Sounds like a plan (*smiles*).

Middle Phase

The middle phase of treatment focused on resolving the interpersonal problem chosen in the first phase, which is complicated bereavement related to the death of Lucky and her mother. The following segment is from session five of our work together.

Zoe: It's good to see you again.

APPN: Likewise (*silence*).

Zoe: During the week, I was thinking about what you said about me having complicated bereavement. I was wondering why you thought it was so.

APPN: I have my ideas, but I'd like to hear from you first what you might have been thinking.

Zoe: Well, when my mom was diagnosed, she seemed the same. It was during my junior year of college and I came home a lot, and even though she was getting chemo, she seemed like her warm, jolly self—except for being tired a lot. She didn't lose her hair or anything like that and she wasn't emaciated. And, she shooed me back to college to finish my senior year. I left in early August for I was involved in a horse show in early September. Anyway, she went down-hill quickly and when I came home about a week before Thanksgiving she died—the day before Thanksgiving. It was all so fast. And, I thought about not going back but knew she would want me to and I was having exams in December, so I just went back. I didn't want to go back home for Christmas break, so I stayed on campus and spent time with a college friend who lived close by. I went over to her house for Christmas. I guess I just pushed it all from my mind.

APPN: That's what it sounds like. What do you think that was about?

Zoe: Well, who wants to hear about the death of a mother—certainly not my college friends. And, I'm not one to talk out loud about things. I keep things to myself most of the time. If I did feel sad, I would just go and study or play with Lucky—he was with me at college.

APPN: Yes. What else?

Zoe: Well, when I got home and found my stepfather remarried and was happy, I didn't want to bring Mom up with him, so I just told myself "Life moves on and you have to as well—that's what Mom would have wanted to see happen." So, I made plans for my next step. And, I was excited to be able to move to my father's farm. He's letting me live in the cottage rent-free and I have Lacey and did have Lucky. It's beautiful country and I get to roam around when I'm not laying in bed doing nothing.

APPN: So, in a way you answered your question as to why complicated bereavement. You moved back to college quickly after your mother's death and had exams and had no time or place or person to cry with and then, when you returned home, everything changed and you needed to focus on first accepting the change and then moving out and moving on to the farm. You also said you are the type of person who holds things in and internally processes rather than expressing your feelings—your grief.

Zoe: Yes.

APPN: I wonder if it would be helpful for you to tell me about your mother. Describe to me your relationship with her—both past and more current memories—both positive and negative memories.

Zoe: Well. Mom was a terrific person. Anyone who met her liked her immediately. She had this way of engaging with people. She listened well and remembered things, so she would ask me as well as others things that were important.

APPN: Can you give me an example?

Zoe: Well. Something small comes to mind. I remember telling her that I had a friend who didn't like to eat off of Fiesta Ware—a type of dishes—for she read somewhere that they are radioactive. I told my mom the story.

My mom told me that they used to put something in the dinnerware— something like uranium oxide but way in the past—and they stopped doing that iaround 1970, so as long as the Fiesta Ware was manufactured after that time, it was safe. Well, we had Fiesta Ware in our home that we use daily, but when my friend from college came over, I noticed my mom used our good china dishes and never used the Fiesta Ware. She never said anything or tried to lecture my friend that she was wrong, but just said to me, well, she has her reasons, so we just won't use the Fiesta Ware while she's here. That was my mom—sensitive to others but never rubbing it in their faces or making fun of them.

APPN: That's a great story. It helps me know what your mom was like. I wonder what you experience when telling me the story?

Zoe: (*Cries*) I feel so sad that she is no longer here.

APPN: If she was here right now, what would you say to her?

Zoe: I miss you so much and wish you were here with me (*cries*).

APPN: (*After a period of time*) Anything else?

Zoe: I don't think I told you that my mother was a vet.

APPN: (*Quizzical look*)

Zoe: I don't mean in the armed service—she was actually a veterinarian.

APPN: How cool is that!

Zoe: Yea. She specialized in large animals—cows and horses mainly. But, after a while, she realized she didn't like the medical side of things and enjoyed raising and riding horses more. So, after I was born, she gave up her career and then after marrying my stepfather, they bought a house with an eight-stall barn and lots of wooded property to ride the horses. I think "horse people" are special.

APPN: In what way was your mother special as a "horse person"?

Zoe: She was very sensitive as I said before. She was good at reading people. And, she was patient and compassionate. I think you learn these things from being around horses. I miss her so much (*cries*).

APPN: (*silence*)

Zoe: And those who ride are disciplined and responsible and have a lot of self-control. They're not all soppy, weepy (*cries*). And, when you are with horses, words don't matter—horses understand voice tone like pitch, intonation, volume, tempo. . . . My mother had that sensitivity to horses and to people around her. And, then she got sick and died.

APPN: I'm wondering about that time period. Would you be willing to say more about that?

Zoe: Well, it was so fast. She was my vibrant mom and then she was sick mom. She was still the same, don't get me wrong, but she was tired that last year when she was getting the chemo and radiation and although she kept up with a positive attitude, it was rough. She couldn't ride anymore the summer before she died and she slept a lot during the day. I never really said goodbye to her for when I came home for Thanksgiving, she was out of it and in and out of consciousness. And, then, she died and I went back to school.

APPN:	So, you never really said goodbye.
Zoe:	Correct.
APPN:	What would you say if she was here now?
Zoe:	What a good person she was.
APPN:	I know you have a picture of her here. Could you imagine she was here now and tell her what you would like to tell her?
Zoe:	(*Puts her picture on the couch next to her*) "You are the best mother a daughter could have. I love you so much. You taught me how to be a loving person—a loving woman and a kind, empathic person. And, you gave me the gift of being a "horse woman" (*cries*). "I wish you were still here, but even though you are not here in body, your memory is always with me and will remain with me forever. I love you and thank you for everything" (*cries*).
APPN:	(*silence*)
Zoe:	That's all I can say today. I'm exhausted.
APPN:	This seems like a good place to stop. Let's just take the last 5 minutes to decide what would be helpful for you to do during the week.
Zoe:	OK.
APPN:	One of the things I think would be useful to do is to create a memory box of your mom. I have some here (*opens closet and shows client a few empty boxes*) that I collected from yard sales and you can take one.
Zoe:	Thanks. What should I put into it?
APPN:	Items that remind you of your mom and in particular things that remind you of times you spent together. For example, in my memory box of my mom, I have photographs, her eyeglasses (she loved to read), a picture of a swimming pool (she loved to swim), a pair of her earrings, and a picture of one of our cats that she loved. I also have a piece of a fur coat that she loved, her favorite perfume, and her favorite CD. And, a few other things too. So, on her birthday or Mother's Day, I open it and she is here with me. That's the idea—to have a place for your special memories of your mom that is concrete—that you can visit and look at and even touch. Would you be willing to do that?
Zoe:	Yes. I would love that.
APPN:	And, would you be willing to bring it to our session next week?
Zoe:	Yes.

Final Phase

The final phase of treatment focused on reviewing the course of therapy, evaluating her symptoms of depression, and planning for the future.

APPN:	Well, this is our next to the last session. Is there anything that happened during the week concerning the loss of your mother that is important to talk about today?

Zoe: Yes. It was her birthday this past weekend. I had my stepfather over for dinner at my cottage and I showed him my memory box.

APPN: What was that like?

Zoe: He cried—we both cried and said how much we miss her and what a wonderful person she was.

APPN: And. . . .

Zoe: It was the first time we talked about Mom and grieved her death together. He told me that he moved on so quickly, and that even though he loves his new wife, he realizes part of moving on so quickly was to numb the pain of his wife's death—my mother. It was a good experience for both of us. And, we talked about our life together—all the vacations and fun things we did and also some of the arguments we had (*laughs*). I sometimes forget about those.

APPN: Like what?

Zoe: Oh, she was always pushing me to get involved with friends—to be more social—to join activities at school. But all I wanted to do was come home and spend time in the barn and ride my horse. She would say that it was not healthy and that I needed to have friends. So, we would fight about that sometimes.

APPN: Do you think she was right?

Zoe: No. I am content with my horse and living alone in my cottage. As you know, I'm working as a vet tech now and I have friends and I sometimes do things with them. We just went to the dog show in New York—that was fun. But I prefer being alone with my animals. And, although no dog will ever replace Lucky, the rescue group I am with fulfills me (*she is volunteering with a dog rescue group*) and maybe one day, I'll get another dog.

APPN: I think that is terrific. Is there anything else that you would like to do?

Zoe: Not really—not now. I am content with Lacey, my rescue group, working as a vet tech, and seeing my friends.

APPN: Is there anything else that happened with you and your stepfather?

Zoe: Oh, we also spoke about our new lives—his with his new wife and three new stepchildren. He said they were not easy kids like I was (*laughs*). And, I talked about my new life on the farm and my job and Lacey. It was good. And, we're going to continue to meet monthly. I'm not ready to go back to the house and he's OK with coming down here or meeting half-way for dinner. That's about it.

APPN: It seems as if you are just about ready "to graduate" from therapy. Let's talk a little about the depression that you came here with originally.

Zoe: Well, I still have my periods of time that I am tearful when I think about my mother—mainly when something triggers a memory, but I get over it fairly quickly. I am sleeping well and eating well. I can be sad at times, but I am not depressed—that place where I feel cut off and everything is gray. And, I have energy and feel motivated to live life each day, which is a good thing, right? I'm glad I never went on medication—that's not my way and I'm glad you didn't push me to do that.

APPN: Well, you did a lot of work in therapy in a very short period of time. Is there anything else about the loss of your mom that you think we need to address?

Zoe: Oh yea. I think you'll be happy to know that a few days ago, my stepfather and I went to the cemetery where Mom's buried—well, she was cremated, but we have a little grave where her ashes are buried and there is a little tombstone. Anyway, it was good visiting her with him and we both spoke to her.

APPN: What did you say?

Zoe: That we missed her. And, we loved having her in our life and we will never forget her and that her memory lives on.

APPN: What are you experiencing as you tell me this?

Zoe: Relief and actually some contentment. I told her about my dog rescue missions—the last one of going to a hoarder's house and rescuing 30 chihuahuas. My stepdad and I had a few laughs. It was actually fun sharing this with him. And, I realize that even though he has remarried, he is still there for me and that's important.

APPN: That's terrific. You've made great progress. Next week will be our last session, and we can examine the end of this increment of work together and see if there is anything we need to plan for the future.

Zoe: Sounds good.

Commentary

Zoe and I worked together for 16 sessions. The assessment and case conceptualization sessions were very important because Zoe came to therapy with more than one interpersonal problem and it was important to choose the one that was most salient. She had experienced the loss of her dog and mother, the difficult change in her home with her stepfather's new marriage and Zoe being displaced, and the role transition of graduating from college, leaving her home that no longer existed, and moving to her father's farm. All three of these were potential interpersonal issues that could have been worked on. Collaboratively, the complicated bereavement was chosen and we worked on grieving the loss of her mother as well as the loss of her dog Lucky. Grieving Zoe's losses was the focus of our work during the middle 10 sessions. During termination, we discussed the successes achieved in the course of therapy, the reduction of her symptoms of depression, and future therapy if she should need further sessions.

IPT is a short-term, structured form of therapy and my bailiwick is long-term therapy. As such, when I conduct short-term therapy, I often feel there is a plethora of material that is not addressed. For example, Zoe's relationship with her biological father was not explored. Her inability to pursue a love-relationship was another area well worth perusal. Zoe's lack of awareness and difficulty expressing emotions in general, and particularly anger, was necessarily skimmed over using a short-term therapy. Accordingly, although her symptoms of depression have decreased and she has grieved the death of her dog and her mother, there is much more work to be done and many more issues to address.

DISCUSSION QUESTIONS

1. IPT, as a short-term, structured, evidence-based treatment, focuses on one interpersonal problem. I chose to look at complicated bereavement in the case presented. Would you have chosen this interpersonal problem? Why or why not?
2. Choose another interpersonal problem to work on for this client. Identify three specific IPT interventions you might use when working with this problem.
3. Identify an interpersonal problem in your own life that is linked to psychological symptoms you may have experienced.
4. How does working with a short-term, structured, evidence-based therapy impact the course of treatment?

REFERENCES

American Psychiatric Association. (2013). *Diagnostic and statistical manual of mental disorders* (5th ed.). Arlington, VA: American Psychiatric Publishing.

Cornes, C. L., & Frank, E. (1994). Interpersonal psychotherapy for depression. *The Clinical Psychologist, 47*(3), 9–10.

Cuijpers, P., Donker, T., Weissman, M. M., Ravitz, P., & Cristea, I. A. (2016). Interpersonal psychotherapy for mental health problems: A comprehensive meta-analysis. *American Journal of Psychiatry, 173*(7), 680–687. doi:10.1176/appi.ajp.2015.15091141

Elkin, I., Shea, M. T., Watkins, J. T., Imber, S. D., Sotsky, S. M., Collins, J. F., . . . Parloff, M. B. (1989). National Institute of Mental Health treatment of depression collaborative research program: General effectiveness of treatments. *Archives of General Psychiatry, 46*(11), 971–982. doi:10.1001/archpsyc.1989.01810110013002

Frank, E., Kupfer, D. J., Perel, J. M., Cornes, C., Jarrett, D. B., Mallinger, A. G., . . . Grochocinski, V. J. (1990). Three-year outcomes for maintenance therapies in recurrent depression. *Archives of General Psychiatry, 47*(12), 1093–1099. doi:10.1001/archpsyc.1990.01810240013002

Klerman, G. L., Dimascio, A., Weissman, M., Prusoff, B., & Paykel, E. S. (1974). Treatment of depression by drugs and psychotherapy. *American Journal of Psychiatry, 131*(2), 186–191. doi:10.1176/ajp.131.2.186

Klerman, G. L., Weissman, M. M., Rounsaville, B. J., & Chevron, E. S. (1984). *Interpersonal psychotherapy of depression*. New York, NY: Basic Books.

Lipsitz, J. D., & Markowitz, J. C. (2013). Mechanisms of change in interpersonal therapy (IPT). *Clinical Psychological Review, 33*(8), 1134–1147. doi:10.1016/j.cpr.2013.09.002

Markowitz, J. C., & Weissman, M. M. (2004). Interpersonal psychotherapy: Principles and applications. *World Psychiatry, 3*(3), 136–139. Retrieved from https://www.ncbi.nlm.nih.gov/pmc/articles/PMC1414693

Markowitz, J. C., & Weissman, M. M. (2012). Interpersonal psychotherapy: Past, present, and future. *Clinical Psychology and Psychotherapy, 19*(2), 99–105. doi:10.1002/cpp.1774

Mufson, L. (1999). Efficacy of interpersonal psychotherapy for depressed adolescents. *Archives of General Psychiatry, 56*(6), 573–579. doi:10.1001/archpsyc.56.6.573

Weissman, M. M., & Markowitz, J. C. (1998). An overview of interpersonal psychotherapy. In J. C. Markowitz (Ed.), *Interpersonal psychotherapy* (pp. 1–33). Washington, DC: American Psychiatric Press.

Weissman, M. M., Markowitz, J. C., & Klerman, G. L. (2007). *Clinician's quick guide to interpersonal psychotherapy*. New York, NY: Oxford University Press.

Weissman, M. M., Prusoff, B. A., Dimascio, A., Neu, C., Goklaney, M., & Klerman, G. L. (1979). The efficacy of drugs and psychotherapy in the treatment of acute depressive episodes. *The American Journal of Psychiatry, 136*(4B), 555–558. doi:10.1176/ajp.1979.136.4b.555

Motivational Interviewing: A Client With Depression

Susie Adams

■ **PERSONAL EXPERIENCE WITH MOTIVATIONAL INTERVIEWING**

Throughout my career as an advanced practice psychiatric nurse, I have relied on Murray Bowen's *Family Systems Theory* as the overarching theory informing my clinical practice. Since the 1970s as a graduate student at the University of California, San Francisco, and as a postgraduate intern for 6 months at the Family Study Unit at Palo Alto Veterans Administration Medical Center in California, I grounded my psychotherapy in Bowen's theory (1978). While aware of William Miller's *Motivational Interviewing* (MI) approach (1983), I learned that it had a broader application beyond the field of addiction from which the theory originally developed during a 2-year faculty fellowship in the treatment of addictions (sponsored by the Association of Medical Educators and Researchers in Substance Abuse [AMERSA]) in the early 2000s. Immersed in learning and teaching MI to interprofessional cohorts of graduate students, I integrated MI into my private practice, treating clients with a variety of mental health disorders. MI enhanced my ability to assess client perceptions of underlying issues, motivation(s) to change, barrier(s) to change, and to facilitate the client's ability to make and sustain a change in his or her patterns of feelings, thoughts, and behaviors. I honed my MI skills by attending workshops and online training offered through the Motivational Interviewing Network of Trainers (MINT; motivationalinterviewing .org). To ensure accurate implementation and treatment fidelity and prevent therapist drift over time, MINT trainers and supervisors review audio and videotaped therapy sessions.

The most common reasons individuals seek counseling are related to major life events (e.g., divorce, relationship breakup, mid-life crisis, aging concerns), disorders related to anxiety and depression, anger management, blended family issues, parenting concerns, addictions, eating disorders, grief or loss, and low self-esteem. Individuals typically seek counseling when they have been unsuccessful in resolving the issue of concern on their own. They typically feel "stuck" and unsure of which direction to turn. Alternatively, individuals referred by their primary healthcare provider for a mental health evaluation are often seeking a quick appraisal with the expectation that medication alone can quickly resolve the issue. In either of these typical scenarios, an MI approach to explore client concerns has proven to be an effective way to engage the client in exploring underlying issues, identifying motivations and barriers to change, and enlisting his or her commitment to change patterns of thinking, feeling, and behaving that contribute to the issue or symptoms of concern.

MI is a humanistic, person-centered approach designed to help individuals resolve ambivalence and empower them to plan for change. It can be used alone to increase motivation for engaging in psychotherapy or in combination with other forms of therapy when resistance is encountered. MI is closely aligned with the Transtheoretical Model developed around the same time (Prochaska, DiClemente, & Norcross, 1992). Although both models concern changing behavior, MI places greater emphasis on getting ready to change. The "spirit" of MI embodies a partnership with clients incorporating the principle of acceptance, belief in individual autonomy, and acknowledgment of the individual's strengths and efforts with empathy and affirmation. The principles of acceptance, conveying accurate empathy, honoring the worth of the individuals, affirming their strengths, and respecting their autonomy are adapted from Carl Rogers' Person-Centered Therapy (1965). W. R. Miller and Rollnick (2013) added the principles of compassion and evocation. Compassion means that therapists give priority to the well-being of clients over their own needs. Evocation is accepting that individuals have within themselves what they need to change and it is the practitioner's job to "draw it out" (W. R. Miller & Rollnick, 2013, p. 21).

MI contains elements of other theories that underlie the change process. Festinger's Cognitive Dissonance Theory (1957) focuses on prejudice, asserting that awareness of discrepancies among beliefs and goals and behavior is an incentive for people to reconcile their inconsistencies. MI highlights dissonance between unhealthy behaviors and the person's values and goals. Bem's (1967) Self-Perception Theory is a refinement of Cognitive Dissonance Theory proposing that hearing oneself argue for change increases the desire to change. In MI it is important for individuals to voice the change they desire, which reinforces motivation for change (Amrhein, Miller, Yahne, Palmer, & Fulcher, 2003). Because MI deals with ambivalence, and resistance, it resembles Reactance Theory (Brehm & Brehm, 1981), the belief that some individuals are more defensive when persuasion or coercion is used because their sense of freedom is threatened. W. R. Miller and Rollnick (2013) prefer to use the word *discord* and believe that discord or differences arise in the context of a relationship and are not an individual trait. However, they concur that taking a directive role and using persuasion to encourage change is the antithesis of their philosophy.

■ FOUNDERS AND LEADERS OF MI

MI was developed by William (Bill) R. Miller and Stephen Rollnick through inductive reasoning based on their clinical practice working with persons with alcohol addictions in the 1980s (W. R. Miller & Rollnick, 1991, 2013). The prevailing treatment approach to addiction at that time was one of confrontation and enlisting family, friends, employer, or other significant members to force the individual to "face their addiction" and seek treatment. Miller did not find this approach to be particularly effective. He took a more supportive, empathic approach in working with patients with addiction. While on sabbatical in Norway working at an alcohol treatment facility, Miller agreed to meet with recently graduated clinical psychologists for supervision. They used role-plays of their most challenging patients and repeatedly questioned Miller to explain, "What are you thinking? Why did you ask that question? Of all the things that you could have reflected, why did you reflect that?" This resulted in Miller articulating his decision rules that guided his style of interviewing. He shared these reflections with colleagues who encouraged him to publish these concepts. Miller and his coauthor, Rollnick, described the process of exploring the individual's ambivalence about the desired behavior change and supporting his or her self-efficacy in implementing desired behavior change. While the emphasis was on exploring ambivalence to elicit "change talk" in the initial two decades of MI, more recently the emphasis has shifted to reflecting and summarizing the individual's thoughts about his or her self-identified concerns (W. R. Miller & Rollnick, 2013).

Since retiring from the University of New Mexico in 2006, Miller continues to lead international workshops, write, volunteer, and compose choral music as Professor Emeritus of Psychology and Psychiatry. His research focuses on four areas of interest: motivation for change; behavioral treatments for substance use disorders; psychology and spirituality; and psychotherapy processes and outcomes.

Rollnick's early experience as a nurse trainee in a hospital addiction treatment setting in the United Kingdom led to his interest in constructive approaches to help people resolve difficult behavior change. This culminated in Rollnick's close collaboration with William Miller on the topic of MI for problem drinkers, the subject of his doctoral dissertation. He currently provides consultation, mentorship, and training on motivation, change, teamwork, and MI as an Honorary Distinguished Professor of Medicine at Cardiff University, United Kingdom.

In 1997 Miller and Rollnick along with a group of their trainees formed the MINT, an international organization committed to promoting high-quality MI practice and training. The MINT website is a public access resource for MI training online and around the world, the latest MI research findings, a library of MI publications and videotapes, and the latest MI news (motivationalinterviewing.org).

■ PHILOSOPHY AND KEY CONCEPTS OF MI

MI is a collaborative, person-centered communication process designed to help individuals resolve ambivalence and plan for change. It is not just a set of techniques for counseling; MI is a way of being with a client based on the following assumptions:

1. Ambivalence about substance use (or any desired change in behavior) is normal and constitutes an important motivational obstacle in recovery (or desired change).
2. Ambivalence can be resolved by working with the client's intrinsic motivations and values.
3. The therapeutic alliance between the therapist and the client is a collaborative partnership to which the therapist brings important expertise.
4. An empathic, supportive, yet directive counseling style provides conditions under which change can occur. (Direct argument and aggressive confrontation tend to increase client defensiveness and reduce the likelihood of behavioral change; W. R. Miller & Rollnick, 1991).

■ DEFINITIONS OF MENTAL HEALTH AND PSYCHOPATHOLOGY IN MI

The ethos of MI is about creating autonomy of "self-responsibility" for the individual (as opposed to imposing by authority), while developing awareness of the gap that exists between where the individual is currently and where he or she wants to be in the future (Gates, 2011). This person-centered approach seeks to empower the individual to make changes in his or her behavior and lifestyle by helping the individual identify personal barriers to change and specific ways to overcome these barriers (A. Miller, 2012). Thus, mental health and psychopathology are concepts that are less important in this approach.

■ THERAPEUTIC GOALS IN MI

The two primary goals of MI are to find a way to increase the client's motivation to change and to facilitate the client's commitment to change. The five principles of MI encompass the following:

1. Express empathy through reflective listening
2. Develop discrepancy between clients' goals or values and their current behavior
3. Avoid argument or direct confrontation
4. Adjust to client resistance rather than opposing it directly
5. Support self-efficacy and optimism (A. Miller, 2012; W. R. Miller, 2018)

■ PERSPECTIVE ON ASSESSMENT IN MI

In MI, assessment is based on expressing empathy through reflective listening to elicit the client's concerns and discrepancy between current problematic behavior and his or her goals, values, and desired behavior. The supportive, nonjudgmental approach fosters client autonomy and empowerment to examine barriers to change and systematically identifies ways to begin modifying behaviors that align with desired goals and values. The therapist does not focus on the past, but evokes the client's examination of what motivates the client within the "here and now." The therapist studiously avoids offering advice, making suggestions, or providing premature or unsolicited solutions. Similarly, the therapist strictly avoids warning, threatening, lecturing, persuading with logic, moralizing, shaming, ridiculing, interpreting, analyzing, questioning, probing, withdrawing, or changing the subject. Somewhat counterintuitive—agreeing, approving, or praising can be an obstacle if the message implies agreement with whatever the client has said. Unsolicited approval may potentially interrupt the communication process and imply an unequal relationship between speaker and listener. Likewise, reassuring, sympathizing, and consoling can interrupt the communication flow and interfere with reflective listening. Miller and Rollnick posit that "if you are not listening reflectively but are instead imposing direction and judgment, you are creating barriers that impair the therapeutic relationship" (1991).

Motivation to change is enhanced when clients perceive discrepancies between their current situation and their hopes for the future. The therapist's task is to help focus the client's attention on how current behavior differs from desired behavior. Reflective listening can increase the client's awareness of the negative consequences his or her current behavior has on current relationships, performance at school or work, enjoyment of life, and physical and mental well-being. The therapist listens carefully for any statement that reflects the client's values and connections to family, friends, significant others, or community. The therapist needs to separate the behavior from the person as the client begins to understand how current behavior undermines his or her personal values and goals. The therapist needs to amplify and focus on this discrepancy until the client can verbalize consistent concern and commitment to change his or her behavior. At this juncture the therapist needs to studiously avoid providing suggestions or possible solutions to modify behavior. The client should present the argument for change!

■ THERAPEUTIC INTERVENTIONS IN MI

Reflectively listening is the essence of MI. Imagine the therapist as a mirror reflecting what the client verbalizes about his or her current situation and what the gaps or discrepancies are between current behavior and desired behavior based on client values and goals. Client-centered interviewing skills that facilitate these principles include (OARS):

- **O: O**pen-ended questions are questions that require more than a "yes" or "no" response. Only 25% of motivational interviews should be open-ended questions.
  - **APPN:** "What do you think about . . .?"
  - **APPN:** "What would your reasons be for . . .?"
- **A: A**ffirmations are statements of support or recognition of clients' strengths
  - **APPN:** "You are certainly determined to get your health back!"
- **R: R**eflections are statements that mirror what the client has said. About 75% of motivational interviews should be comprised of reflections.
  - **Client:** "What do you know about drugs? You probably never even smoked weed!"
  - **APPN:** "It's hard to imagine how I could possibly understand you."
- **S:** Summaries are a collection of reflections.
  - **APPN:** "To make sure I'm understanding what you've been telling me, let me sum up . . . ."

There are three levels of reflective listening:

- Repeat or rephrase: repeat key words, staying close to what the client has said.
- Paraphrase: restate the essence of what the client has said in a more concise, clear way.
- Reflection of feelings or values: identify key emotions and feedback to the client for clarification.

There are different types of reflections:

- Simple Reflection: Restate, mirror, and economize what the client has said.
  - **Client:** "I'm feeling pretty depressed today."
  - **APPN:** "It sounds like you're feeling down."
- Complex Reflection: Restate content and additionally identify underlying emotion.
  - **Client:** "I had a fight with my roommate because she forgot to take the recycling out and that's one of her jobs."
  - **APPN:** "It sounds as if you are frustrated with her because she fell down on her agreed upon responsibilities."
- Reframing: Offers a new and positive interpretation in order for the client to see his or her perception in a different light.
  - **Client:** "My mother is always nagging me."
  - **APPN:** "She must really care a lot about you to tell you something she feels is important, even though you might get angry with her."
- Using Metaphors or Similes: Helps to take the client's issues out of a personal context.
  - **Client:** "It feels like a bunch of crows pecking at you."
  - **APPN:** "With all of your responsibilities, you must feel like a rope pulled in a bunch of different directions."
- Reflection with a Twist: Involves either a reflection or a statement of agreement, followed by a reframe.
  - **Client:** "Nobody can make me go to school."

- – **APPN:** "You're right; nobody can make you go to school. But, you will need to complete school in order to reach some of your goals that we've discussed (such as living on your own)."
- Amplified Reflection: Involves taking the client's side of the argument to the extreme, but be careful not to communicate endorsement of negative behavior.
  - – **Client:** "I need weed to relax."
  - – **APPN:** "Smoking weed is the *only thing* you can do to relax."
- Double-Sided Reflection: Ties into the idea of developing discrepancy, which is the act of helping clients look at the difference between where they currently are and where they want to be.
  - – **APPN:** "So, you really enjoy a lot of things about smoking, but at the same time it's interfering with your skiing and other sports."
  - – **APPN:** "On the one hand you like sleeping late, on the other being late to school is getting you in trouble"

(A. Miller, 2012; Rollnick, Miller, & Butler, 2007; Rosengren, 2017).

Employing these interventions, summarized by the pneumonic OARS, while adhering to the principles of MI gently empowers the client to make choices that move him or her in the direction the client envisions. The emphasis is on guiding the client to identify cognitive dissonance between the *facilitators of* and *barriers to* a desired behavior change based on the client's values and beliefs.

■ CASE STUDY

Background

I first met Kathy 20 years ago, referred by her primary care provider (PCP) for her depression, anxiety, and anger that emerged 18 months earlier after her husband's new job in the agricultural industry brought the family to middle Tennessee from Jefferson City, Missouri. At the time of the initial visit, Kathy was age 37, married 15 years, and the mother of three children—Rachel, age 8; Elizabeth, age 6; and William, age 2. She acknowledged prior times of anxiety and depression—at age 5 when her parents divorced, during stressful times at college, and after the birth of her second child—but "never as bad" as this current episode. Her PCP had initiated antidepressant medication (a selective serotonin reuptake inhibitor) with only partial symptom response. As part of my initial evaluation, I was able to rule out bipolar disorder, confirm recurrent major depression, and change medication to a different antidepressant medication (selective serotonin and norepinephrine reuptake inhibitor). However, the medication adjustment alone would not address the underlying issues fueling Kathy's depression.

Kathy attributed the progressive worsening of her symptoms to her unhappiness since relocating to middle Tennessee, missing her friends, her church, her life as the wife of a university professor in agricultural sciences, her part-time work as a research assistant for another faculty member, and her extensive support system. She bitterly resented her husband's new job for tearing her away from a lifestyle and close-knit community in Missouri that she now idealized. She worried that her depression, anxiety, and anger were affecting her relationship with her children and that she was a "bad mother." She struggled with guilt for being short-tempered with the children, feeling paralyzed by her depression and unmotivated to unpack boxes and organize their new home, or make any effort to build new relationships with neighbors or at her daughter's elementary school. She was withdrawn and resentful, verbalizing that the family would be "better off without me."

I share this case study because it offers an example of a client who had considerable difficulty in changing her feelings of resentment about relocating the family for her husband's career, her idealized feelings about her former life in Missouri, and her reluctance to engage in meaningful activities to build relationships in her new community. MI enables me to sustain a nonjudgmental, empathic approach while seeking to identify what values and beliefs she held that would fuel her willingness to change. How could I empower Kathy to take personal responsibility to "bloom where you are planted" rather than remaining bitter, angry, depressed, and "stuck"—blaming her unhappiness on her husband's career choice which she originally supported?

I combined MI with medication management for Kathy over the past 20 years to initially support her small yet steady steps in changing her perspective on the move to Tennessee and later on her relationships with her children, her husband, and her neighbors, as well as, most importantly, her sense of personal accountability for her life choices. At one point, I also conducted 12 weekly sessions of Eye Movement, Desensitization, and Reprocessing (EMDR) to work through childhood trauma and perceived abandonment by her father (Shapiro, 2002). Although medication has proven effective in achieving symptom remission for her episodes of major depression and comorbid dysthymia, MI has proven to be most helpful to her in working through her psychological issues and coping with ongoing life stressors.

Transcript of MI Sessions

The transcripts presented here were selected from segments of the beginning, middle, and maintenance phase of therapy.

Beginning Phase

The early sessions focused on building a therapeutic relationship, understanding the client's perception of the problem, and eliciting the client's values and beliefs that potentially could motivate change.

APPN:	Hello. I understand your doctor (PCP) referred you to see me. How can I be of help?
Kathy:	Yes. I've been struggling with anxiety and depression for the past year and a half, but it's getting worse, not better. I've been miserable since we moved to Tennessee 18 months ago. Nothing's gone as we expected. I wish we'd never left Missouri.
APPN:	How so?
Kathy:	We had lived in Jefferson City for 12 years. My husband was a professor in the agricultural sciences program and I worked as a part-time research assistant for another faculty member in his department. Our children were happy there . . . I loved our home, our neighbors, our friends at Mizzou, our church . . . (*begins to softly cry*).
APPN:	Leaving that close-knit community of friends has been more difficult than you expected.
Kathy:	Yes . . . I didn't realize all that I was giving up or how much having a third child would change my daily life. William was only 6 months old when we left Missouri and I was still up at night nursing him at 2:00 a.m. and 6:00 a.m. He was a fussy baby—more so than the girls.
APPN:	Tell me about your children.

Kathy:	We have three now. Rachel is 8 years old in third grade. Elizabeth is 6 years old in first grade. And William just turned 2 *(years)*. I decided when we moved here that I'd home school the girls. Without my part-time research position, I thought I'd be bored at home alone with the baby. I have a B.S. in biology and loved teaching middle school before I met John, my husband. I continued teaching full time until we had Rachel. That's when I left teaching. I joined another faculty colleague's research team part-time and worked in the lab. It gave me the flexibility I needed to raise our kids. Rachel had just finished first grade in the public school and Elizabeth had been in pre-K just before we moved to Tennessee.
APPN:	How is the home schooling going?
Kathy:	Well . . . I've been so disorganized . . . we've been living out of boxes since coming to Tennessee. The first house we bought had foundation problems. We had to sue the builder and never really unpacked everything. Then we moved to a second home about 10 months ago, and it needs new flooring and carpets. Why unpack things when we know the flooring needs replacement? So, I can't seem to get lesson plans organized for the girls. They're both eager to read and learn . . . but I'm so overwhelmed, I don't know where to start. I find myself snapping at them all the time . . . sometimes I explode in a rage. Then I break down in tears. I'm ashamed of the mean things I've said to the kids and blaming everything wrong on their dad. I retreat to my bedroom for hours because I don't want them to see me upset or crying all the time. Sometimes I think they'd be better off without me as a mother.
APPN:	That must be scary . . . when your anger escalates to rage at your children.
Kathy:	Yes. Sometimes I think I'm going crazy. That I'll lose control and do something I'll regret.
APPN:	Tell me, have you had thoughts of hurting your children? Or hurting yourself or ending your life at those times?
Kathy:	No! I've thought it might be better if I just went to sleep and didn't wake up, but I'd never do anything to end my life. I wouldn't do that to my kids and I believe that it's up to God when your time on earth is finished. And, I'd never hurt my kids.
APPN:	I'm glad to hear your reasons for not taking your life. Both are valid. I do need to ask if you've ever had a plan of how you would take your life.
Kathy:	No. Never. I wouldn't do that.
APPN:	Sometimes depression can be so painful that people see no other way out. Would you be willing to tell me or seek emergency help if that should ever happen to you in the future?
Kathy:	Yes. I can do that. I want to get over this depression. I want to be a better mother.
APPN:	Then, being a better mother is what we'll focus on. Tell me about your depression the past 18 months. What symptoms did you notice initially and how have these or additional symptoms progressed?

Kathy:	Initially after William was born—about 6 months before we moved to Tennessee—I was always tired from nursing him every 3 hours. I'd try to catch naps between feedings but I never could fall asleep. We knew we were moving by the time he was 3 months old, so every day I'd try to pack things we didn't use, but I had trouble concentrating and organizing the packing. I had no energy and no motivation. I realized then I didn't want to leave. I was sad and tearful packing things up, saying good-bye to church and neighborhood friends, saying good-bye to my lab coworkers. I didn't have much appetite, though I tried to drink lots of milk and fluids and eat small meals throughout the day because I was nursing. But I still dropped below my usual weight of 125 pounds.

When we got to Tennessee in July, we realized the house we had bought had serious foundation problems. We sued the builder while we lived in a small rental condo. The kids were bored, cooped up inside to stay in air-conditioning with no pool, no friends, and nothing to do except watch TV, read, or play games . . . that's when I started gathering materials and curriculum to home school Rachel and Elizabeth. We didn't know what school district they'd be in as we couldn't start looking for another house until the lawsuit was settled. I also thought it would give me something to focus on and pull me out of my slump. It only made things worse for me . . . I was stressed out and John was no help as he was spending 10-hour days acclimating to his new position in industrial agriculture. He had to travel frequently—visiting customers all over the mid-south consulting on pesticides and fertilizers for cotton crops. I had no one to turn to for help with the kids or to get any relief.

APPN:	What's been the most difficult part of your depression?
Kathy:	Feeling alone. That there's no one who can help me with the kids. Missing my friends from Missouri. I've called some of them, but who wants to listen to someone who only complains? And John helps some on weekends but we've grown distant as well. He's tired of hearing me complain. I know I sound like a broken record. John encourages me to get out and meet the neighbors or even enroll the girls in public school to relieve my stress. But the neighbors already have their cliques and don't include us. There aren't many school-age kids in the subdivision . . . mostly middle school and high school. So, the girls play together in our back yard or indoors when they're not working on a lesson or learning module.
APPN:	And enrolling the girls in public school?
Kathy:	Maybe when they're older—in high school—but not now. I think they're ahead of their age group in all of their subjects—spelling, reading, math—I don't want them in public school right now. What would I do without them at home?
APPN:	You're proud of your daughters' spelling, reading, and math proficiency being home-schooled, and would miss them were they to go to public school.
Kathy:	Exactly.

APPN:	Do you see any disadvantage to home-schooling the girls? Do you worry that they may be missing any experiences that kids in public or private schools have?
Kathy:	I suppose they might miss activities with classmates, but they enjoy playing together most of the time . . . occasionally Rachel gets tired of Elizabeth following her around. I suppose when they're older they'll want to have friends over, play on sports teams, and go to sleepovers— but that's years down the road. For now—I want to home-school the girls even though I feel disorganized and overwhelmed at times.
APPN:	You link the onset of your depression to your family's move to Tennessee and the most difficult aspect of the depression for you is "feeling alone." Is there anything that helps you feel less alone?
Kathy:	If I was in Missouri, I'd have any number of close friends to talk to, but here I know no one and I don't feel welcome. I'm not a southerner. The neighbors have made no effort to get to know our family or us.
APPN:	How did you build those friendships when you first moved to Missouri?
Kathy:	People are different in the Midwest. They're more neighborly. When we moved to our first apartment before we had kids, the neighbors stopped by, introduced themselves, some even brought us a plate of cookies, and they invited us over to watch Mizzou football games. When we moved to our first home—the same thing happened—people stopped by, introduced themselves, invited us to cookouts, brought cookies or bread by the house, and welcomed us to the neighborhood. No one has done that here!
APPN:	So you're wondering "What happened to southern hospitality?" . . .
Kathy:	Well, yes, you could say that.
APPN:	What options do you see to make friends here?
Kathy:	We've tried going to different churches, but we haven't found anywhere we feel comfortable. I've pretty much given up on finding a church. I suppose I could march over to a neighbor's house with a plate of cookies for them (said with sarcasm) . . . but how many plates of cookies would it take? They seem busy with their own lives.
APPN:	You seem hurt by the neighbors not making the first step when you moved into the neighborhood. How could you hit the "re-start" button? What might you say if you initiated an introduction?
Kathy:	I suppose I could start with, "Hello, I'm Kathy, your neighbor next door. I've been so busy getting settled in the house and home-schooling our two daughters that I hadn't had a chance to come over and introduce myself. We moved here from Missouri. My husband, John, is in the agriculture industry and travels a lot. It's a Midwest custom to bring cookies to new neighbors. I thought I'd bring cookies to *my* new neighbors."
APPN:	Caution! You wouldn't want to insinuate that they weren't "neighborly" . . . but that will depend on your tone of voice. That's a good start. Would you be willing to try this approach with one or two of your neighbors?
Kathy:	I don't see any harm in trying.

Kathy did initiate several introductions to neighbors who were generally pleasant, although it did not develop into any close friendships for several years. This only further confirmed her appraisal that her southern neighbors were not hospitable and she missed her Midwestern friends. The theme of her efforts to initiate friendships periodically resurfaced throughout our counseling sessions with her increasing self-awareness that it was difficult for her to initiate a reason to get together and her dislike of "small talk" as she phrased it. When a new family moved to the neighborhood after 3 or 4 years, Kathy brought a plate of cookies and welcomed them to the neighborhood. Much to Kathy's surprise, Julie, her new neighbor, reciprocated and so ensued a friendship that flourished and helped Kathy connect with other families in the neighborhood.

Middle Phase

I have included transcripts from two different sessions in our middle phase of therapy.

Middle Phase, Session 1

APPN: It's been a few months since I last saw you for medication renewal. Is there anything you need to work on today? *(This was her cue to identify any counseling issues.)*

Kathy: The girls are arguing more, especially Rachel. She complains that she's not learning enough science and advanced math at home. She wants to join the science and math classes at the community home-school center in Franklin. I not sure I like that idea.

APPN: How old are the girls now?

Kathy: Rachel is 15 and Elizabeth is 13.

APPN: What do you see as the *pros* and *cons* of Rachel joining the science and math classes at the home-school center? I understand that the center operates like a "co-op" with parents volunteering their time to teach subjects in which they have college undergrad and doctoral degrees. They use standardized curricula and widely used textbooks.

Kathy: I know that the home-school center is accredited and the people teaching different subjects are qualified. I just don't think it's necessary. I have a biology degree and I took all the advanced calculus and trigonometry and differential equation classes in high school and college. I think I'm well qualified to teach those subjects.

APPN: What else may be motivating Rachel to take classes at the home-school center?

Kathy: She says she doesn't have any friends and the home-school center would give her a chance to have friends . . . (long pause of silence).

APPN: And?

Kathy: And, *(long pause)*, I think she'll go "boy crazy" . . . she's also pushing to get her learner's permit to drive. I'm not ready for that either. She has gymnastics and dance classes. She has friends there.

APPN: Rachel is growing up and beginning to show an interest in relationships outside her home. She has her younger brother, Will, who's 9, but I imagine Rachel is curious about boys her age. At age 15 or 16, what were your interests?

Kathy:	I was focused on school to be able to get a scholarship and a career. Remember, I was growing up in Appalachia with my mom and sister. Education was the only way out of poverty. I watched many of the girls where I grew up get pregnant at 14, 15, or 16 years old and drop out of school. I want Rachel to stay focused on her schoolwork, not chase after boys.
APPN:	You're afraid that Rachel will not use good judgment spending time with boys her age and you want to protect her. On the other hand, how long can you realistically keep her from any interactions with boys her age? And, will this really protect her?
Kathy:	You raise a valid point.
APPN:	May I offer an additional perspective to consider?
Kathy:	Of course. I tend to get stuck in my own way of seeing things. You've helped me see other ways to look at situations.
APPN:	If you forbid a person from pursuing something, often that person desires it even more. Even if it means breaking rules and taking risks. Might it be better to allow Rachel to develop friendships with boys and girls her age, while encouraging her to set healthy, safe boundaries, than preventing her from having relationships with boys by insisting she finish her high school studies at home with you?
Kathy:	You're suggesting that allowing Rachel to interact with boys at the home-school center provides a safe and supervised environment? That she's less likely to rebel against me and her dad by going "boy crazy"? Hmmmm . . . certainly something to think about.

Kathy and John eventually decided to let all three of the children (Rachel 15 years, Elizabeth 13 years, and William 9 years) enroll in classes at the home-school center that fall. Rachel and Elizabeth developed friendships with both boys and girls their age, later attended their respective junior and senior proms sponsored by the home-school center, and neither of the girls went "boy crazy" as Kathy had feared. Rachel graduated from college with a baccalaureate degree in nursing, is self-supporting, and has had several boyfriends, but no one that she's chosen to marry. Elizabeth graduated from college with a marketing degree, married a fellow she met in college, and they are expecting a first child. William will soon graduate from college with an engineering degree. All three are pursuing independent lives and gather as an extended family at holidays and birthdays.

Middle Phase, Session 2

APPN:	How are you? What do we need to focus on today?
Kathy:	Things are generally going well. The girls are in college. William will graduate from high school in a couple years. John is happy with his work. I keep busy with the house and garden. I enjoy my monthly book club and weekly Bible study group, but I've gradually gained 25 pounds over the past 3 years. I'm only 5 feet tall, so 25 pounds is a lot! Now I'm in menopause and that makes it worse . . . the emotional eating. I've tried diets, I've tried to exercise, but I never stick with it. I feel fat and ugly (tears up).
APPN:	You're discouraged about your weight gain and appearance.

Kathy:	Yes. None of my clothes fit any more. I've been buying baggy sweat pants and sweatshirts for winter and loose jogging and sportswear for summer to hide my weight.
APPN:	Your weight has fluctuated by 15 to 20 pounds during the 15 or so years I've known you. What has been most helpful in the past in losing weight?
Kathy:	My jazzercise class at the Y (YMCA)—but it's not working like it used to. I've quit going I'm so discouraged. Usually, if I'd go to jazzercise three to five times a week, I could lose 5 to 10 pounds in 2 to 3 months, but menopause has changed my metabolism I think. I can just look at a cookie or sweet and gain weight.
APPN:	When is the last time you went to jazzercise?
Kathy:	Well, truthfully, probably 8 or 9 months ago. I've just given up and told myself I'll just have to get used to being fat and ugly.
APPN:	You sound resigned. What motivated you in the past to lose weight?
Kathy:	I feel better when I'm around 130 to 135 pounds. I have more energy. My clothes fit and I feel more attractive. Not to mention it's better for my health. As I put on this 25 pounds my blood pressure went back up and I had to go back on my blood pressure medicine . . . and that makes me nauseous and have muscle cramps in my legs. I don't like it.
APPN:	What are the most difficult aspects of resuming jazzercise and staying on a regular exercise routine?
Kathy:	When I go for a straight month or more and don't see any weight loss I get frustrated and just give up. Sometimes, especially in winter when it's cold or rainy or gray outside, I just don't want to get out of my pajamas or leave the house. It's easier to stay home. Sometime I get bored with the jazzercise—especially if I'm not losing weight or feeling like I have any energy.
APPN:	What other options do you think might help sustain your motivation when you want to quit exercising?
Kathy:	I think having some variety of exercise would help. And having a buddy to exercise with me. Avoiding sweets and heavy fats; eating more veggies, fruits, and salads wouldn't hurt either. When I get discouraged, I eat more sweets and fast food burgers.
APPN:	What might the variety of exercise look like?
Kathy:	When the weather's nice, I could ask Charlotte and Joan if I could join their morning walk in the neighborhood. They've invited me several times over the years. I also could see if they have any interest in joining me for the jazzercise classes at the Y. I could try some of the other classes at the Y such as yoga, Zumba, water aerobics, and any of their cardio and strength classes. Now that I'm not home-schooling, I can arrange my schedule to do what I want.
APPN:	Rather than tackling multiple new exercise classes, what one new exercise sounds the most appealing to add to your jazzercise that you have enjoyed for years?

Kathy:	I think walking with Charlotte and Joan would lift my spirits and give me something to look forward to on a daily basis. Then, I could still go to jazzercise three times a week after my morning walks.
APPN:	Are you willing to commit to that plan for a month and then reevaluate?
Kathy:	I have nothing to lose . . . (laughing) . . . except some extra pounds.
APPN:	As for your nutrition, what are the greatest challenges to eating balanced meals? I know you've met with a nutritionist in the past and have menus and meal plans to reduce weight and maintain a healthy weight once you get to your goal. I also recall that you had success using the Weight Watchers program and weighing in weekly. I recall you used an online app, right?
Kathy:	Yes. I did use the Weight Watchers online app (www.weightwatchers .com/us/how-it-works/tracking). It's been awhile, but it did keep me motivated. The biggest hurdle to nutritious meals is the meal planning, grocery shopping, and meal prep time. You know I'm a fast food junkie and with John out of town, it's easier to buy frozen pizza or prepackaged meals for one.
APPN:	It is hard to do all the meal planning and prep for one or two people—isn't William still at home?
Kathy:	Yes, he is. That boy lives on milk, sandwiches, and pasta dishes.
APPN:	How did you manage the meal planning and prep when you used Weight Watchers in the past?
Kathy:	The key was doing the grocery shopping Sunday after church, and the chopping and prep Sunday afternoon for meals for the rest of the week. I need to get back to that routine.
APPN:	So . . . you're committing to daily morning walks with your friends, Charlotte and Joan, in addition to jazzercise three times a week. You're committing to grocery shopping and meal prep for the week on Sundays. And you're going to enroll in the online Weight Watchers mobile app. That's a lot to commit to . . . are you sure this is not overcommitting?
Kathy:	No. I've got to get back to a healthier weight. I know I'll have more energy. And . . . (slight pause—smiling), John and I are talking about a Mediterranean cruise in the fall for our 30th wedding anniversary—I want to feel good about how I look.
APPN:	That's a wonderful incentive! We'll track your progress monthly to help you sustain your motivation.

Kathy has struggled with her weight throughout the two decades I have known her. When she gained 10 or more pounds, it was usually an indication that she had a recurrent episode of depression requiring medication adjustment. She did lose 20 pounds the year of her 30th wedding anniversary and thoroughly enjoyed the Mediterranean cruise.

Final Phase

I still continue to work with Kathy. This last transcript is part of a recent session.

APPN:	Hello, Kathy. What do we need to focus on today?

Kathy:	*(starts quietly crying)* . . . I'm sorry . . . I don't know why I'm crying.
APPN:	Kathy, you don't need to apologize for your feelings. I hope you know that by now. Tell me about your feelings.
Kathy:	I'm just profoundly sad, when I should be happy. Rachel's loving her work as an ICU nurse. Elizabeth and Scot *(her husband of 2 years)* are expecting a baby in 6 months. And, William will graduate from engineering school in the spring.
APPN:	Tell me about the sadness.
Kathy:	I've been thinking about my life. I was such a bad mother . . . my children had to fend for themselves when I'd lock myself in my bedroom during my worst periods of dark depression. I was awful to them at times—irritable, angry, sometimes I'd fly into a rage. I remember slapping Rachel so hard in the face when she back-talked me one time. She was just 7 or 8 years old. She didn't deserve that. She probably hates me. The children probably all hate me . . . .
APPN:	You're feeling guilty and perhaps embarrassed about how you sometimes treated the children when they were young.
Kathy:	I'm ashamed of some of the things I said and did. The kids were so young. They didn't deserve to be treated that way. I know it happened when my depression was at its worst . . . before I started seeing you . . . but I probably emotionally scarred them for life. I can't stop thinking about it.
APPN:	This was the focus of some of our earliest counseling sessions during the first few years that I saw you. You were able to see that you weren't a "bad person" or "bad mother," but a person who, in the depth of a depression, said and did some things she regretted. You were able to move beyond that severe depression and be more responsive to the emotional needs of your children.
Kathy:	I realize I've fallen back into my negative thinking again.
APPN:	I wonder what's triggering these negative thoughts at this time. Any ideas?
Kathy	The kids are all grown up and moving forward with their lives. They don't need me anymore. I've found myself looking back and reflecting on my life so far and all the regrets I have . . . .
APPN:	And it sounds like you're dwelling on some of the regrets you have as a mother rather than a more balanced self-appraisal. No mother is perfect. How do you evaluate whether someone is successful as a parent?
Kathy:	That you've raised your children to be honest, reliable, trustworthy . . . to be a person of integrity . . . to be sensitive to the feelings and needs of others . . . to work hard and give your best effort . . . to be able to have a career and financially support yourself . . . and to be happy with your life.
APPN:	That's a pretty tall order. As you think about each of your children, how well do you think you and your husband have done overall as parents based on those criteria?

Kathy:	Well, Rachel and Elizabeth are already living independently and supporting themselves. William soon will be as an engineer. Sometimes I think Rachel is too self-centered, but then I consider how much she enjoys caring for others as a nurse. The kids have never given us any reason to doubt their honesty or trust. I guess overall I'm pretty proud of them.
APPN:	Sounds like you've been successful parents using your own criteria or standards. You can take pride in knowing that your children are successfully "leaving the nest" and are becoming self-sufficient young adults.
Kathy:	I hadn't thought of it from that perspective.
APPN:	You also mentioned feeling sad, that your children "don't need you." They may not need you to fix their meals, drive them to school or activities, or navigate the ups and downs of life, but they still need your emotional support and parental adult guidance. The task you face now is transitioning from an adolescent and parent relationship to a young-adult and parent relationship. The other task you face is finding purpose and meaning in this next chapter in your life.
Kathy:	That's where I need to focus next . . . .
APPN:	How would you like to begin?
Kathy:	Perhaps taking inventory of things I've put off doing while the kids were still living at home. I love animals and always wanted to work with a veterinarian or train seeing eye or service dogs. John and I have never had much time alone together. We've talked about trips we'd like to take and maybe joining our neighborhood friends for a cruise they're planning next year.
APPN:	You've mentioned your interest in working at a vet's office in the past and training service dogs, yet you've never pursued either interest. What have been the biggest barriers?
Kathy:	I know I used the excuse that I needed to be available for anything the kids might need from me, but truthfully, I didn't want to commit to anything on a weekly basis. I worried that I might not get along with people in a vet's office. I'm not good at customer relations. I'd be better at assisting the vet with exams and procedures. Becoming a vet's assistant would mean I'd have to go back to school for training. I'm not sure I want to go back to school. As for training service dogs to be placed with other people, I'm not sure what that entails as far as the types of training programs, what's a reputable organization that trains the animal trainers, whether it's a volunteer or paid service. I just have no idea where to start. And then my inertia kicks in and I don't follow through. I just daydream about it.
APPN:	How can you approach this "dream" differently now that the kids aren't at home?
Kathy:	Training service dogs seems more appealing than working for a vet. But I need to do a lot of homework. I could start by asking our family vet about reputable training programs and go from there.
APPN:	Sounds like a reasonable first step.

Commentary

Kathy has been a client of mine for two decades where a MI approach was used to facilitate growth and resilience throughout the critical issues in her life—the loss of her idealized community and lifestyle following the birth of her third child and relocation to a different region and state, the challenges of home schooling and raising a family, her struggle with weight gain and menopause, her reckoning with an "empty nest" after her children launched into adult life, and the recent search for meaning and purpose in her life—all while coping with recurrent episodes of depression and persistent dysthymia. I have selected a session from her initial visits, a session from her struggle with weight gain, a session during a period of acute loneliness once her children were all successfully launched as young adults, and most recently her reflections on current life choices that provide connection and purpose. At the time of her sister's death (long history of drug addiction with comorbid bipolar disorder) and her mother's death (history of alcohol dependence in sustained recovery with lifelong depression), we engaged in 12 EMDR sessions to process long-buried childhood trauma. Her father had divorced her mother for another woman and left the two girls (Kathy and her sister) to live in poverty with their mother in rural Appalachia. Once she was able to grieve and process the trauma of her lost childhood and the recent deaths of her sister and mother, Kathy focused on her current family life and desire to be a good mother and wife. Kathy has gradually developed the ability to evaluate her thoughts, feelings, and behaviors regarding situations and relationships by examining her ambivalence and pursuing a path guided by her values and beliefs. At times she finds it difficult to sustain those choices and struggles for a time before she recommits to a behavior change. Kathy befriended one neighbor while she weeded her flowerbed by offering to share a cutting when the neighbor commented how much she admired Kathy's flowers. This small introduction led to Kathy being invited to a neighborhood potluck. She felt welcomed at the potluck and discovered others who shared similar interests. Ever since then, she has been included in neighborhood activities and gatherings—monthly book club meetings, holiday potlucks, morning walks, chats over coffee, and even a "girl's getaway trip to the beach in Alabama" each spring. Kathy stays in touch with one of her former neighbors who moved to Florida and is still included in their annual beach trip. Kathy recently reflected, "I guess I've finally learned to 'bloom where I'm planted.'"

DISCUSSION QUESTIONS

1. If you were counseling a patient who had long-standing resistance to change or difficulty seeing his or her role in self-defeating behaviors, what resources can you identify as a therapist to help you engage the patient more effectively?
2. What are the traps that therapists using MI need to avoid when they encounter patient resistance or ambivalence?
3. At what points in the therapy sessions presented would you suggest different reflections and affirmations to increase the patient's self-awareness of the choices she is making and how it affects her life?
4. How do you envision using MI in your practice setting and role?

REFERENCES

Amrhein, P. C., Miller, W. R., Yahne, C. E., Palmer, M., & Fulcher, L. (2003). Client commitment language during motivational interviewing predicts drug use outcome. *Journal of Consulting and Clinical Psychology, 71,* 862–878. doi:10.1037/0022-006X.71.5.862

Bem, D. J. (1967). Self-perception: An alternative interpretation of cognitive dissonance phenomena. *Psychological Review, 74,* 183–200. doi:10.1037/h0024835

Bowen, M. (1978). *Family therapy in clinical practice.* New York, NY: Jason Aronson.

Brehm, S. S., & Brehm, J. W. (1981). *Psychological reactance: A theory of freedom and control.* New York, NY: Academic Press.

Festinger, L. (1957). *A theory of cognitive dissonance.* Evanston, IL: Row, Peterson.

Gates, A. (2011). Motivational interviewing and empowering patients to make lifestyle changes. *Exercise works!* Retrieved from http://www.exercise-works.org/latest-news/2011/12/11/motivational-interviewing-and-empowering-patients-to-make-li.html

Miller, A. (2012). *Instructor's manual for core concepts in motivational interviewing with Cathy Cole, LCSW.* Mill Valley, CA: Psychotherapy.net. Retrieved from https://www.psychotherapy.net/data/uploads/51103cc9a11b0.pdf

Miller, W. R. (1983). Motivational interviewing with problem drinkers. *Behavioural Psychotherapy, 11,* 147–172. doi:10.1017/S0141347300006583

Miller, W. R. (2018). *Listening well: The art of empathic understanding.* Eugene, OR: Wipf & Stock.

Miller W. R., & Rollnick, S. (1991). *Motivational interviewing: Preparing people for change.* New York, NY: Guilford Press.

Miller, W. R., & Rollnick, S. (2013). *Motivational interviewing: Helping people change* (3rd ed.). New York, NY: Guilford Press.

Prochaska, J. O., DiClemente, C. C., & Norcross, J. C. (1992). In search of how people change: Applications to addictive behaviors. *American Psychologists, 47,* 1102–1114. doi:10.1037/0003-066X.47.9.1102

Rogers, C. R. (1965). *Client-centered therapy.* New York, NY: Houghton Mifflin.

Rollnick, S., Miller, W. R., & Butler, C. C. (2007). *Motivational interviewing in health care: Helping patients change behavior.* New York, NY: Guilford Press.

Rosengren, D. B. (2017). *Building motivational interviewing skills: A practitioner workbook* (2nd ed.). New York, NY: Guilford Press.

Shapiro, F. (Ed.). (2002). *EMDR as an integrative psychotherapy approach: Experts of diverse orientations explore the paradigm prism.* Washington, DC: American Psychological Association.

Harm Reduction Psychotherapy: A Client With a Substance Use Disorder

Michelle Knapp and Adam Kozikowski

■ PERSONAL EXPERIENCE WITH HARM REDUCTION PSYCHOTHERAPY

Problematic substance use and its sequelae of interpersonal and social problems are common among individuals seeking psychotherapy. In 2017, the National Survey on Drug Use and Health found that more than 8.5 million adults have both a substance use disorder (SUD) and other psychiatric disorder, and trends show that SUDs are not decreasing (Lipari & Van Horn, 2017; Substance Abuse and Mental Health Services Administration, 2018). SUDs can cause significant psychological and physiological turmoil for those affected. Unfortunately, few people receive adequate treatment for these disorders. Some reasons may be related to the stigma of substance use, limited specialized treatment facilities, and lack of providers who are comfortable or knowledgeable in the long-term management of SUDs—conditions that are unlikely to change anytime in the near future.

Historically, substance use treatment has focused on an "abstinence-only" model of care. This all-or-nothing approach to treatment places emphasis on the SUD and the client's "choice" to avoid change. Though abstinence may be one goal of treatment, focusing on this alone may predispose clients to failure. Clients often experience shame or defeat in relapse and are reluctant to face providers and continue with treatment. Harm Reduction psychotherapy is a more contemporary and successful approach to helping clients in their treatment of substance use (Marlatt, 1998).

As the authors of this chapter, we have over four decades of combined years of experience working with clients having substance use issues. Initially, we worked as psychiatric nurses on substance use detoxification units and short-term rehabilitation units of general hospitals. The majority of our experience at that time involved working with practitioners who subscribed to the abstinence-only model of treatment. Nevertheless, we rarely found the expectation of abstinence helpful for our clients. In consequent review of the literature, we were astonished by the poor outcomes of the abstinence-only model of care. As a result, we began to seriously question and ultimately rethink the abstinence-only approach.

In general, we have always found our clients with substance use issues to be a diverse group of stimulating, captivating clients who are flexible and open to participating in psychotherapy. Nonetheless, with the abstinence-only model, the philosophy prevails that clients cannot benefit from psychotherapy while they are using substances. Hence, the belief that when clients articulate their psychological issues while still using substances, they are designated as being in denial; therefore, the fundamental notion is their substance use must be addressed prior to embarking on any psychological work. In those early days, early on when we worked with the "abstinence-only" model, it was our role to encourage clients to accept abstinence as the goal of treatment and to discourage them from working on their other psychological issues until the substance use was addressed.

Our exposure to the Harm Reduction model of treatment occurred when we began working as psychiatric nurses at Roosevelt Hospital's Addiction Institute in New York City with some of the world's foremost thinkers in substance use treatment. In this setting, we developed an in-depth understanding of Harm Reduction philosophy as well as the techniques of Harm Reduction psychotherapy and the benefits it could provide clients suffering from SUDs. We also received high-level supervision from physicians certified in addiction psychiatry.

While working at Roosevelt Hospital's Addiction Institute, we began graduate school at New York University (NYU) to become psychiatric nurse practitioners. At NYU, we received in-depth training in Carl Rogers' Person-Centered Therapy approach as well as William Miller and Stephen Rollnick's Motivational Interviewing (MI) approach. Both approaches are incorporated into Harm Reduction psychotherapy. After becoming psychiatric nurse practitioners, we received further training in Harm Reduction psychotherapy as well as different therapeutic modalities including Gestalt therapy, Cognitive Behavioral therapy, and Somatic therapies. We incorporate aspects of these approaches into our Harm Reduction psychotherapy as well.

As psychiatric nurse practitioners, we have worked at a number of inpatient and outpatient facilities over the past decade. We have developed specialties with a variety of populations having SUDs including the forensic population and the LGBTQ population. Within these populations, we have been able to treat clients with acute and chronic SUDs across many cultural and socioeconomic backgrounds. Dr. Michelle Knapp also currently works in a specialized opioid agonist therapy setting providing Harm Reduction psychotherapy and medication-assisted treatments to pregnant women who use substances. In addition to our extensive clinical experience, we have taught graduate level courses in SUDs and behavioral addictions and have conducted numerous workshops on Harm Reduction psychotherapy at major universities, psychotherapy training institutes, and at national and regional conferences. Dr. Michelle Knapp is also the director of the Substance Use Sequence at NYU, which awards students a certificate in SUDs after completing three courses and an internship with clients having SUDs. The courses teach students how to treat SUDs and related addictions from a Harm Reduction philosophy and provides them training in both MI and Harm Reduction psychotherapy. Adam Kozikowski currently works as an adjunct faculty at NYU where he teaches brain stimulation approaches for clients with SUDs as well as individual, group, couples, and family psychotherapy supervision. In addition, he teaches at the Center for Gestalt Psychotherapy and Training.

■ FOUNDERS AND LEADERS OF HARM REDUCTION PSYCHOTHERAPY

There are three important researchers and clinicians who are considered to be important in the development of Harm Reduction psychotherapy. They are Elvin Morton Jellinek, Edward John Khantzian, and Gordon Alan Marlatt.

The "abstinence-only" model of treatment for clients with SUDs assumes that change cannot be achieved in any area of life until the client stops using substances. There is an assumption made that the substance user is in denial about the "real" problem. This model is grounded in the belief that addiction is a moral disease. In 1960, E. Morton Jellinek, a physiologist, alcoholism researcher, and founder of the Yale Center of Alcohol Studies, challenged this idea in his breakthrough book, *The Disease Concept of Alcoholism*. He proposed that individuals labeled as alcoholics should be treated as physiologically sick people and that alcoholism is a disease with pathophysiological origins.

Jellinek coined the expression "the disease model of alcoholism" and significantly altered the belief that addiction is a moral disease to the belief that alcoholism is a medical disease (Jellinek, 1960).

In 1985, Edward John Khantzian, a psychiatrist, psychoanalyst, and professor of psychiatry at Harvard University, published his landmark article, "The Self-Medication Hypothesis of Addictive Disorders," where he further challenged the "abstinence-only" model of substance use. Khantzian originated the self-medication hypothesis of substance use, identifying substances as external modifiers of emotions. Thus, individuals who use substances are not moral failures, but are attempting to self-medicate and thus ameliorate unbearable states of distress rooted in psychological suffering, rather than for pleasure seeking or self-destruction. He believed that it was unreasonable to expect individuals to forfeit what may be the only thing helping them cope (Khantzian, 1985). Khantzian is considered a pioneer in substance use studies and treatment. In his latest book, *Treating Addiction: Beyond the Pain*, he describes individual and group treatments for clients with substance use issues as well as accessible resources for mental health professionals working with this population (Khantzian, 2018).

Alan Marlatt (1941–2011), a clinical psychologist, is often identified as the seminal founder of the Harm Reduction psychotherapy approach. For 30 years he directed the University of Washington in Seattle's Addictive Behaviors Research Center with the philosophy of compassionate pragmatism rather than moralistic idealism (Snyder, 2011). At the Center, he pioneered research in the Harm Reduction psychotherapy approach for treating substance use and addictive behaviors as well as understanding and preventing relapse. Marlatt acknowledged that the only way to therapeutically engage a client using substances was to encourage some degree of personal control. This was a paradigm shift—a view that respected clients' capacity for unlimited change. His methodical research connected the physiological and psychological aspects of addiction. Marlatt rejected the assumption that change was all-or-nothing and theorized that there exists a complex relationship between the mind and body that requires helping clients who are "intrinsically unique" find their own "intrinsically unique" starting points. For example, if a client wanted to drink only three beers per day instead of quitting altogether, he would work with that goal. While abstinence is likely the best possible outcome for clients with a history of heavy and problematic substance use, he saw a person-centered approach as key to addiction treatment.

Marlatt is considered to be a maverick in the field of substance use treatment—a man who went against the zeitgeist of his time as the philosophy of Harm Reduction had not yet been recognized as a viable option for substance use problems. His classic book, *Harm Reduction: Pragmatic Strategies for Managing High-Risk Behaviors*, was published in 1998, and is the first major Harm Reduction book. In this book, rather than insisting on abstinence as a prerequisite to continued treatment, he describes the principles of Harm Reduction and the strategies to minimize self-destructive consequences of substance use and other addictive behaviors. The book discusses meeting substance users "where they're at" and includes community-based services that empower clients to set and meet their own treatment goals. It gives examples of Harm Reduction strategies such as needle exchange programs, alternative alcohol interventions, and AIDS prevention campaigns. An understanding into the often contentious philosophical and policy-related debates surrounding harm reduction are also addressed in his book.

■ PHILOSOPHY AND KEY CONCEPTS OF HARM REDUCTION PSYCHOTHERAPY

Harm Reduction as a philosophy is viewed as a social justice and human rights approach to risky behavior as opposed to a moralistic and criminalizing one. The central tenet is the recognition that many individuals engage in behaviors that carry risk; it seeks to alleviate the potential harm associated with risky behaviors rather than attempting to prohibit them. It supports the view that individuals should not be denied treatment merely because they take risks. The Harm Reduction philosophy encompasses a range of public health practices and has been applied to a number of risky behaviors such as unsafe sex, problematic gambling, and distracted driving. It is characteristically associated with problematic substance use because most of the research and clinical interventions are with this population (Carrico et al., 2014; Gilchrist et al., 2017; Tatarsky & Marlatt, 2010).

As applied to substance use, the Harm Reduction philosophy focuses on positive change. It does not require that individuals stop using substances as a precondition of treatment. Additionally, it does not assume that abstinence is the only acceptable goal, but focuses rather on the reduction of harmful consequences both to the individual and to society. Harm Reduction strategies have been developed for community intervention, such as needle exchange and overdose prevention programs, and have had a positive impact on individual and community health.

Harm Reduction psychotherapy encompasses concepts and interventions to reduce the problematic effects of substance use (Marlatt, 1998). Clients with substance use present a unique challenge to the psychotherapist as the substance use is frequently exacerbated during the course of psychotherapy. Since Harm Reduction psychotherapy is still in its early stages of development, its key concepts will certainly be further developed as the approach progresses. The following are some key concepts in Harm Reduction psychotherapy.

Person-Centered

Harm Reduction psychotherapy is a person-centered approach that views the relationship between the client and therapist as a collaborative partnership. Drawing from the person-centered principles of Carl Rogers, Harm Reduction psychotherapy seeks to address the needs of the client while following the best practice principle of keeping the client engaged in treatment. Trust and respect for the client are central, as well as an open-minded and a nonjudgmental attitude toward substance abuse. A person-centered approach supports the client to work through his or her psychological and substance use issues at his or her own rate of speed (Rogers, 1961). It seeks to acknowledge the client's strengths and efforts with compassion and acceptance. The approach closely tracks the client. For example, if issues related to substance use emerge in therapy, these become the point of discussion; likewise, if psychological issues emerge in therapy, these become the focus of discussion. A person-centered approach recognizes that clients make mistakes and need to have reasonable consequences (Marlatt, 1998).

Incremental Change

Harm Reduction psychotherapy assumes that harm is decreased when individuals are empowered to make small changes in their behavior, specifically designed to reduce harmful consequences. Harmful consequences are seen as varying on a continuum, and the approach encourages and supports small, incremental steps forward in the reduction of these consequences. Incremental behavioral changes can have startlingly positive outcomes in other aspects of the client's life. It encourages and facilitates the client to change and grow psychologically in stages. Harm Reduction psychotherapy meets clients where they are in regard to level of motivation. It returns the locus of control to the client (Logan & Marlatt, 2010).

Therapeutic Progress

A striking difference between Harm Reduction psychotherapy and an abstinence-only model is the definition of therapeutic progress (Logan & Marlatt, 2010). In the abstinence-only model, clients are considered failures if they use any type of substance. As such, clients are denied the gradual development of coping skills implicit in harm reduction. Harm Reduction psychotherapy disregards the notion of a "failed attempt" and instead follows clients' ongoing accountability without a termination philosophy (Hawk et al., 2017). From this position, some degree of recidivism is expected and a "slip" may actually be a helpful learning point rather than a failure (Marlatt & Gordon, 1985).

Psychological Issues

Harm Reduction psychotherapy provides access to underlying psychological issues. As clients make small incremental yet significant changes to their substance use (e.g., a decrease in substance consumption), a point of entry is opened for access to psychological issues. Furthermore, neurobiological changes occur in the brain with incremental changes in substance use, thus opening neural pathways, which facilitate affective and cognitive change (Khantzian, 2018).

■ DEFINITIONS OF MENTAL HEALTH AND PSYCHOPATHOLOGY IN HARM REDUCTION PSYCHOTHERAPY

Harm Reduction psychotherapy does not define mental health and psychopathology in traditional terms. Mental health is defined when clients become aware that they have a problem and that the substance serves some purpose for them, but also has negative outcomes. Eventually, clients desire to change the behavior and begin to move in a direction of decreasing substance use, which decreases negative consequences and improves life quality (Khantzian, 1985). Thus, mental health is a process, and small incremental behavioral changes in substance use precede awareness of underlying psychological issues. As clients continue behavioral change, self-efficacy in the area of substance refusal increases, facilitating them to simultaneously devote time in psychotherapy to these underlying psychological issues.

In Harm Reduction psychotherapy, psychopathology can be defined as using substances as a coping mechanism without an awareness of the problematic nature and consequences of the use. Psychopathology can be viewed as on a continuum as well. The further down the spectrum of use that clients move, the greater the harm, and the more stunted the psychological and physiological health. In this case, perspectives on well-being and functionality of clients become distorted and irrational, and the underlying psychological issues become inaccessible.

■ THERAPEUTIC GOALS IN HARM REDUCTION PSYCHOTHERAPY

Harm Reduction approaches are facilitative rather than coercive, and aim to reinforce positive change in a client's life, no matter how small the increment of change may be. The overarching aim of Harm Reduction psychotherapy is to return the client to a higher level of functioning by decreasing harm caused by substance use. Most important, the clinician has no preconceived notions about the degree of change. The clinician's goals are secondary to what the client wants (Logan & Marlatt, 2010). Ambivalence predominates as part of the stages of change and the clinician rolls with the client's resistance through the ambivalence (Marlatt, 1998; Miller & Rollnick, 2013). While the clinician has an opinion, he or she maintains respect for the client's decisions in regard to change. The treatment plan is the ideal substance use plan, as delineated by the client; it allows the client to define maximum use while concomitantly minimizing harm. Some short-term goals may include the following:

- To change the type of substance consumed
- To decrease the frequency and amount of substances consumed
- To reduce the days and times of consumption
- To reduce the amount of money spent on substances

A long-term goal is often created, but is not required as it may be overwhelming or unnecessary for the client. In Harm Reduction psychotherapy, clients who engage in heavy and problematic use of substances benefit from the development of externally rather than internally motivated short-term goals. Some external goals may include the following:

- To resecure employment
- To make it to work on time
- To reduce debt and get finances in order
- to stop fighting with family members about use

The clinician's responsibility is to help the client estimate the relative reduction in harm that a specific change in substance use or specific change in a behavioral pattern would create. The clinician pays particular attention to harmful outcomes that the client articulates, which have motivated the client to change the consumption pattern. This is done in a stepwise fashion and goals are reviewed in every session. The goals typically change during the course of therapy.

▪ PERSPECTIVE ON ASSESSMENT IN HARM REDUCTION PSYCHOTHERAPY

A robust Harm Reduction assessment aids the client more than the therapist. The clinician's interview encourages the client to perform a self-assessment on patterns of use that are causing harm. Harm is operationalized as any outcome of use that has negative consequences. Harm is both psychological and physiological and often manifests as detrimental to the client's potential success and achievement. Each client will assess different patterns causing harm. For example, one client of Adam Kozikowski's stated that smoking caused him to have difficulty swimming laps at his local Young Men's Christian Association (YMCA), while another client of his stated that smoking caused him to have interpersonal problems with his partner. The assessment helps the client develop a reasonable plan that he or she can implement. The clinician gains an understanding of where the client is now, and where he or she wishes to be on the spectrum of use and functional domains. Patterns of use are identified so that reasonable techniques for change are incorporated into the substance use plan.

The clinician gleans an understanding of the client's relationship with the substance. We always follow Khantzian's rule of empathy and relationship building by asking, "What does the drug do for you?" (Khantzian, 2017). Other key questions include:

- What is the frequency and route of use?
- Is the substance used alone or socially?
- What feelings are elicited with use?
- How much time is spent thinking about the substance?

If we have a client who is binging on a substance such as alcohol, we might ask the question: Does the thought of consumption occur when walking by a liquor store or does it start on Thursday night, when you are anticipating that cold beer after work on Friday? This is a subtle way to encourage the client to consider the role of the substance in anticipatory emotions. If we have a chronic user, we ask about prior attempts to quit and if medication has ever been prescribed to assist in the treatment.

Goals and motivation for change are always assessed. There may be particular problems with outcomes related to the pattern of use that drive the client's desire for change. We often ask, "If there is one thing that you could change about the problems related to your use, what would it be?" It is important for the *client* to identify, in the *here and now*, what is driving the desire to change.

■ THERAPEUTIC INTERVENTIONS IN HARM REDUCTION PSYCHOTHERAPY

Harm Reduction psychotherapy encompasses interventions to reduce the problematic effects of substance use and addictive behavior (Marlatt, 1998). As Harm Reduction psychotherapy is in its early stages of development, additional interventions will undoubtably be added as the therapy advances. The following are some standard interventions in Harm Reduction psychotherapy.

Therapeutic Relationship

Developing a positive therapeutic relationship is essential in Harm Reduction psychotherapy. It is founded in the nonjudgmental approach of Carl Rogers' Person-Centered Psychotherapy and stresses the three facilitative conditions for change: unconditional positive regard, empathic understanding, and genuineness. These conditions help to build rapport and strengthen the therapeutic relationship (Rogers, 1961). The focus is on the subjective reality of the client—the therapist needs to ask himself or herself the question: *Do I understand the client's phenomenological experience?*

Motivational Interviewing

Harm Reduction psychotherapy utilizes the MI techniques of William Miller and Stephen Rollnick and their four central phase processes: engaging, focusing, evoking, and planning. Engaging is the process of establishing a helping connection and working relationship. Similar to Carl Roger's Person-Centered approach, it is nondirective and seeks to understand the client's perspective by using empathic listening and simple and complex reflections. The next three phase processes (focusing, evoking, and planning) are more directive in approach. Focusing is helping the client develop a specific agenda and direction for change in the session. Evoking is eliciting the client's own motivations and arguments for change. Planning is developing a commitment to change and formulating a specific plan of action (Miller & Rollnick, 2013). Other important skills in MI are developing discrepancy (perceiving the difference between what is desired and what is currently occurring as a result of the substance use), rolling with resistance (realizing that the client views the situation differently and understanding the client's perspective and changing direction or listening more carefully and responding in a new way), and promoting self-efficacy (increasing the client's belief in his or her ability to make a change; Miller & Rollnick, 2013).

Redefining Success

Harm Reduction psychotherapy inherently redefines success as it rejects the assumption that any return to use of a substance stops progress. As the abstinence-only model has exposed many clients to judgment, trust is a major problem for many clients. It is important for the client to have a clear understanding that the therapist does not have preconceived ideas about what the client wants or needs. The client is asked to identify his or her perspective on harm. To get to a place of comfort, the client needs to know that the therapist will work with him or her on whatever route the client decides to take. There is one question that is paramount to all others: What do *you* want to do? The client is often incredulous to be asked this question, but it helps to strengthen the therapeutic alliance and for the client to be able to determine the path that he or she chooses.

Identifying Motivating Factors

Motivation to use substances and to change are interwoven. Motivation to consume substances and change behavioral patterns vary based on a variety of factors related to the continuum of use and negative consequences. The therapist's role is to help the client develop an understanding of both the driving force of use—commonly a feeling associated with the use—and the actual outcomes of use. For example, a college-age client may be motivated to binge on alcohol with an anticipatory feeling of excitement during social events and experience few negative outcomes, or a client who consumes an opioid chronically may be motivated to consume in order to avoid withdrawal. The motivation to change may be more internal for the binge-using client, but more external for the addicted client, where use has led to harm in one's social well-being and sense of security. The client with a greater degree of physiological harm may derive more benefit from medication-assisted treatment to bring him or her to a place where there is greater control of behavior.

Gradualism

Gradualism is a hallmark strategy of Harm Reduction skill building and refers to the idea that any change in a positive direction demonstrates a change toward a healthier life (Hawk et al., 2017). Gradualism can be thought of as incrementalism and is an active technique with cognitive, affective, and behavioral components. It is especially advantageous for recovery, for if clients understand the concept of making small changes, they are less likely to revert to old patterns when and if recidivism occurs. It may also significantly impact self-efficacy. Substance users are taught to incorporate incremental changes in many areas of their lives (Boucher et al., 2017).

Incrementalism is also beneficial for therapists for there are not unreasonable expectations, which makes working with the client more rewarding. Therapists and clients work together to develop a substance use plan that incrementally decreases the amount of substance used, thus decreasing the overall harm. Therapists assist clients with incrementalism through skill building, practicing refusal skills, identifying alternative behaviors, redefining success, and considering relapse prevention (Logan & Marlatt, 2010). The therapist explores how much a client wants to use and the problems related to the current use pattern. Then, a reasonable plan is made during therapy. Initially the plan may include changing the time and days of consumption or changing the amount used. During each visit, change is reviewed and the plan is incrementally revised based on the client's needs and desires. The therapist reviews what worked and what did not work, and adjusts the plan with the client. This review of the plan is not rigidly formatted; rather, the Harm Reduction discussion is woven within the context of the session's material.

Practicing Refusal Skills and Relapse Prevention

Refusal skills are key for effective Harm Reduction psychotherapy. Cue cravings and social pressures are very powerful threats to a client's recovery. Refusal skills are developed throughout the course of Harm Reduction psychotherapy and become stronger as the client makes changes. It is believed that perceptions of threat and the efficacy of a health message can influence the client's intention to engage in healthy behaviors (Witte & Allen, 2000). When a client's perceived self-efficacy is greater than the threat, the client often avoids the behavior (Choi, Krieger, & Hecht, 2013). Part of practicing refusal skills is learning to replace the harmful behavior with a healthier behavior. The clinician helps the client choose alternative behaviors in which the client has a strong self-efficacy (Bandura, 2006). As the client sees he or she is able to engage in alternative behaviors, self-efficacy is strengthened. The pivotal question for the therapist to determine is this: What does my client enjoy, is good at, and is healthy for him or her?

■ CASE STUDY

Background

Sally was introduced to me (Dr. Michelle Knapp) as a referral from a colleague who felt Sally needed psychotherapy to address her problematic substance use. An overdose on prescription opioids was the precipitating event that pushed Sally to seek professional care although she had been in denial about her problem for many years. Sally was a high-functioning client with a bachelor's degree in psychology working as an executive producer of a well-known real-life television series on addictions. She had just moved to New York City from the West Coast after a failed marriage in which she and her husband had engaged in infidelity. Sally had no children and felt relatively isolated given that her only living relatives were her mother and father—both of whom had mental illness—living 2,000 miles away. Sally had many resentments from her childhood as her father had untreated bipolar disorder and "put us through hell." Throughout the course of treatment, Sally came to share with me that much of her adolescence was spent moving around the country with her depressed mother in an attempt to escape her father. She developed rather superficial relationships with people and had very few friends; that pattern followed Sally to New York.

At the time I met Sally, she was 38 years old and identified herself as an "existential thinker" who questioned "the purpose" of her life. She had no higher power and did not believe in God, nor did she suspect that the universe had any sort of energy that influenced her existence. Sally had an overwhelming sense of guilt and shame about being addicted to prescription opioids, which she had started using about a decade prior to treat her migraine headaches. She would commonly refer to herself as an "undercover addict." There was a degree of paranoia that she would be "found out for a fraud" and had even requested that the initial screening be performed via a private, untraceable application on a smartphone.

At the beginning of treatment, it was clear that Sally did not like who she was at her core. Although her mother was physically present, she was overly anxious and controlling during her childhood. Sally often assumed the parental role given that her mother had frequent decompensations for which her mother was hospitalized. Sally developed poor patterns of self-regulation yet wanted to control her life without any assistance. She was a lonely person with a tough exterior facade. Sally felt guilty about her infidelity and more guilty about not being able to control the substances she consumed. In fact, during her course of treatment, she would try to manage her own medication regimen by changing her doses and had poor boundaries, often approaching me as her coworker rather than her therapist.

We chose to present this client as her course of treatment is rather typical for a high-functioning client using substances to relieve feelings related to unresolved inner conflict: She had difficulty with self-control, made attempts to abstain believing that abstinence is the ultimate self-control, experienced relapse, struggled with further guilt and shame, and suffered the consequences of subsequent use. With Harm Reduction psychotherapy using a person-centered approach, she was engaging in some degree of self-control, making incremental and gradual changes to her use which ultimately helped her to change. Throughout the course of treatment, the door was never closed and Sally left treatment and returned about five times.

■ TRANSCRIPT OF HARM REDUCTION PSYCHOTHERAPY SESSIONS

Beginning Phase

The first session focused on developing a relationship with the client, identifying the substance use problem and related psychopathological processes. The client was assessed for readiness to change and insight into how substance use has affected her.

APPN:	Hello, I'm glad you were able to make it today.
Sally:	Hi. It's so nice to meet you finally.
APPN:	Can you tell me what led you to come in today?
Sally:	People have been telling me for a long time that they are worried about me. And I've finally gotten to the point where I'm worried about myself.
APPN:	Tell me more about what you are worried about.
Sally:	I feel like I can't get through my day without taking these pills. (*Takes pills out.*) I started taking these pills for a headache years ago, and when I got divorced last year, my use really took off.
APPN:	It sounds like taking these pills does something to help you get through the day. Can you tell me more about what you experience when you take them?
Sally:	Well, when I started using them, it just made the world feel like a better place. Like nothing could go wrong. It was a constant feeling of ease, everything was good. I felt high on life. When I started having problems in my marriage, I would take them, so I didn't feel anything at all—but I wasn't high anymore. That's the problem now, I just don't feel anything. But when I *don't* take them, I feel horrible.
APPN:	When you say you don't feel anything, what's that like for you?

Sally:	That's a good question. I guess it's not that I don't feel anything—I feel lifeless. And without them I feel dead. I guess I feel depressed—if this is what depression feels like.
APPN:	It sounds like it's very uncomfortable to experience these feelings of depression which you are describing. When did you start experiencing the depressed feelings?
Sally:	To be honest, I'm actually not quite sure. But, I think it happened when my husband discovered me in an affair. We had always relied on each other and no one else. Neither one of us believed in any kind of God or higher power, and I started to feel depressed, so I took more pills and one day I almost died. But I don't want to die.
APPN:	That sounds scary. It sounds like you are describing experiencing a great deal of emotional pain. So much that the relief you got from the pills was more important in the moment than your life.
Sally:	I guess that's why I'm here. I feel like I can't live without these pills now. But the scary part is I'm not really sure I *want* to live without these pills.
APPN:	So, you don't want to live without taking these pills, and at the same time it might not be possible to live *with* them. Do you think you really want to stop taking them?
Sally:	I'm not sure. It feels like I'm stuck either way.
APPN:	Tell me how you imagine what your life would be like if you weren't taking these pills.
Sally:	Like I said before, I would just feel depressed. Like it was too painful to do anything—to function.
APPN:	What if we were able to work through these feelings of depression together?
Sally:	That's fine, but I feel like I can't sit in my own skin. I want to crawl out. Can you help me now?
APPN:	Ah . . . I've heard this many times from people. It's very difficult to be uncomfortable. We can certainly give you medication to help you through the discomfort, and it may be helpful to understand that the discomfort is part of the healing process. By working through the feeling, you can learn different ways to manage your feelings, without the medication.
Sally:	I am not so sure that I want to dig that deep. I have a lot of skeletons in my closet.
APPN:	What kind of skeletons?
Sally:	Well, I *was* having an extramarital affair. I am an awful person. And now I am alone and not so sure that I want to be. I never thought I needed anybody. Here I am—successful, have a great career, and money to live. I just moved to NYC. I pretty much have the dream life as others would see it. But I'm not happy. What have I done to f--- up my life? I am not so sure that this can be undone.
APPN:	This is all very distressing.

Sally:	(Crying) Yes. I just don't think I want to talk about my problems. It's too difficult to hear myself.
APPN:	Would you be willing to start looking at these problems, if there was even a small chance that you could feel better? And you control the pace?
Sally:	I don't want anybody to know I am in treatment.
APPN:	And, you don't have to tell anybody.
Sally:	And, I can't really guarantee that I will quit these pills. They work like magic for me . . . but I would be willing to hear you out—at least for a while.
APPN:	I look forward to exploring these experiences further with you. Perhaps together we can gain further insight into your experiences, which could ultimately help you to feel better.
Sally:	I appreciate that. Thank you for listening.
APPN:	It is my pleasure. I look forward to continuing next week.

Middle Phase

The middle sessions function primarily to help the client work through the primary material. Importantly, substance use often reemerges and may worsen during the middle sessions; therefore, integration of MI remains essential.

APPN:	Welcome back. Where would you like to start today?
Sally:	You're going to be so angry with me, I messed up last weekend.
APPN:	Tell me about how you feel you messed up.
Sally:	Things were going so well—I had done all that work to stop. I cut down over all those weeks and was taking my medication (*silence*).
APPN:	(*silence*)
Sally:	But my ex-husband was coming to town and all those feelings came up.
APPN:	Tell me more about *those* feelings. What were you experiencing?
Sally:	I realized I couldn't blame him anymore for our failed marriage. And I heard he was bringing his new girlfriend with him. And it really took me to a dark place. And, I picked up again. I'm really angry with myself. You must be angry with me too.
APPN:	I can hear your disappointment, though I do not feel anger toward you. You have done some deep work here. Let's go back to that moment where you decided to pick up. Give me, in one word, how you felt.
Sally:	Alone. I felt all alone in the world. And we, you and me, we've talked about this. I seem to push people away. Why do you think I do that?
APPN:	So let's go back to the word "alone." I've heard you bring up this idea of being "alone" several times in the past few months. Was there ever a time in your life when you didn't feel alone?
Sally:	Hmmm . . . I can't quite recall.

APPN:	Do you feel alone right now?
Sally:	Not sitting here in front of you, but when I walk out the door I will. And then I want to pick up that bottle. My ex-husband coming here just reminded me, I guess, of how lonely I really am. That maybe all this time I have needed others, but it's easier to get that from a pill.
APPN:	What's "that"? What do you get from the pill?
Sally:	(*silence*)
APPN:	And you might not have that answer.
Sally:	Now that you say this, I have to tell you. The pill didn't do for me what it used to do.
APPN:	You mean that it did not make you feel less alone?
Sally:	No. I actually felt worse.
APPN:	More alone?
Sally:	Yes, and on top of it, I was so angry with myself.
APPN:	And you're still angry with yourself?
Sally:	And I am pissed at my ex for bringing his new girlfriend. It really makes me want to go out again and use.
APPN:	Sally, I am going to push this a bit. We have been working on this for quite some time. What does using do for you?
Sally:	It gives me an escape from my head.
APPN:	So, "it" is using and "it" makes you feel more alone.
Sally:	I am just always looking for that escape.
APPN:	And, what are you escaping from?
Sally:	That's a good question. I just don't know. Myself, I suppose. I just can't seem to get it right, can I? What if I use but just less than I used to?
APPN:	It sounds like that's what you did the other night.
Sally:	(*silence*)
APPN:	Sally, you've stopped and then gone back out to use a few times. Besides feeling more alone, what else can you say came from those experiences?
Sally:	(*crying*)
APPN:	(*silence*)
Sally:	I was more depressed and I almost overdosed at dinner. My friends were there and I had changed my medications up so I could use again— get high. I knew exactly what I was doing. My friends saw me nearly overdose.
APPN:	You mean, your friends saw you nearly *die*?
Sally:	Yes, and I didn't make it to work for 2 days and almost got fired.
APPN:	So, it seems that you've shown you *can* use, but I am curious—do you think it might be more helpful overall *not* to use?

Sally: I haven't really thought of things that way.

APPN: On the flip side, perhaps using is so important to you that you won't give it up, no matter the cost.

Sally: Perhaps . . . but I don't want to feel like my life is controlled by these pills any more. I don't want to struggle with the guilt. I don't want to feel depressed either.

APPN: I hear that. I recall you saying that you were looking for an escape from the difficult feelings. I also hear that the pills can lead to difficult feelings.

Sally: Yes, that's true, I guess. I suppose the negative feelings are there whether or not I use the pills now. They don't really bring that positive feeling, that euphoria.

APPN: I wonder if it's possible to work through those difficult feelings, in this space, in order for them to feel less painful.

Sally: Yeah, that sounds great. Also difficult . . . and scary. I don't want to open something that feels too raw.

APPN: We will move at your pace.

Sally: That idea feels better. I mean, I suppose what I'm getting at is that I would love to feel less depressed about things in my life. And be able to feel that on my own, without taking pills.

APPN: I believe that could be possible.

Sally: It feels too hard to fully believe. But I think there is a part of me that feels like that could be true.

APPN: We can continue to explore this further.

Sally: Yes. I have to be honest that I have been using about three oxycodones every day now. I stopped my other medication.

APPN: Okay. Do you think you want to go back to cutting down?

Sally: Yes. I definitely do.

APPN: What do you think is reasonable for you? How have you been using them? Are you reaching for them at a particular time or when something comes up at work that is particularly stressful, for example?

Sally: (*sighs*) I usually take one at work—when those thoughts start. And then a few more when I get home.

APPN: Okay. Do you want to try taking one less per day until our next session?

Sally: That sounds okay with me.

APPN: So, perhaps one less at night when you get home?

Sally: Sure.

Final Phase

This termination session provides the client an opportunity to reflect on successes and continued work necessary for recovery. And, most important, it provides an open door for the client to return.

APPN:	Hello, I know this will be our last session, and I want to make open the space to reflect on our time together and the work you have accomplished.
Sally:	Hi, I am excited about all I have done. And also a little nervous about moving away from here. From you too.
APPN:	Tell me what comes up for you?
Sally:	Well, I'm extremely proud of my sobriety. But I know I have to keep working on it. I guess I'm still afraid of going back—relapsing. I've had a few along the way.
APPN:	Yes, that is sometimes part of the recovery process, and normal. What I noticed has been your resiliency in managing when you relapsed. Does this resonate with you?
Sally:	I do feel more resilient. . . . Like it has been easier to bounce back. But I do fear that the next time I encounter something difficult, it could lead to me using again.
APPN:	I hear that. I also know that you have developed a greater insight into your experience.
Sally:	I do feel more connected to myself.
APPN:	How so?
Sally:	Well, I guess I just feel more aware of my emotions. I know when I am in a bad mood, and I feel like I have some other ways to manage it— which does not include medicating with opiates. I also know I have a support system—people who I can go to for real support.
APPN:	You've certainly accomplished a lot.
Sally:	Yes, it does feel that way. (*Some noticeable tears*)
APPN:	As you reflect on the great progress you've made, I notice you appear sad.
Sally:	Sometimes I feel like an imposter. Like I can't keep this up. Almost like . . . I don't deserve to be happy or doing well.
APPN:	I still see that either way you've shown a lot of courage. That feels real to me.
Sally:	I suppose so. Sometimes I still need reassurance.
APPN:	I hear that you will need reassurance. I also hear how you've been able to provide support for yourself.
Sally:	True. I know I'm still vulnerable though.
APPN:	Recovery is a process. And you are taking that on. And I also know that the possibility of relapse is very real for many people.
Sally:	Yes, I know.
APPN:	How are you preparing for that possibility? And managing the risks?
Sally:	Well, I have my friend. She has gone through a similar struggle and has been sober for many, many years. She has been a big source of support for me. Also, I do still have my Narcan kit. Just in case. Though

sometimes it is a reminder of my failure. I have already had a chance to tell a few friends, "No." I am practicing that, as you suggested.

APPN: I hear how your kit reminds you of past use. I also see an insight and realistic measure to set yourself up to do well. I see you know the dangers of an overdose, especially after a period of sobriety. I also see how you are supporting yourself in maintaining that sobriety.

Sally: I never really thought about it that way. I guess it feels good to be taking care of my body in that way.

APPN: I feel warm when I reflect on the work you have done.

Sally: I appreciate that. I feel grateful that you challenged me in a gentle way, and never judged me for my choices.

APPN: The space in which we did our work together was only possible by both of us showing up. You have shown some great strengths.

Sally: I am sad about our time together ending. But I am hopeful for the future.

APPN: I acknowledge your sadness and it touches me. Though our time is ending and you are moving away, I believe you have the tools to continue doing great work if you choose to.

Sally: You mean with someone else?

APPN: Yes.

Sally: I hadn't really thought of that. Though I do feel it would be good to continue with my own self growth. I don't really want to lose the progress I have made.

APPN: And what incredible growth.

Sally: Thank you.

Commentary

Sally's presentation is very typical for a client with substance use problems as she arrived with a myriad of reasons for seeking treatment that, in her mind, were not necessarily related to substance use. I (Dr. Michelle Knapp) had worked with Sally for 3 years when she reentered treatment postrelapse to illicit opiate use. The previously described sessions were taken from her initial treatment. The sessions collectively illustrate the typical pattern of recidivism in clients who attempt to abstain: She cut back several times, abstained from use for substantial periods of time, and relapsed to heavy use several times over the course of a few years. Her ambivalence to change during the first session was palpable, which cautioned me against developing a specific, outlined plan to decrease her use. For Sally, Harm Reduction psychotherapy did not incorporate a written taper schedule as that would likely not have worked for her. Negative consequences (relationship problems, near-death experience) were highly motivating for Sally and the content was used as a tool rather than punishment. Sally, like others who have long-term substance use problems, could easily become wary speaking only about the use as she struggles with her role in relationship dynamics. It was important for Sally to address those other issues as she worked to regain her internal locus of control. Gradualism, rolling with the resistance, and practicing refusal skills were all incorporated in subtle ways. Most importantly, while Sally may choose to end psychotherapy at any time, she knows she can return at any time.

DISCUSSION QUESTIONS

1. Can you identify a particular life event, perhaps an outcome of a series of detrimental behaviors, that ignited within you a desire for change?
2. If you were to inventory habits that you have wanted to change for a considerable amount of time, how successful do you believe you would be without making incremental change?
3. Were there any times during the session that you might have felt discouraged by Sally's ambivalence? Would you have handled the session differently?
4. Person-centered, humanistic psychotherapy techniques were used as part of Harm Reduction psychotherapy during Sally's sessions. Are there any other forms of therapy that you might choose to integrate with Harm Reduction psychotherapy?

REFERENCES

Bandura, A. (2006). Guide for constructing self-efficacy scales. In F. Pajares & T. Urdan (Eds.), *Self-efficacy beliefs of adolescents* (pp. 307–337). Greenwich, CT: Information Age.

Boucher, L. M., Marshall, Z., Martin, A., Larose-Hébert, K., Flynn, J. V., Lalonde, C., . . . Kendall, C. (2017). Expanding conceptualizations of harm reduction: Results from a qualitative community-based participatory research study with people who inject drugs. *Harm Reduction Journal, 14,* 18. doi.org/10.1186/s12954-017-0145-2

Carrico, A. W., Flentje, A., Gruber, V. A., Woods, W. J., Discepola, M. V., Dilworth, S. E., . . . Siever, M. D. (2014). Community-based harm reduction substance abuse treatment with methamphetamine-using men who have sex with men. *Journal of Urban Health: Bulletin of the New York Academy of Medicine, 91*(3), 555–567. doi:10.1007/s11524-014-9870-y

Choi, H. J., Krieger, J. L., & Hecht, M. L. (2013). Reconceptualizing efficacy in substance use prevention research: Refusal response efficacy and drug resistance self-efficacy in adolescent substance use. *Health Communication, 28*(1), 40–52. doi:10.1080/10410236.2012.720245

Gilchrist, G., Swan, D., Widyaratna, K., Marquez-Arrico, J. E., Hughes, E., Mdege, N. D., . . . Tirado-Munoz, J. (2017). A systematic review and meta-analysis of psychosocial interventions to reduce drug and sexual blood borne virus risk behaviours among people who inject drugs. *AIDS and Behavior, 21*(7), 1791–1811. doi:10.1007/s10461-017-1755-0

Hawk, M., Coulter, R. W., Egan, J. E., Fisk, S., Friedman, M. R., Tula, M., & Kinsky, S. (2017). Harm reduction principles for healthcare settings. *Harm Reduction Journal, 14,* 70. doi:10.1186/s12954-017-0196-4

Jellinek, E. M. (1960). *The disease concept of alcoholism.* New Haven, CT: Hillhouse Press.

Khantzian, E. J. (1985). The self-medication hypothesis of addictive disorders: Focus on heroin and cocaine dependence. *American Journal of Psychiatry, 142*(11), 1259–1264. doi:10.1176/ajp.142.11.1259

Khantzian, E. J. (2017, February 21). The theory of self-medication and addiction. *Psychiatric Times, 34*(2). Retrieved from https://www.psychiatrictimes.com/addiction/theory-self-medication-and-addiction

Khantzian, E. J. (2018). *Treating addiction: Beyond the pain.* Lanham, MD: Rowman & Littlefield.

Lipari, R. N., & Van Horn, S. L. (2017, June 29). *Trends in substance use disorders among adults aged 18 or older. The CBHSQ report.* Retrieved from https://www.samhsa.gov/data/sites/default/files/report_2790/ShortReport-2790.html

Logan, D. E., & Marlatt, G. A. (2010). Harm reduction therapy: A practice-friendly review of research. *Journal of Clinical Psychology, 66*(2), 201–214. doi:10.1002/jclp.20669

‍

Marlatt, G. A. (Ed.). (1998). *Harm reduction: Pragmatic strategies for managing high-risk behaviors.* New York, NY: Guilford Press.

Marlatt, G. A., & Gordon, J. R. (Eds.). (1985). *Relapse prevention: Maintenance strategies in the treatment of addictive behaviors.* New York, NY: Guilford Press.

Miller, W., & Rollnick, S. (2013). *Motivational interviewing helping people change* (3rd ed.). New York, NY: Guilford Press.

Rogers, C. R. (1961). *On becoming a person: A therapist's view of psychotherapy.* New York, NY: Pearson.

Snyder, A. (2011). Obituary. G. Alan Marlatt (Ed.). *The Lancet, 377*(9781), 1914. doi:10.1016/S0140-6736(11)60801-5

Substance Abuse and Mental Health Services Administration. (2018). *Key substance use and mental health indicators in the United States: Results from the 2017 National Survey on Drug Use and Health* (HHS Publication No. SMA 18-5068, NSDUH Series H-53). Rockville, MD: Center for Behavioral Health Statistics and Quality, Author. Retrieved from https://www.samhsa.gov/data/sites/default/files/cbhsq-reports/NSDUHFFR2017/NSDUHFFR2017.pdf

Tatarsky, A., & Marlatt, G. A. (2010). State of the art in Harm Reduction psychotherapy: An emerging treatment for substance misuse. *Journal of Clinical Psychology, 66*(2), 117–122. doi:10.1002/jclp.20672

Witte, K., & Allen, M. (2000). A meta-analysis of fear appeals: Implications for effective public health campaigns. *Health Education Behavior, 27*(5), 591–615. doi:10.1177/109019810002700506

Eye Movement Desensitization and Reprocessing Therapy: Healing Trauma

Kathleen Wheeler

■ PERSONAL EXPERIENCE WITH EYE MOVEMENT DESENSITIZATION AND REPROCESSING PSYCHOTHERAPY

Soon after completing my master's and doctoral degree in advanced practice psychiatric nursing at New York University in the mid-80s, I wanted to start my own private practice. However, I knew that in order to gain the clinical skills and confidence for this enterprise, I needed first to get more training in psychotherapy. I decided to enroll in a 4-year psychoanalytic program at the Training Institute for Mental Health Professionals in New York City. Notably, I was the first nurse to apply and be accepted by this institute. Following the rigorous program, which required 4 years of coursework, my own personal analysis three to four times per week, a 10-hour caseload of clients at the Institute weekly, and supervision three times per week, I was ready to see clients on my own. Although I found my clients interesting, sometimes the sessions seemed tedious and unfocused as the client free associated and I strived to understand dynamically what was happening in this process and what, if any, interpretation was appropriate at this time for this person. As a nurse, I had worked in acute care and ICUs, so the pace of change for clients in psychotherapy seemed laborious.

After 5 years of a part-time private practice in psychoanalytic psychotherapy and teaching psychiatric nursing at Hunter College, I heard from a colleague and friend about a new, strange therapy from which she said her clients were getting amazing results, Eye Movement Desensitization and Reprocessing (EMDR). I was skeptical but curious and decided to take Part 1 of Basic Training in EMDR, which involved a 3-day weekend with lecture in the morning and practice in the afternoon. Trainees in EMDR are invited to experience EMDR by identifying something disturbing to work on in the afternoon practice sessions with a trainee partner; thus, the power of the process is experienced first-hand.

This training was the beginning of my passion and excitement that has led me on a remarkable healing and intellectual journey for the past 20 years. Three months later, I enrolled in Part 2 of EMDR training, another 3-day weekend, and began consultation with an approved EMDR International Association (EMDRIA) consultant, becoming first certified in EMDR, then an approved consultant, a facilitator for the trainings, and finally an EMDR trainer. The EMDRIA community has been my professional home for the past 20 years and I continue to sponsor EMDR scholars and clinicians at workshops at my university. As an EMDR trainer, I have been privileged to train many licensed mental health professionals in the community, and as the director of our Psychiatric Mental Health Nurse Practitioner (PMHNP) program at my University, I include EMDR trainings in our curriculum in order that our graduate PMHNP students all receive basic training in EMDR therapy.

The power of this remarkable therapy has continued to amaze and fascinate me! When facilitating the process of EMDR in sessions, I cannot predict where the person's associations will go once the desensitization phase of EMDR begins. I am a witness in awe of each person's unconscious and his or her ability to make personal idiosyncratic connections and associations as dysfunctional memory networks are accessed and reconnected. EMDR clinicians learn to stay out of the way and allow the person's own innate self-healing to occur. At first glance, EMDR therapy seems simple and user friendly to the eager therapist who follows the scripted protocol. However, I have found that there is always more to learn as each person is unique, trauma is often complex, and there are nuances to treatment for different client populations and problems. For those with little or no trauma history and only one single distinct trauma, EMDR therapy can resolve the trauma in three to five sessions. However, most clients do not seek out therapy because of a single traumatic incident that has happened. More often, the client comes in with layers of historical trauma and problems of anxiety, depression, relationships, pain, and, in general, difficulties in living that are long-standing that have compromised his or her ability to live fully in the present. Helping others to be all they can be and could have been without the burden of adverse life experiences and trauma is exciting and a profound honor and privilege.

■ FOUNDER OF EMDR PSYCHOTHERAPY

Francine Shapiro, a brilliant humanitarian, developed EMDR in 1989 after her famous "walk in the park" when she noticed that disturbing thoughts seemed to disappear as her eyes tracked back and forth horizontally. As a newly trained behavioral psychologist, she was curious and began experimenting with eye movements with her colleagues and friends. Her subsequent randomized clinical trial (RCT) on veterans with posttraumatic stress disorder (PTSD) was published in 1989 and introduced Eye Movement Desensitization (EMD) treatment as a behavioral technique to be integrated into other therapies. She changed EMD to EMDR once she realized that more was happening than just desensitization. Memories were actually being reprocessed because of the cognitive restructuring, the spontaneous insights, and the increase in self-efficacy. This led to a more integrative information processing paradigm that Shapiro subsequently developed, the Adaptive Information Processing (AIP) model.

Dr. Shapiro recognized early on the importance of research to validate efficacy and to disseminate this powerful treatment. She dedicated her life to advocating for EMDR research; developing EMDR therapy; mentoring and training colleagues; encouraging the establishment and leadership of numerous national and international EMDR organizations, the EMDR Humanitarian Assistance Programs, the EMDR Institute, and the EMDR Research Foundation; and writing articles and books on EMDR therapy. Her intelligence, commitment, compassion, generosity, and humanitarian ideals inspired the EMDR community throughout the world.

Dr. Shapiro died in 2019 at the age of 71 having shepherded EMDR from a simple behavioral technique to a full-fledged psychotherapy approach with established efficacy not only for PTSD but also for a wide range of clinical disorders. At close to 6 feet tall, Dr. Shapiro was an imposing figure and her shyness and humility were sometimes misinterpreted as aloofness. Clinicians, myself included, who were lucky enough to be mentored and trained by her were both in awe and fear of her as she expected no less than excellence from her trainees. Dr. Shapiro's energy, integrity, vitality, and guidance provided a powerful role model for all those who knew her. She continues to live on in the professional standards she set, the research rigor she demanded, and the EMDR protocol she developed to guide practice.

Since EMDR's origin in 1989, there are more than 44 RCTs validating EMDR therapy in the treatment of PTSD and acute trauma and another 28 RCTs for other disorders such as depression, anxiety disorders, substance use, and pain (Maxfield, 2019). EMDR therapy has been included in numerous national and international practice guidelines (de Jongh, Amann, Hofmann, Lee, & Farrell, 2019) and there are EMDR organizations all over the world. EMDR protocols have been translated into Chinese, Danish, Dutch, French, German, Indonesian, Italian, Japanese, Norwegian, Polish, Portuguese, Spanish, Swedish, Thai, and Turkish (Wheeler, 2013). Francine Shapiro's remarkable legacy has been a gift to the world.

▪ PHILOSOPHY AND KEY CONCEPTS OF EMDR

EMDR therapy is a therapeutic approach that emphasizes the brain's information processing system of how memories are stored. EMDR therapy is guided by AIP theory, which Dr. Shapiro developed as foundational to understanding and guiding EMDR therapy. AIP posits that each person has an inherent information processing system that strives for a state of adaptive resolution; that is, information from the environment normally and naturally is taken in and integrated into existing adaptive memory networks. However, when a trauma or distressing event occurs, the memory is stored dysfunctionally and does not get linked up to other adaptive memory networks; instead, the memory is fragmented and stored in its disturbing state as an image, an emotion, a sound, or a sensation.

AIP provides the clinician a conceptual model for practice even if EMDR therapy is not used (Wheeler, 2022a). EMDR therapy is considered an integrative psychotherapy as components of EMDR are compatible with other orientations such as psychodynamic, cognitive, experiential, behavioral, and somatic therapies.

▪ DEFINITIONS OF MENTAL HEALTH AND PSYCHOPATHOLOGY IN EMDR

Shapiro coined the terms *"large t" traumas* and *"small t" traumas*. "Large t" traumas are those that meet Criterion A events for PTSD such as war, incest, natural disasters, and rape, while "small t" traumas are those events that are quite distressing such as humiliations, bullying, loss, and rejections that can be maladaptively stored in memory (Shapiro, 2018). These "small t" traumas can manifest in the present as chronic feelings of being unworthy as well as other false-negative beliefs that permeate all aspects of one's personality. In EMDR therapy, once the past events are processed, then the present triggers are processed, and finally future templates are processed; consequently, the cognitive distortions are replaced with adaptive beliefs, thus resolving the presenting symptoms.

Thus, mental health is viewed as a by-product of neurophysiological processing of traumatic experiences with adaptive resolutions. Connections to appropriate associations are made and information is integrated and available for future use (Shapiro, 2018).

Most psychopathology, not organically based, is conceptualized as originating from past traumatic experiences that have been inadequately processed and consequently maladaptively stored as information in dysfunctional memory. These traumatic experiences retain a high level of sensory and emotional intensity, even years after the original traumatic event occurred. The person's memory can be triggered by present-day internal or external reminders, resulting in activating symptoms such as emotional dysregulation, hyperarousal, intrusive thoughts, and sensory flashbacks that result in mental health problems such as anxiety, depression, dissociation, and PTSD. These symptoms and mental health problems are driven by earlier experiences that are inadequately processed (Shapiro, 2018).

■ THERAPEUTIC GOALS IN EMDR PSYCHOTHERAPY

The goals of EMDR therapy are to

1. identify and reprocess memories informing current problems,
2. strengthen access to adaptive memory networks,
3. eliminate dysfunctional memory networks,
4. incorporate needed skills, behaviors, and beliefs about self/other,
5. achieve effective and efficient treatment effects while maintaining client stability and safety, and
6. bring contentment, satisfaction, and well-being into client's life.

EMDR therapy processes disturbing events and integrates dysfunctional memory networks into adaptive memory networks. The power or influence of these negative experiences is weakened and positive experiences are strengthened in the person's life. Once this is accomplished, the person can be who he or she is meant to be in a healthy life affirming manner.

■ PERSPECTIVE ON ASSESSMENT IN EMDR PSYCHOTHERAPY

Although there is an official Assessment Phase, which is Phase Three in the EMDR protocol, assessment actually begins in Phase One with history taking and treatment planning in order to assess the client's stability and clinical symptoms. Screening for dissociation is usually assessed with the Dissociative Experiences Scale (DES) because if the client is dissociative or in crisis, EMDR therapy should not be initiated. EMDR therapy melts dissociative barriers so that the client who is highly dissociative can quickly destabilize during Phase Four, the Desensitization Phase. Assessment of the client's stability, as well as his or her ability to manage intense emotions and to develop a therapeutic relationship, is essential and ongoing throughout all phases of treatment. A longer Preparation Phase, which is Phase Two, may be needed, especially if the client has suffered significant childhood trauma.

There is an eight-phase protocol for EMDR therapy. Assessment is ongoing and occurs in all of the following phases (Box 14.1).

BOX 14.1 Eight-Phase Protocol for EMDR Therapy

One	History and Treatment Planning—assessment of stability and current life constraints; evaluation of clinical symptoms (affect tolerance and dissociation); screening for use of EMDR; identification of targets including small traumas and big traumas; developing a treatment plan
Two	Preparation—establish therapeutic alliance; educate the client about AIP and EMDR; evaluate secondary gains; practice relaxation and imagery of a safe/calm place; resource development if needed
Three	Assessment—identify components of the target; client identifies an image that represents the experience or worst part of it; an NC associated with the incident or image and a PC that represents what the person would like to feel about himself or herself now; the client then rates the PC on a 1 to 7 VOC scale that represents how true the PC feels now; then the emotions associated with the event are identified with SUD scale on a 0 to 10 rated scale; finally, the person is asked where he or she feels the disturbance in his or her body
Four	Desensitization—begin sets of bilateral stimulation with eye movements, sound, and/or tapping and continue until the SUD is 0 or 1
Five	Installation—install PC with bilateral stimulation
Six	Body Scan—note tension and sensations in body for any residual
Seven	Closure—instruct about keeping a log and educate about disturbances that may occur post session
Eight	Reevaluation—reassess and review targets that were processed at the beginning of the next session

AIP, adaptive information processing; EMDR, eye movement desensitization and reprocessing; NC, negative cognition; PC, positive cognition; SUD, subjective unit of disturbance; VOC, validity of cognition.

The Assessment Phase, Phase Three, begins after the History and Preparation Phases. Targets have been identified through history taking which might include instances recalled from the past of humiliation, rejection, loss, nightmares, or "big t traumas" of disasters, war, and sexual and physical violence. The Assessment Phase asks the client to identify components of the particular target chosen by the client to work on. See earlier Phase Three of EMDR Therapy. Shapiro states that working on the first, worst memory/ event is often the best way to proceed since the generalization effects from reprocessing this memory will spread to other distressing instances, resulting in an overall decrease in fear and anxiety in the client's overall disturbance level (Shapiro, 2018).

■ **THERAPEUTIC INTERVENTIONS IN EMDR PSYCHOTHERAPY**

EMDR therapy is an integrative eight-phase psychotherapy based on a comprehensive three-pronged approach that includes earlier life experience, present-day stressors (i.e., triggers), and desired thoughts and actions for the future. The memory is activated and the therapist guides the client in processing affective, cognitive, and somatic material with procedures and protocols that include some form of bilateral stimulation (BLS) during a session. The BLS may take the form of eyes moving horizontally back and forth, sounds alternating in each ear, or alternate tapping on each hand or knee. Eye movements are preferable because research supports this type of bilateral stimulation as effective (Lee & Cuijpers, 2013).

The bilateral stimulation is thought to decrease the arousal level so that relaxation occurs, allowing for the linkage of the dysfunctional material with more adaptive memory networks (Shapiro, 2018). However, the exact mechanism of action of EMDR therapy is unclear just as other psychotherapies' action/s are unknown, but because EMDR is such an unusual and powerful therapy, there have been many studies designed to understand how it works. It is the first psychotherapy to demonstrate a neurophysiological effect of altered brain wave activity in response to treatment (Pagani, Högberg, Fernandez, & Siracusano, 2012).

■ CASE STUDY

Background

Jean is a 58-year-old woman who was referred to me by her friend because her current therapist, who she had seen for several years, was making her feel "crazy." Jean was told by her therapist that she was too unstable to come only once a week for her psychotherapy sessions and had to come twice a week because she was highly dissociative and that she might try to hurt herself in a dissociated state. Jean had thrown away all of her old prescriptions at the urging of her therapist to ensure that she was safe from herself. Jean had a pervasive feeling of being unsafe and was concerned that she was not perceiving reality correctly. Jean denied any past self-harm or current suicidal ideation. Her goals for therapy with me were to decrease dissociative episodes and her anxiety about safety issues. She scheduled twice a week sessions for 6 months and then decreased to once a week sessions once she felt safe enough and connected enough to trust herself and me.

Phase One: History and Treatment Planning

Since Jean had come to therapy after a betrayal by her previous therapist, special attention was paid in the early months of treatment on developing a therapeutic alliance with her. Supportive psychotherapy techniques were used with open-ended questions, reflections, and summarizing the main points of her sessions, and by carefully listening to Jean's story and concerns. Ensuring good boundaries, being present, and maintaining the frame are essential in cultivating trust and safety in the therapeutic relationship.

A timeline was drawn to illustrate Jean's resources and traumas with a straight horizontal line demarcating chronologically each decade of her life with important positive events and people on the top of the line for each decade and disturbing events and traumas below the horizontal line (see Wheeler, 2022a). Disturbing events were rated on a 0 to 10 Subjective Units of Disturbance Scale (SUDS). Jean was encouraged during her narrative about her history to only give the highlights without the details so that she would not be activated by these disturbing memories during history taking. Alternating the disturbing events with the resources for each decade was a helpful way to help Jean stay emotionally regulated. Jean rarely showed emotion and she intellectualized most events, which kept her safe and on an even keel. However, she was aware of her body sensations, which helped her to access emotions and boded well for processing trauma with EMDR therapy. Many victims of early trauma have difficulty feeling body sensations and need to work to track internal sensations.

Jean reported that she became aware of her early emotional and sexual childhood abuse in her therapy over the past few years. She is the youngest of four children. Her mother was angry, critical, erratic, and distant; hence, Jean's older sister, Doris, played a maternal role in Jean's life. Jean has vague memories of her older brother sexually abusing her when she was around 4 years old as well as her sister Doris and Doris' boyfriend sexually abusing her starting around age 12 and throughout her adolescence. Jean suffered chronic bladder infections as a child for which she received painful medical treatment aimed at dilating her urethra between ages 4 to 6. As a teenager, Jean drank and took drugs and was sexually promiscuous. Despite her tumultuous history, Jean graduated from college cum laude with a degree in accounting and began working at an accounting firm where she met her husband with whom she had two children. Ten years later, she divorced her husband because he was emotionally abusive. Jean has raised her children on her own with minimal help and involvement from their father, and has been a stay at home mom for the past 20 years.

Jean is estranged from her family of origin. Her father and brother are now deceased and her mother and two older sisters live near each other where she grew up in Tennessee. Fourteen years ago, Jean quit drinking alcohol and now attends three to four Alcoholics Anonymous (AA) meetings a week. She serves as a sponsor in AA and has a wide network of female friends as a support system. Two years ago, Jean was diagnosed with an autoimmune disorder, which causes her a lot of joint pain and fatigue. Medications at intake included topiramate (Topamax) 100 mg and vilazodone (Viibryd) 30 mg for the past 10 to 11 years.

For clients like Jean who have suffered pervasive childhood trauma, there may not be one specific event to target. Target is the term used to identify memories for reprocessing in EMDR therapy. For clients with complex trauma, it is often helpful to identify clusters of events that have similar negative beliefs as a starting point. Jean said she had a fear of being abducted, raped, and disappearing. Jean did not identify her memories of sexual abuse as highly disturbing during history taking. She wanted to feel safer, decrease her dissociation, and decrease current triggers in the many situations that increased her anxiety. The most disturbing experiences were current triggers of threats to her safety such as walking her dogs past two men or fears of safety in her own home. It was decided that these would be appropriate first targets for EMDR therapy once Jean was stabilized, and this was discussed with Jean. In addition, how EMDR works was explained in order for Jean to decide if she wanted to see if EMDR therapy would decrease her anxiety around safety issues. The following statement was made to Jean and is typical for all clients seen for EMDR therapy:

APPN: When a disturbing event occurs, it can get locked in the brain with the original picture, sounds, thoughts, feelings, and body sensations. This material can combine factual material with fantasy and with images that stand for the actual event or feelings about it. EMDR seems to stimulate the information and allows the brain to process the experience. That may be what is happening in REM or dream sleep—the eye movements (or tones or tactile stimulation) may help to process the unconscious material. It is your own brain that will be doing the healing and you are the one in control.

Phase Two: Preparation

Due to Jean's early childhood trauma and the betrayal by her last therapist, the first 6 months of Jean's therapy focused on stabilization and building up resources through an imagery of a calm place exercise, circle of friends, deep breathing, light stream container, butterfly hug, and other imagery in order to strengthen her window of tolerance or resilient zone (Wheeler, 2022a). Slow BLS with eye movements were used to further strengthen her resources. This gave Jean a demonstration of what the eye movements would be like when the disturbing experiences were reprocessed later. Since Jean identified dissociation as a problem, special attention was given to grounding strategies such as noticing her feet on the floor and the couch supporting her body. It is particularly important for clients with complex trauma to remain oriented to the present when accessing traumatic memories. She was taught "the back of the head" technique that gives the therapist information about the client's present orientation during sessions. This technique and script to assess moment-to-moment dissociation is included in Knipe's *EMDR Toolbox* (2019).

The DES (included in Chapter 3 of Wheeler, 2022b) was administered. Most items were not significant except for one item where she indicated that she had no memory for some important events in her life, such as her graduations from high school and college and her wedding. She indicated that these memory lapses occurred 70% of the time. Jean was reassured that she was not highly dissociative as other items on the scale were not significant, and she did not exhibit significant symptoms of dissociation such as being slow to respond, spacing out during conversation, or feeling out of touch with her surroundings. Since her score on the Beck Depression Inventory was 16, indicating only mild depression, the Topamax and Viibryd were tapered and discontinued as her resources were enhanced and other strategies to manage anxiety and depression, such as exercising, walking, music, and Pilates, were integrated into her life. These activities decreased her overall sympathetic arousal, so Jean could stay in the "window of tolerance" (her resilient zone).

Phase Three: Assessment

The initial EMDR Therapy processing sessions (Phases Three to Eight) were successful for the targets of safety and Jean experienced subsequent decreased anxiety about safety issues. Previously, she had been afraid to walk outside in her neighborhood for fear of being attacked and she also had an elaborate alarm system installed in her house but now noted that she did not feel the need to turn it on and she could walk her dogs without fear. Other initial targets included her joint pain when she experienced flare-ups of her autoimmune disorder. These sessions left her remarkably pain free for short periods of time, but her pain returned periodically, limiting her mobility but much less frequently than before. A number of RCTs have found that EMDR therapy deceases pain for many different pain conditions (Tesarz, Wicking, Bernardy, & Seidler, 2019).

The following session is reported here to give the reader an idea of how a typical EMDR therapy session unfolds. Jean began the session by stating that she felt physically better since starting a 1-month trial dose of steroids for her autoimmune disorder. She said that when she was in so much pain before, she felt that she had to put a barrier between herself and her pain so that she did not acknowledge her pain and that somehow she felt she was responsible for her pain and autoimmune disorder because she had been sexually abused as a child. Jean also recounted how she felt about a friend who had recently betrayed her and that somehow even though she knew it wasn't true, she felt that it was her fault.

From an AIP perspective, the current triggers of pain and betrayal are often due to earlier past memories that the person is either unaware of or only dimly aware of that are not fully conscious. Once these are known and processed, the triggers for the pain and betrayal will decrease. A float back was initiated to see if she could access any past memories that may be triggering her current symptoms with her false negative beliefs about herself: "I'm doing something wrong." and "There's something wrong with me." We began with the trigger of the friend's betrayal as that seemed to be the most activated memory at the moment.

APPN:	As you bring up the recent experience of June betraying you, notice the image that comes to mind, the negative thoughts you're having about yourself (*negative cognition [NC]*) "I've done something wrong" along with the sadness (*emotion*). Where do you feel that in your body (*sensations*)?
Jean:	My throat is tightening and in my stomach.
APPN:	OK, let your mind float back to an earlier time in your life when you thought "I'm doing something wrong," felt sad, and had that same feeling in your throat and stomach, and just notice what if anything comes to mind . . . ."
	(*Silence for a few moments while Jean reviews earlier memories.*)
Jean:	Mom used to shake me when something bad happened to me; like one time I got hit by a bike and my mom grabbed me and shook me.
APPN:	Is it OK to do some bilateral eye movements as you think about this memory?
Jean:	Yes.
APPN:	What picture represents the worst part of the experience as you think about it now?
Jean:	The look on her face like she was really mad.
APPN:	What words go best with that picture that express the negative belief you're having about yourself as you think of it now?
Jean:	I'm doing something wrong. (*NC*)
APPN:	So now as you think about this memory of Mom shaking you after the bike hit you, what would you like to think about yourself instead of "I'm doing something wrong"?
Jean:	I did the best I could. (*positive cognition [PC]*)
APPN:	How true does that feel to you on a 1 to 7 scale with 7 being the most true? (*validity of cognition [VOC]*)
Jean:	I guess I do think that now.
APPN:	But when you float back to that memory, how true does "I did the best I could" feel for you now on a 1 to 7 scale with 1 not true at all and 7 absolutely true? (*VOC*)
Jean:	Hmmm, maybe a 2 or 3?
APPN:	And the emotion?
Jean:	Sadness.

APPN:	On a 0 to 10 scale with 0 being no disturbance at all and 10 being the highest disturbance you can imagine, how disturbing does it feel to you now? *(SUD)*
Jean:	A 6 maybe.
APPN:	Where do you feel that in your body?
Jean:	My throat and stomach.

Phase Four: Desensitization

APPN:	Often we will be doing a simple check on what you are experiencing. I'll ask you to give me brief feedback as to what is happening. Sometimes things will change and sometimes they won't. There are no supposed to's in this process. So just give as accurate feedback as you can as to what is happening without judging whether it should be happening or not. Just let whatever happens, happen. Remember, you have your STOP signal should you need it.
APPN:	I'd like you to bring up that image and the words "I'm doing something wrong" *(NC)*, the sadness, and notice where you feel it in your body; and follow my fingers. *(20 to 24 BLS are directed by APPN facilitating horizontal eye movements.)*
Jean:	Another time I got lost in the mall and she did the same thing . . . started shaking me.
APPN:	Just notice . . . go with that . . . *(BLS)*.
Jean:	We weren't allowed to laugh or run in the house or Mom would get mad; I spent a lot of time at the neighbor's house.
APPN:	Just notice . . . go with that . . . *(BLS)*.
Jean:	I was a bed wetter; . . . just existing is doing something wrong . . . .
APPN:	Go with that . . . *(BLS)*.
Jean:	It's too painful to think people would hurt me now so if I cause it, then it's not so hurtful.
APPN:	Go with that . . . *(BLS)*.
Jean:	*(crying)* I just thought about when my mom told me that I was a surprise and unplanned.
APPN:	It's OK, it's old stuff, just go with that . . . *(BLS)*.
Jean:	*(crying)* Like me being born was a problem . . . I did something wrong by being born . . . .
APPN:	Go with that . . . *(BLS)*.
Jean:	*(crying)* I'm still in the way . . . she didn't want me to visit last year because I'm not wanted . . . .
APPN:	Go with that . . . *(BLS)*.

Jean:	I do everything so differently with my kids; I got such a nice note from Louis after he visited for the holidays . . . I always wanted to feel close to him so getting that sweet note made me feel so great.
APPN:	Go with that . . . (*BLS*).
APPN:	OK, so go back now . . . what do you get now?
Jean:	Now I have a headache; I did feel loved by my father but he didn't stick up for me.
APPN:	(*BLS*) (*switched to tappers from eye movements because of headache*)
Jean:	I was surprised when she said that about me not being planned since I was the youngest, my mom usually picked on my older brother and father, not me.
APPN:	Go with that . . . (*BLS*).
Jean:	No one said anything when Mom said that . . . Doris, my older sister, was usually kind to me but I don't remember her saying something nice to me like: "Don't worry sweetie, you are loved."
APPN:	Go with that . . . (*BLS*).
Jean:	(*crying*) Thinking now of Doris betraying me when I was 12 and making me have sex with her boyfriend . . . .

Jean had accessed another disturbing memory network and we only had 10 minutes left in the session so I needed to close down this session so Jean could leave the session in a calm state. This is called Closure of an Incomplete Session.

APPN:	It is so sad. I'm sorry Jean but we only have 10 minutes left and I want to make sure that we can put away some of these sad feelings that have come up today. How big a container would you need to put all these disturbing feelings away?
Jean:	Not big, really, I am OK.
	(*Silence while Jean composes herself*)
APPN:	You did a really good job sticking with some very painful feelings here today. Processing may continue after our session. You may or may not notice new insights, thoughts, memories, physical sensations, or dreams. Some people find it helpful to journal between sessions. We'll talk about it at our next session. Remember to use your resources such as calm place or exercise as needed this week.

Although a float back was used at the beginning of the Assessment Phase for this session, a float back is usually done in Phase Two, Preparation, when targets are identified for processing. However, often clients with complex trauma such as Jean do not have specific memories of trauma but have many experiences of trauma so that it is difficult to identify a discrete trauma to target. Thus, the present trigger can be the portal of entry leading to the most significant past memory for processing (Figure 14.1).

The earlier session was an incomplete session as Phases Five to Eight were not completed since we ran out of time. Once the SUD decreases to a 0 or perhaps a 1, Phases Five to Seven can be completed. When Jean came in the following week, we reevaluated the work from the previous session. Often, processing continues after the EMDR session, so it is important to evaluate when the person comes to his or her next session

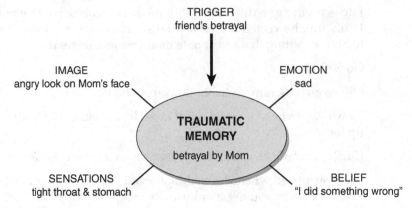

FIGURE 14.1 Components of floatback memory.

because the target memory may be completely reprocessed between sessions. It is important to complete all eight phases of the protocol and then to install a future template so that the person will not be triggered in the future. Sometimes education is needed in order for the person to incorporate a future positive action. For example, if there has been early sexual abuse, education about sexual safety and assertiveness may be needed before the person feels comfortable dating.

Phase Eight: Reevaluation at the Next Session

APPN:	As you bring to mind the memory we focused on during our last session, what are you noticing now?
Jean:	I never realized I felt that way before.
APPN:	What do you mean?
Jean:	How sad I was that my mom said that and how me just being born made me feel that I had done something wrong.
APPN:	OK, bring up that memory now of your mom saying that. What emotions are you experiencing now?
Jean:	Sad.
APPN:	On a scale from 0 to 10, how disturbing is it?
Jean:	Hmmm . . . I know it isn't good but I don't feel upset about it now. My mom was horrible and mean and that wasn't my fault.
APPN:	So how disturbing is that to you now on a 0 to 10?
Jean:	Maybe a 1. Like it happened but I know my father loved me and Doris too. I know my kids love me and I bend over backward to let them know that they are loved so they don't feel like I did.

Phase Five: Installation

APPN:	So last week you wanted to think "I did the best I could." Is that still the way you would like to feel when you think about this?

Jean:	No, I think I would like to feel "I am lovable" as I know I did the best I could.
APPN:	Think about the memory and the words "I am lovable" (*PC*). On a 1 to 7 scale, how true do those words "I am lovable" feel to you now? (*VOC*)
Jean:	A 7. I do know I am lovable.
APPN:	Hold the memory in mind and the words "I am lovable" together and follow my fingers . . . (*BLS*).

Phase Six: Body Scan

APPN:	Now close your eyes and keep in mind the original experience and the words "I am lovable." Bring your attention to the different parts of your body, starting with your head and working downward. Any place you find any tension, tightness, or unusual sensation, tell me.
Jean:	Nothing . . . am I supposed to feel something?
APPN:	There are no supposed to's but last week you felt tightness in your throat and stomach. Just think of the memory and scan your body to make sure it is OK . . . (*BLS*).
Jean:	No, there is nothing there. I am OK even though that happened.

Phase Seven: Closure

APPN:	(*Jean's calm place exercise completed the session*) You did a really good job today revisiting this. Other memories, thoughts, or feelings may come up this week. Journaling can be helpful as well as being sure to take good care of yourself.

Commentary

These transcripts illustrate EMDR therapy with a client with complex trauma. Jean taps into emotions of sadness as she remembers how unloved and betrayed she felt as a child. She tends to intellectualize and rarely expresses emotion so this was an important step for her to be able to feel deeply her sadness. This session illustrates how memories are connected by emotion as she then remembers being betrayed by her mom and her sister. Her initial goal for therapy to feel safe was met during the first 6 months of therapy. Her feelings of responsibility/defectiveness then came to the foreground and involved pervasive feelings of guilt and thoughts that she did something wrong. As Jean realizes during her processing: "It's too painful to think people would hurt me now so if I cause it; then it's not so hurtful." This is common thinking among children who are abused and often persists into adulthood with deep feelings of guilt that they have done something wrong without any understanding why. Jean's insight during the session *"that blaming herself kept her from the painful awareness that she was hurt by those who were supposed to love her"* seemed to have helped her to move away from her pervasive feelings that she is doing something wrong, as she then changes her positive cognition from one of self-blame: *"I did the best I could"* to that of *"I am lovable."* Jean's spontaneous insight is common in EMDR therapy as is her emotional catharsis. Through desensitizing and processing these dysfunctional memories, she was able to link into more adaptive memory networks and mourn the loss of the love she never felt from her mom.

Present triggers of betrayal by her friend were then targeted with the EMDR protocol and a future template, which is the last prong of the EMDR therapy, was installed. This involves identifying a future situation similar to the present trigger where a more adaptive response occurs. Jean imagined her friend betraying her in the future and responding as she would like to respond without being triggered and remaining calm. This imagery was reinforced with BLS. Jean has made good progress in therapy this past year and collaborative goals for EMDR resourcing and processing will continue to guide our future work together.

DISCUSSION QUESTIONS

1. Can you think of clients who would benefit from EMDR therapy?
2. Do a timeline on yourself as described earlier and then write a summary paragraph about your resources and what you feel still needs to be worked on so you can live a full life.
3. Keep a log of triggers (disturbing experiences) for a week and for each trigger, state the image/incident, thought, emotion, and body sensation to deepen your awareness of your own triggers.
4. Fill out DES (online) and score it. Keep track with a log how many times you notice yourself dissociating over the course of the week.

REFERENCES

de Jongh, A., Amann, B. L., Hofmann, A., Lee, C. W., & Farrell, D. (2019). Status of EMDR therapy in the treatment of posttraumatic stress disorder 30 years after its introduction. *Journal of EMDR Practice and Research, 13*(4), 261–269. doi:10.1891/1933-3196.13.4.261

Knipe, J. (2019). *EMDR toolbox: Theory and treatment of complex PTSD and dissociation* (2nd ed.). New York, NY: Springer Publishing Company.

Lee, C. W., & Cuijpers, P. (2013). A meta-analysis of the contribution of eye movements in processing emotional memories. *Journal of Behavior Therapy & Experimental Psychiatry, 44*, 231–239. doi:10.1016/j.jbtep.2012.11.001

Maxfield, L. (2019). A clinician's guide to the efficacy of EMDR therapy. *Journal of EMDR Practice and Research, 13*(4), 239–246. doi:10.1891/1933-3196.13.4.239

Pagani, M., Högberg, G., Fernandez, I., & Siracusano, A. (2013). Correlates of EMDR therapy in functional and structural neuroimaging: A critical summary of recent findings. *Journal of EMDR Practice & Research, 7*(1), 29–38. doi:10.1891/1933-3196.7.1.29

Shapiro, F. (2018). *Eye Movement Desensitization and Reprocessing (EMDR)* (3rd ed.). New York, NY: Guilford Press.

Tesarz, J., Wicking, M., Bernardy, K., & Seidler, G. H. (2019). EMDR therapy's efficacy in the treatment of pain. *Journal of EMDR Practice & Research, 13*(4), 337–344. doi:10.1891/1933-3196 .13.4.337

Wheeler, K. (2013, September). *25 years of EMDR.* Presented at EMDRIA Annual Conference, Austin, TX.

Wheeler, K. (Ed.). (2022a). *Psychotherapy for the advanced practice psychiatric nurse: A how-to guide for evidence-based practice* (3rd ed.). New York, NY: Springer Publishing Company.

Wheeler, K. (2022b). Stabilization for trauma and dissociation. In K. Wheeler (Ed.), *Psychotherapy for the advanced practice psychiatric nurse: A how-to guide for evidence-based practice* (3rd ed., pp. 000–000). New York, NY: Springer Publishing Company.

The Trauma Resiliency Model®: A Client With Chronic Trauma

Linda Grabbe

■ PERSONAL EXPERIENCE WITH THE TRAUMA RESILIENCY MODEL®

My first exposure to the Trauma Resiliency Model (TRM) came when I was a post-master's certificate program student in a psychiatric-mental health nurse practitioner program. I had 20 years of experience as a family nurse practitioner taking care of a highly traumatized population in Atlanta: homeless women, children, and young adults as well as impoverished women in addiction treatment. Because the mental health needs of this population were largely unmet, I was seeking a form of therapy that could be helpful and healing from trauma. By far the kindest approach that I found was TRM, which, although a trauma-processing model, does not require that a trauma story be told. I participated in both level one and level two TRM trainings, offered through the Trauma Resource Institute in California. I was doubly attracted to this model because of the large emphasis placed on self-stabilization skills, which can be taught separately as the Community Resiliency Model® (CRM).

■ FOUNDERS AND LEADERS OF THE TRM

The origin of TRM was serendipitous. A number of international, natural disasters occurred in the early 2000s, resulting in a worldwide effort to offer emergency assistance. In response to the tidal wave in Southeast Asia, to earthquakes in Haiti and China, and to hurricanes in the Philippines and the United States, many healthcare providers and mental healthcare providers lent their assistance. A number of the mental healthcare practitioners were trained in Somatic Experiencing®, a long-term, body-oriented approach to healing trauma developed by Peter Levine. Due to the necessity for brief interventions under disaster conditions, many of these therapists simply provided basic sensory awareness, self-regulation skills to trauma survivors, usually in one or two encounters. Research published subsequently on these survivors demonstrated reduced incidences of posttraumatic stress disorder (PTSD; M. L. Leitch, 2007; M. L. Leitch, Vanslyke, & Allen, 2009; Parker, Doctor, & Selvam, 2008). These sensory awareness, self-regulation skills evolved and were taught to hundreds of Sichuan earthquake first responders, that is, physicians, nurses, teachers, and social workers, who used the skills for their own well-being and to teach to the trauma survivors (L. Leitch &

Miller-Karas, 2009). Elaine Miller-Karas, Geneie Everett, and Laurie Leitch went on to co-develop TRM and CRM.

Miller-Karas recognized that the stabilization skills of CRM might work effectively for survivors with chronic trauma exposure. Under a grant from the state of California, CRM skills were taught to members of several marginalized groups, who subsequently demonstrated beneficial mental health effects, including decreases in depression, hostility, anxiety, and somatic symptoms and increases in relaxation, contentedness, and somatic well-being. The vast majority of participants used the stabilization skills of CRM daily to manage their stress (Citron & Miller-Karas, 2013). A study of a single CRM class for impoverished women in addiction treatment reveled that somatic complaints, anger, and anxiety symptoms declined significantly with a moderate to large effect size (Grabbe, Higgins, Jordan, Gibson, & Murphy, 2020). CRM's first randomized controlled trial found that nurses who received a 3-hour CRM class demonstrated improved well-being, resilience, secondary stress, and physical symptoms (Grabbe, Higgins, Baird, Craven, San Fratello, 2019).

TRM has taken its place alongside other body-based psychotherapies including Levine's Somatic Experiencing (Levine, 1997, 2010; Payne, Levine, & Crane-Godreau, 2015), Heller and LaPierre's NeuroAffective Relational Model (Heller & LaPierre, 2012), Ogden's Sensorimotor Psychotherapy (Ogden & Fisher, 2015; Ogden, Minton, & Pain, 2006), Rothschild's Somatic Trauma Therapy (Rothschild, 2000, 2010, 2017), and Steele, Boon, and Van der Hart's Integrative Therapy for Complex Trauma and Structural Dissociation (Steele, Boon, & Van der Hart, 2017). These innovative, body-centered psychotherapies all use the perception of body sensations to treat symptoms of PTSD and other trauma-related problems. TRM addresses the diagnosis of Complex PTSD (CPTSD) with its six symptom clusters: the three PTSD criteria of reexperiencing, avoidance, and hypervigilance and the three self-organization disturbances of emotional dysregulation, interpersonal difficulties, and negative self-concept included in the *International Classification of Diseases-11* (Jowett, Karatzias, Shevlin, & Albert, 2020).

TRM is an individual psychotherapy comprised of nine self-stabilization and trauma-processing techniques. The first six of these techniques are considered standalone, self-care interventions and may be taught as the CRM wellness skills to community groups, with significant public health implications. The last three techniques are for trauma processing. These do not take place until the ability to stabilize emotionally is firmly in place and the client has learned the first six wellness skills.

■ PHILOSOPHY AND KEY CONCEPTS OF THE TRM

Somatic therapies have evolved over time from the cathartic approaches of Wilhelm Reich's Character Analysis (1945/1980) and Alexander Lowen's Bioenergetics Analysis (1958) to the contemporary approaches of Peter Levine's Somatic Experiencing (Levine, 1997) and Pat Ogden's Sensorimotor Psychotherapy (Ogden & Fisher, 2015). All of the somatic, body-based therapies have a belief that trauma impacts the body, especially the nervous system, and that psychotherapeutic approaches need to work with the body in order to heal. Body-based therapies give clients a chance to rewire their nervous system and learn more adaptive ways to deal with traumatic triggers (van der Kolk, 2015). TRM is based on the following key concepts:

- Human responses to threat are primitive, instinctual, and physiological in nature. Threat, stress, and trauma may overwhelm the normal cognitive processes that allow for reasoned decision-making and reflection. TRM's body-based approach focuses on conscious awareness of autonomic nervous system responses to stress as a preventative and healing modality.

- Responses to trauma may be persistently lodged in the mind and body, to the extent that emotion regulation is extremely difficult or impossible. In particular, subcortical regions of the brain (amygdala, thalamus, hippocampus, hypothalamus, and brainstem) may be deregulated by trauma (van der Kolk, 2015).
- Attempts to cope with the residual effects of trauma may include maladaptive behaviors and psychiatric disorders. These may include mood and anxiety disorders, somatization disorders, obsessive-compulsive disorders, eating disorders, and substance use problems as well as self-injurious behaviors and violence. Nevertheless, even in cases of severe and long-lasting trauma, resilient individuals are often able to survive and thrive.
- Positive biological adaptations in the brain are a feature of resilience; however, they depend on multiple factors and mediators (Gröger et al., 2016; Horn, Charney, & Feder, 2016). Resiliency, a skill that may be learned, is the ability to identify and use individual and collective strengths to live fully in the present moment and to thrive while managing the tasks of daily living (Miller-Karas, 2015). The body has an inherent but unarticulated healing capacity if individuals can learn how to draw on it.
- Sensory awareness of internal bodily states (also called interoception or "felt sense") may be cultivated and offers opportunities for preventing and treating stress and trauma disorders (van der Kolk, 2015; van der Werff, van den Berg, Pannekoek, Elzinga, & van der Wee, 2013). Van der Kolk states that sensory awareness may be the most fundamental way to redevelop a sense of self, live life fully again, and regain self-mastery by "allowing the body to have experiences which deeply and viscerally contradict the helplessness, rage, or collapse that result from trauma" (van der Kolk, 2015, p. 3).

▪ DEFINITION OF MENTAL HEALTH AND PSYCHOPATHOLOGY IN THE TRM

Mental health in TRM is defined as being aware of one's responses to stress and trauma, noticing where in the body emotional distress registers, and having the present-moment awareness skills to shift into a more resilient state of well-being. Psychopathology occurs in hyper- or hypo-aroused autonomic states without the understanding that these states are the result of a destabilized nervous system. TRM depathologizes psychiatric conditions of anxiety (agitation, anger, panic), depression (sadness, isolation, anhedonia), and dissociation (disconnection, derealization, depersonalization) by educating patients about symptoms of excess sympathetic or parasympathetic discharge, using the concept of the Resilient Zone (RZ). The RZ is the bandwidth of stress tolerance—the state where individuals are capable of dealing with whatever is thrown their way and can think clearly, and, if challenged, think through options and make decisions based on rational thought processes (see Figure 15.1).

Physical, emotional, and behavioral responses to stress and trauma are explained as normal biological processes, and unhealthy coping behaviors (e.g., substance use, self-injurious behavior, violence) are viewed as attempts to adapt. Clients who practice TRM self-regulation skills view themselves more compassionately, and with this greater self-understanding spend more time in their RZ and develop a wider zone over time. Clients learn that all persons (including the therapist) are sometimes "bumped-out" of their RZ due to stressful and traumatic events and triggers (Figure 15.2) and that these responses are about biology, not moral or psychological weakness and failure. As traumatic stress symptoms are normalized, feelings of shame and self-blame are reduced or eliminated.

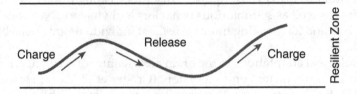

FIGURE 15.1 The resilient zone. When functioning within one's resilient zone, flexibility and adaptability in body, mind, and spirit can be achieved at the highest capacity. CRM skills help widen the resilient zone.

CRM, Community Resiliency Model.

Source: Reproduced with permission from Elaine Miller-Karas, MSW, LCSW. Trauma Resource Institute.

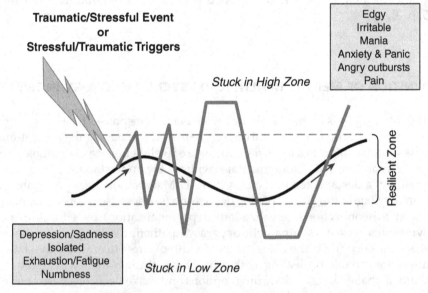

FIGURE 15.2 Stressful and traumatic events and triggers. Depiction of stressful and traumatic triggers and events influencing one's Resilient Zone. Individuals may become stuck in a "high zone" or "low zone," and exhibit behaviors indicative of one zone or the other.

Source: Adapted by Elaine Miller-Karas from an original graphic by Levine/Heller. Reproduced with permission from Elaine Miller-Karas, MSW, LCSW. Trauma Resource Institute.

■ THERAPEUTIC GOALS IN THE TRM

Healing occurs through the release of blocked energy held in the body after overwhelming stress and trauma. TRM aims to bring healing to clients through invitation, respect, and choice and by helping them identify resources that are their own internal strengths. Clients learn that they can reset their own nervous system and return to feeling more in control through the TRM self-care techniques of self-soothing and self-compassion. Clients who understand their stress and trauma responses, in particular body symptoms of distress, are able to identify resources from within to feel better and return to a state of resilience. In essence, clients produce their own "best medicine" to deal with distress (Miller-Karas, 2015). Clients' own sensory awareness is the key instrument of therapy. One of the most important goals of TRM is to help clients recognize and identify sensations connected to their RZ. When clients actively use TRM skills, they become empowered and hopeful about the future.

■ PERSPECTIVE ON ASSESSMENT IN THE TRM

In TRM, the establishment of a therapeutic relationship based on an atmosphere of trust and comfort is essential. The model is explained in the first session, along with the assurance that TRM skills may be practiced only to the extent that is acceptable and comfortable to the client. While some clients may be more aware of sensations in their body and readily learn to localize and name these sensations, the skill may be new to other clients. These clients may feel uncomfortable at first with practicing the skills and that is fine. It is important to state upfront that although TRM assists clients in healing from trauma, specific trauma stories do not need to be told for trauma processing to occur. If it seems appropriate, the Adverse Childhood Experiences (ACEs) screening tool may be used. When using this instrument, it is the number of ACEs that is more important than the specific events that occurred (Felitti et al., 1998).

Once the therapeutic relationship is established, a more detailed history can be obtained including a mental state exam and health history. One way of gathering important life information is by using an Event History Calendar (Yi, Lori, & Martyn, 2008). This calendar elicits life events in a timeline, and includes successes and losses. A chronologic horizontal line identifies the life span in increments of years while the vertical line identifies variable life categories (see Table 15.1). The client completes this timeline on his or her own, or with the advanced practice psychiatric nurse (APPN), who can add notes when discussing it.

TABLE 15.1 EVENT HISTORY CALENDAR

	0–10 Years	11–20 Years	21–30 Years	31–40 Years	41–50 Years +
Living situations					
Relationships					
Life events					
Health					

(continued)

TABLE 15.1 EVENT HISTORY CALENDAR (*CONTINUED*)					
	0–10 Years	11–20 Years	21–30 Years	31–40 Years	41–50 Years +
Health risk behaviors					
Etc.					

Source: Data from Yi, C. H. (Gina), Lori, J, and Martyn, K. (2008). Development of prenatal event history calendar for Black women. *Journal of Obstetric, Gynecologic & Neonatal Nursing, 37*(4), 464–473. https://doi.org/10.1111/j.1552-6909.2008.00255.x.

▪ THERAPEUTIC INTERVENTIONS IN THE TRM

Therapeutic Relationship

TRM focuses on establishing a trusting and comfortable therapeutic relationship. A primary aspect of this relationship is for the therapist to be the vehicle for the client to identify his or her own resources and sensations. The therapist listens to the description of the client's resource (a person, animal, place, memory, activity, belief, or personal strength that brings peace, safety, joy, or calm) and then, by asking for more detail about the resource, strengthens it (Grabbe & Miller-Karas, 2018). The social connection between therapist and client is paramount in TRM. For example, when the client shares a meaningful memory, the therapist asks for more detail, especially sensory elements of the memory. Thus, the memory becomes a shared, mutually understood video clip of that moment. The therapist repeats his or her understanding of the memory to ensure that the account of it is correct. And, when the client is in agreement, the therapist asks what the client is sensing in his or her body while talking about the memory. The encounter is characterized by an immediate, deep, mutual understanding. The APPN needs to be mature and empathetic, but curious to learn what clients bring forth from within—not only the client's resource or memory, but also the sensations that are experienced when describing it to the APPN.

Presence

TRM cultivates the quality of presence, both in the therapist and client. While it is common for clients to simply say, "It feels good," the APPN should try to steer clients away from words such as *good, bad, positive, negative,* and even the word *feeling*—because of dual meanings of sensation or emotion. Rather, the simple TRM technique is to help the client get into the habit of being able to notice sensations that accompany emotions and to differentiate between those that are pleasant or unpleasant. These physical responses to stress, excitement, or dismay are nearly universal (Nummenmaa, Glerean, Hari, & Hietanen, 2014), and may occur prior to cognition and emotion. The therapist needs to maintain full presence to the client's experience in the moment and remain attuned to nonverbal expressions and the client's reported immediate experience.

Reflection

The client's experience with TRM is meant to shore up his or her sense of being alive in the most fundamental manner by experiencing present moment awareness during the therapy session and at moments in the client's day-to-day life. The habit of paying attention to body sensations and naming them, and focusing on sensations of well-being, may come to be effortless. Each time the client engages in this experience, he or she is bolstering neural pathways, bringing the restorative parasympathetic nervous system into dominance, reducing the wear and tear of the sympathetic discharge, and providing an opportunity for the cortical areas to come on board for reasoned decision-making. Essentially, the techniques are allowing the cortical and subcortical brain regions to come into synchrony. Often, the experience of TRM basic skills in a therapeutic session will engender new meanings of the client's experience. After resourcing, for example, a conflict or problem will seem smaller and more manageable. Although TRM does not ask specific questions about life meaning, freedom, or choices, these may spontaneously emanate from discussing difficulties and using the self-regulation skills or through processing in sessions using the three last TRM skills.

Nine Skills of the TRM

In TRM, clients learn to pay attention to their internal impulses and sensations. The therapist gently guides, but does not make suggestions or impose meanings or interpretations (Miller-Karas, 2015). TRM uses a set of nine skills for stabilization and reprocessing traumatic experiences.

The first six skills of TRM (tracking, resourcing, grounding, gesturing, help now!, and shift and stay) are the self-regulation skills, which are fundamental throughout TRM therapy. They are also called "wellness skills" and are learned for the purpose of self-care as well as self-regulation. The skills help to not only regulate emotions, but also uncomfortable physical sensations. The skills may be taught by non–mental health professionals, reaching a broader audience, and are called the CRM. Clients do not need to tell their trauma story, unless they want to, but rather learn to become aware of physical sensations associated with traumatic memories and to use these first six TRM stabilization skills to reduce and release the traumatic stress. Resiliency questions, such as "What helped you get through that?" or "What is helping you now?", serve to shift the trauma narrative to a narrative of survival and resilience.

The last three skills of TRM (titration, pendulation, and completion of survival response) are for reprocessing traumatic experiences (Grabbe & Miller-Karas, 2018). Trauma processing occurs only by "going to the edge" of profoundly difficult experiences (titration), and either shifting back to a pleasant or neutral sensation or a resource (pendulation) or recognizing uncompleted urges within the body and verbalizing or enacting them "in vivo" in the therapy setting (completion of survival response). The nine skills of TRM are as follows:

Skill 1 Tracking. Tracking is conscious awareness of body sensations used for all of the TRM skills. This awareness can direct clients to locate pleasant or neutral sensations in the body or to notice sensations associated with the five senses.

Skill 2 Resourcing. Resourcing is a person, animal, place, memory, activity, belief, or personal strength that brings a sense of peace, safety, joy, or calm (Grabbe & Miller-Karas, 2018). Clients are asked to identify a resource and then to describe a few of its qualities. Clients are then asked to describe the sensations they are experiencing in their body when talking about the resource. If unable, clients are asked about the sensations of breathing, heart rate, and muscle tension/relaxation. When clients experience future stress, they can purposefully access their resource to return to a resilient state.

Skill 3 Grounding. Grounding is somatic awareness of the sensations of support and security in the present moment. Grounding can take place at rest or during physical movement, such as walking. Clients notice the sensations of their feet on the floor or paying attention to the texture, temperature, and other features of the surfaces with which they are in contact such as a table or chair, one's crossed hands, or the clothes they are wearing.

Skill 4 Gesturing. Gesturing is spontaneous movements and natural, involuntary motions of the body that occur as expressions of internal sensations of distress or well-being. Most people have spontaneous, comforting gestures that help bring them back to their RZ. By slowing down gestures and repeating comforting movements to absorb and track the sensations they generate, clients may be able to return to a resilient state. The APPN helps clients identify self-soothing gestures that are not self-harming and then encourages them to bring awareness to the gesture with intention.

Skill 5 Help Now! Help now! techniques are used when a client is in a very dysregulated or distressed state. These include a quick, focused activation of the senses (temperature, colors, textures, objects, and sounds) to environmental stimuli. Techniques such as counting steps while walking, counting backward, and slowly pushing the arms against a hard, flat surface are emergency strategies for clients to use in these difficult states.

Skill 6 Shift and Stay. Shift and stay selects from the menu of tracking, resourcing, grounding, gesturing, or help now skills, depending on the needs of the situation, and intentionally lingers with the experience until the unpleasant sensation and emotion abate. It is essential for clients to stay with the pleasant or neutral sensations for approximately 15 seconds to experience the shift successfully and transfer the experience into long-term memory (Hansen, 2016).

Skill 7 Titration. Titration is becoming aware of the sensation connected to the traumatic event by drawing attention to a smaller, more manageable part of the sensation. Clients are invited by the APPN to describe in specific detail the size, shape, color, and so on, of the sensation in order to concretize the sensation. The APPN then asks the client to notice a smaller piece of the activation. As a smaller part of the sensation is identified, the image of the sensation often changes and becomes smaller. Clients are asked if they notice any change in breathing, heart rate, or muscle tension. The APPN also remarks on any changes that are noticed, such as clients taking deeper breaths or clients having a more relaxed posture.

Skill 8 Pendulation. Pendulation is moving or shifting back and forth between sensations of distress and sensations of greater well-being within the body. The APPN guides the client to pendulate away from distress to neutral or pleasant sensations and then to describe them. Then, the APPN guides clients back to the distressing sensations and gently asks if the sensations remain the same or if they have changed. If there is a change, clients are invited to notice the difference in order to reinforce the "felt-sense" of the change. By guiding clients to notice less distressing, neutral, or pleasant sensations, pendulation interrupts the negative feedback loop in the brain and supports a more resilient pathway. When a sensation is titrated, a natural shifting occurs, bringing the nervous system back into balance. The APPN invites clients to bring awareness to the change as the nervous system comes back into balance and a lessening of the distressing sensation occurs. As the distressing sensations abate and clients return to balance, new meanings or understandings will often emerge as well. This is considered a "bottom up" shift. The skills of titration and pendulation are often used together.

Skill 9 Completion of Survival Responses. Completion of survival responses is completing the survival skills that were thwarted when the trauma originally occurred. In the face of threat to a client's existence, the nervous system responds with heightened energy to fight or flee. If the survival responses are completed, the nervous system returns to balance, and clients are left with no untoward post-traumatic effects. But if clients experience extreme fear coupled with an inescapable attack, they may freeze and be unable to complete the survival response. The freeze response is characterized by profound motor inhibition; yet, there is a powerful sympathetic nervous system response set off with its dramatic rise in respiration, heart rate, and blood pressure and a surge of neurohormones. The APPN's goal is to help clients complete the survival responses that were thwarted. As clients recount the traumatic experience, the APPN asks them if they have an impulse within the body to do something. Clients may notice a restlessness in their legs or arms and the desire to run or swing their arms. The APPN invites clients to complete the response in the present moment while sitting, standing, or moving. The APPN can also invite clients to experience the impulse to move in their "mind's eye" and to notice what happens on the inside when they make the movement now in the present moment of their imagination. As the survival response is completed, the nervous system may return to a balanced state. Nervous system releases can include shaking, trembling, burping, and yawning as equilibrium is restored. Often new meanings emerge laced with self-compassion and empathy.

■ CASE STUDY

Background

I first met Kara, a 55-year-old African American woman, 5 years ago when she was in a homeless shelter and sought mental healthcare at the shelter's free clinic. This was her first experience in therapy. She has been in therapy with me since then, but with few visits over the last 2 years. Kara experienced multiple traumatic events in her life, including childhood sexual abuse by an uncle. Her ACEs score was four, which put her at risk for chronic physical and psychiatric illnesses. As an adult, she had experienced physical and emotional abuse by a partner, long-term drug addiction, prostitution, homelessness, and incarceration. She smoked cigarettes and had numerous relapses of her drug addiction. Her psychiatric diagnoses included PTSD, bipolar disorder, and dissociative identity disorder. Under severe stress, she heard the voices of two distinct parts of self: a child named Zoe, who either played happily or cried, and a harsh, tough adult named Crystal, who was always angry and violent, especially if Zoe was crying. Kara was fully aware that others did not hear these voices. She stated that she wanted therapy to figure out "who she was." In therapy, she has learned that her parts of self have served to protect her at different times in her life and these parts need to cooperate, support, and understand each other. Since Kara has learned to help her parts of self cooperate with one another, she reports hearing their voices much less often. I have had guidance since the beginning of my work with Kara from my mentor, Kathy Steele, a psychiatric clinical nurse specialist who is a world-renown expert in trauma and dissociation.

Kara is currently stable on her psychiatric medications. She lived for a time with Meline, with whom she did not get along, but currently has permanent housing with a good friend, Sally, as her roommate. She receives disability and regular medical and psychiatric care, and is in contact with her family. She has worked in fast food restaurants in the past, but is currently unable to work. She is obese and has diabetes and arthritis. She is a gifted artist, and makes money by selling pictures or decorative items that she sews. I first introduced TRM to this client after I had known her for about 1 year. She has integrated the first six self-care skills of TRM into her daily life and has shared them with others. Each time I see her, I ask how she has been using the skills, and we sometimes listen to an "ichill" of TRM developer Elaine Miller-Karas explaining the skills for reinforcement (www.ichillapp.com/index.html) or to the associated application on a smartphone. In therapy meetings, we have used the last three TRM skills when discussing difficult issues.

Beginning Phase

This segment from an early session of our work was focused on understanding the RZ and TRM wellness skills, particularly on developing awareness.

APPN:	Kara, I attended a course recently and discovered some skills which may be really helpful to you. Would you be willing to try them out? (*nods*) I'd like to teach you one of the main concepts of the Trauma Resiliency Model, which we call TRM.
Kara:	Okay.
APPN:	So, this is a picture that shows the Resilient Zone (*see images in the free "ichill" app*). So, that's an internal state of feeling pretty good. You can call it the "okay" zone, that zone of well-being when you're your best self.
Kara:	Oh yeah, okay.
APPN:	We go through our ups and downs through the day and sometimes you're a little irritable, upset, or sad, but basically you will cope with the things that happen every day. The upswing of the line—that's where you have the increase in heart rate, blood pressure, and that is to respond to some need. For example, if you are anxious about something or need to rush somewhere, you're going to have this boost of energy, and expenditure of energy, and then this downswing is when you sit down and relax and restore. So, the nervous system has an accelerator and a brake. You can't have them both on at once. One dominates. So, what you learn in TRM is the techniques to stay in your RZ. Okay?
Kara:	Yeah. It's like a battery.
APPN:	And then this other picture shows that sometimes something happens that really throws us off. This is something that either accumulates or it could happen once and quickly—maybe witnessing some violence, or somebody being aggressive to you such that you're really unhappy and upset. So, you can see that that normal wavy line gets jagged and you end up sort of going back and forth and the accelerator or the brakes can actually get stuck and force you out of your RZ. The fact is we all get knocked outside our zone. So, what you learn in TRM is to widen your zone. You widen it so you can tolerate stress better. And then sometimes we actually get stuck outside the zone, and that's bad news because it doesn't feel good to be outside the zone and people try all kinds of things to get back, even drugs or fighting or something like that. It's an attempt to let out some of that trauma and stress. If you have too much of the accelerator, you end up outside the zone, and we call it being "stuck on high." So that's where you're going to have racing thoughts, maybe agitation, irritability, anxiety, anger. You're all hyped up in your body. You've got that heart rate going fast, fast, fast. Now, the opposite can happen and that is also a stress reaction. If somebody insults you, for example, and you're really hurt by it, you could have excess brakes, or "stuck on low." That's the other part of this automatic nervous system.
Kara:	Um-hm.
APPN:	Okay, so if you get thrust out on low, everything goes slow. You can feel tired, sad, disconnected. You may feel numb, you want to be isolated, and

just stay in bed. And this is where you may dissociate. That means that you're just disconnected completely with what's going on around you.

Kara: Yeah, I get that way a lot.

APPN: So, the CRM skills that you are learning are techniques that you can use either when you're outside your zone to get back into a balanced, comfortable place, or just off and on during the day as a habit, and that will widen your zone over time. It's also called sensory mindfulness or awareness of sensations in the body. So, let's talk about those skills now. Let's start with a little practice. Take this stress ball in your hand (*pause*). Can you name the sensations that you notice? You can close your eyes if you like.

Kara: Oh, squishy, rubbery, squishy, rubbery. It's cold.

APPN: Okay. You did a few things there. You were sensing with your hands, and you named what you were noticing.

Kara: Yeah. I like this. It's easy on the hands.

APPN: Those textures, how would you describe those textures?

Kara: Plastic. Squishy. Mmm. Soft.

APPN: Okay. You can keep this and tomorrow if you hold it, you may come up with some new words. And you can even make up words to describe it.

Kara: Oh my gosh, I just noticed, I just seen it. It's sort of like, oh my gosh. There's like colors coming out of it. It looks like little pumpkins popping out.

APPN: You were just tracking sensations that were coming from your senses, and that is the first TRM skill. Now what I want you to do is track some sensations inside your body. So, can you notice your breathing if that is comfortable for you?

Kara: Yeah, it's slow. Relaxed. That's the only way I can describe it.

APPN: Now, can you notice your muscle tension? In your body, can you notice the state of your muscles?

Kara: They're not tense, but they're not relaxed either. All this in here is like warm because I've been using my muscles.

APPN: Alright, now can you maybe notice your heart beating? Try paying attention to your heart.

Kara: (*Long pause*) It's not beating fast. It's just beating normal right now.

APPN: Where do you feel it do you think?

KARA: Right here.

APPN: In your chest, okay. So, when we do TRM, we ask you to "sense in" to your body, if you are comfortable doing that. Notice what's going on in your body and it's actually a very powerful way to build up your RZ.

APPN: Okay, now what I'd like to do is move to the second TRM skill, which is called resourcing. So, what I would like you to do is think of a person or a place or some activity that you like to do. Or a memory that is special for you, but brings you some sense of peace and calm and safety, and maybe joy. It could be something about yourself that is a strength—something

	about your body or your personality. So just think for a minute and see if you can come up with something that we could use (*pause*).
Kara:	Being on the phone with my mother and my stepfather at the same time.
APPN:	Being on the phone with your mother and stepfather?
Kara:	Yeah, because I can be on the phone with them for hours. And when my momma calls me, I'll put her on speaker and her and dad will be cooking their dinner and talking to me and I'll be talking to them here, while I sew or do my artwork. Like 2 or 3 hours.
APPN:	When was the last time you got to do that?
Kara:	Yesterday. I talk to them every day now. And then now my little sister and me are finally talking too, on messenger, when she's off. We talk for 2½ hours, and that was the first time I've ever talked to her like that. We're starting up a relationship, you know what I'm saying?
APPN:	Can you tell me more about that?
Kara:	Oh, I'm just glad that's she talking to me now. You know what I'm saying? We started talking about Mom and Dad. Dad with his heart problems.
APPN:	Okay. So, it sounds like there was some important things you had to talk about.
Kara:	Yeah. And we talked a little bit about how she's doing. I told her how I'm doing.
APPN:	Can you describe her to me?
Kara:	Tall. Big. She like grows. Big, tall like her daddy. I'm short like our Mom. I got the short gene and she got the tall one.
APPN:	Now when you're talking about your sister and the fact that you got to talk to her for so long, or about doing your work, listening to your parents as they are cooking and just talking for the longest time with everyone on speaker, can you tell me what it is you notice happening inside your body? Do you notice any sensations as you are talking to me now?
Kara:	Yeah, I feel safe.
APPN:	Safe. Can you tell me where you feel that safety?
Kara:	Everywhere.
APPN:	Mm-hm. Anywhere in your body in particular?
Kara:	Everywhere. Here (*pointing to her chest*). I feel safe when I talk to my parents.
APPN:	I'm so glad. What do you notice there?
Kara:	Right in here. It feels warm inside here.
APPN:	Do you notice any change in your heartbeat or breathing?
Kara:	It feels light.
APPN:	So just notice that and stay with those sensations for a few moments and enjoy that safe feeling.

Kara:	OK (*nodding*).
APPN:	(*pause*) And you can use that resource if you are outside your RZ. Remember the details of the experience and the warm sensation of safety in your chest, and see what happens.

Commentary

This sample of a conversation with Kara shows how TRM self-stabilization skills are first introduced. The first encounter should include learning tracking and resourcing skills, so that the client comes away with the experience of feeling better, or less bad, and possibly with the notion of hope and an awareness that a sense of well-being is possible. The client is invited to notice and report sensations, both external and external. Asked to come up with a "resource," a menu of types of choices is offered. Suggestions are not made, because a resource will simply emerge naturally and fairly quickly. If an unhealthy resource is selected, for example, "smoking weed," the client is asked to come up with a different resource or to describe some aspect of the resource that is healthy, such as the friend he or she was with. The therapist plays a critical role as a listener, at times gently guiding the client to identify physical sensations, characterize them, and name them. Given a moment's time to reflect, clients produce a resource that is uniquely theirs and the therapist validates the client through careful listening and asking questions about the details of the resource. When clients cannot notice body sensations, they are asked about the sensations of breathing, heart rate, and muscle tension/relaxation, if they are comfortable doing so.

Middle Phase

This segment from the middle phase focuses on a skill to use under duress.

APPN:	So how are you doing and are you using the TRM skills?
Kara:	Last week, I had a really bad scene with my roommate, Meline. She was trying to break down my door. I don't know what got into her. She went crazy. I stayed in my room and kept my phone near me to call the police. My boyfriend was with me.
APPN:	What did you do?
Kara:	My roommate was yelling and screaming. I kept my phone by me, but Zoe was crying and crying, so scared.
APPN:	What about Crystal?
Kara:	She was yelling too, mad at Zoe for being so weak, and yelling to open the door and punch the f****** b******'s teeth out.
APPN:	What did you do?
Kara:	I was noticing the floor under my feet and the feel of the blanket on the bed where I sat. I was grounding and just stayed still till she actually did break that door down. I had called 911 and they came fast. They took her to jail but not me since I never touched her.
APPN:	How did you handle the voices?
Kara:	They were OK. Well, I get them to get along now. Remember I agreed to get them to cooperate with each other? Anyway, that women isn't never coming back here. That's what my program told me.

Commentary

This experience was a huge step forward for Kara, who in the past had gotten into fights easily, and on occasion had been jailed herself. She was practicing the basic TRM skills. This example shows that while her dissociative parts reacted to a situation of danger, she was able to apply specific grounding and tracking techniques to stay in a clear enough state of mind to not succumb to her impulse to fight with her roommate. In TRM, we teach a three-part model of the brain, and when outside the RZ we teach that the "thinking" brain is off-line. In this very difficult experience, Kara remained in her zone, with her capacity to respond in a rational way "on-line." She never saw this roommate again and had confidence that she could manage a crisis.

Final Phase

This segment from the final phase occurred after a hiatus of 6 months. It focuses on the emergence of themes.

APPN:	I wonder if we could do another resourcing exercise today. Can you think of a place, some place that you've been to that is special for you?
Kara:	I haven't been anywhere, but to the doctors.
APPN:	Okay, well, what about a memory that you have of something that was a good time.
Kara:	When me and Sally went to do the laundry at her laundromat over by her job.
APPN:	Okay.
Kara:	We had a good time.
APPN:	Why was that? Tell me more.
Kara:	We went across the parking lot and got something to eat. And it was fun being out and about, because I don't get out that often. So, yeah, I had a good time.
APPN:	Okay. So, you and Sally were at the laundromat, and after you got your clothes started, you went and got something to eat. And what was the best part?
Kara:	The eating. Just a hamburger and French fries. Nothing special. But, oh my god their hamburgers are delicious. Sally took me there, they were gigantic. I said oh my god, you could sink your teeth into them. They were so juicy, and oily, and good.
APPN:	I can see that you're smiling and laughing. When you do that—when you're smiling and laughing—what do you notice? As you think about that trip and the special meal, and that juicy hamburger with Sally, what do you notice happening on the inside of your body?
Kara:	My face feels warm and my cheeks feel a little tight from smiling. But I feel good.
APPN:	What happened to your heart rate or your breathing?
Kara:	It's kind of fast because I was laughing.

APPN:	That's a good resource, because you're thinking already about the sensory elements. And you noticed your warm face and your heart beating. Can you just stay with those sensations for about 15 seconds now? (*pause*)
Kara:	It's like Zoe is having fun, my inner child is having fun.
APPN:	And how about Crystal?
Kara:	Crystal isn't in right now. She's still hurting.
APPN:	Still hurting?
Kara:	You know he left me. He got his check and he left me.
APPN:	He got what?
Kara:	His check, his disability. And then he left me.
APPN:	I am so sorry. That was a very long-term relationship.
Kara:	Yeah, that just ended like that, you know. He didn't say nothing to me. No f*** you. See you later, b****, or thank you, but I don't need you anymore. Nothing. No closure. Just left. He wouldn't answer his phone, so I went and I took him off my thing. I was paying a hundred twenty bucks a month for both of our phones.
APPN:	That must really hurt.
Kara:	Yeah it does. I just don't understand. It hurt my feelings.
APPN:	I can see it's upsetting for you.
Kara:	I'm just now getting used to being by myself.
APPN:	When you're stressed like that, where does it, where in your body does it register?
Kara:	I mean I was, I was really stressed thinking, I couldn't even cry. I just, I was like scared because I was alone again, but then I'm not alone. I still got my parents. I still got my sister. I still got Sally. I still got friends around here. I'm not alone. I'm just single again. And then after I figured that out, I was like fine after that. But the thing about being alone, I fear dying alone, and nobody know until I, you know I'm too stinky for them to find me (*laughing*) you know.
APPN:	I know it's upsetting for you to talk about dying alone and being left. How long has it been?
Kara:	Six months. Yeah, 6 months . . . after 4½ years.
APPN:	You had said this was one of your first relationships.
Kara:	You know what, I'm going to see him one day and be able to tell him how I feel. By that time, I hope I'm not really, I'm not going to curse him out. I'm not going to raise my voice. I'm just going to say, you know, the way you did me, that was wrong. You know. And the thing that hurt was that I had to tell my parents in a way where they wouldn't be . . . I mean, you know, my mom and dad got close to him.
APPN:	I know.
Kara:	I never brought any man home. He was the first one and my mom and dad loved him. My mom and dad would call him on his phone too. If I

didn't answer mine, they'd call his and talk to him and find out where I'm at. The last Christmas before he left me, last Christmas my mom and dad was hugging him. You know my dad embraced him. And I was like yeah, they're getting closer to him. I mean you know he was saying I'm not going nowhere. I'll never leave you. Anyway, I don't want to talk about it. It's past tense. It's over. I don't have to worry about nobody but me now. Me and Sally.

APPN: So, you know if you get to thinking about it and you get . . . .

Kara: Yeah. You know. I still don't wish him bad you know. I don't wish nothing bad on him. But I miss him. I miss my best friend. He was my best friend you know. We could never be together again though. I could never trust him again you know.

APPN: As you are talking about him, I wonder if you can notice what happens in your body?

Kara: It hurts here in my chest and in my eyes.

APPN: I notice your eyes are wet (*pause*). Can you describe what you notice in your chest?

Kara: It hurts across here. Dull.

APPN: Does it have a shape?

Kara: It's big and feels heavy. Like a heavy ball.

APPN: You say it is shaped like a ball. Does the sensation have a color?

Kara: It feels like a big, grey, heavy ball.

APPN: Can you sense just an edge of the sensation that you described as a large, grey ball on your chest?

Kara: I can try. Just the edge? OK.

APPN: Let's try to practice the tracking again to see if that helps you feel better. Okay now. Can you notice somewhere in your body that feels strong or pleasant or neutral, but not unpleasant?

Kara: My head. Cause today my head, my body is so sore because it's raining outside. My arthritis. It just hurts.

APPN: Now can you shift to somewhere else in your body that doesn't feel that much pain, or feels okay? Is there a place inside that is less painful, tense, or distressing?

Kara: My head. It feels good. I mean I'm awake. Oh, (*sighing*) relaxed. My mind isn't racing right now like it usually is. I'm focused.

APPN: Can we go back to that sensation in your chest? I wonder if you can tell me if that has changed?

Kara: Oh, the ball is gone now. It is OK now (*sigh*). I'm OK. I'm OK, just me and Sally. I'll be OK without him. I don't need him. Considering I'm single. Pretty happy. I don't have to worry about nobody but myself.

APPN: Well, you can be very proud of that.

Kara: Just me and Sally, you know. That's a good thing. I'm glad of that (*laughing*). I guess that's what I'm telling you. Thank you. Thank you so much.

Commentary

Kara was devastated by the loss of what she thought was a relationship that would last for the rest of her life. Moreover, she had had the approval of her parents regarding this man and could not summon the courage to tell them that she had lost him. She is able to talk about the hurt she feels and is angry that he simply disappeared suddenly from her life. Just as TRM is exquisitely trauma-sensitive, so is the therapist, protecting the client from having a retraumatizing experience, and even from delving into negative emotions. Although it is useful for clients to become aware of sensations connected to difficult emotions such as anxiety or anger, time is not spent digging into these. As the APPN invited the client to titrate the unpleasant sensations, the sensation's intensity lessened. She found new meanings about her boyfriend leaving. When a person accesses the "felt-sense" of well-being, there are often more compassionate meanings that emerge. TRM skills seemed to have helped her cope and she has not relapsed and restarted her drug use. She knows that her artwork and her connections with others sustain her. Kara continues to need supportive therapy.

DISCUSSION QUESTIONS

1. If you were to look at the RZ images, can you think of times when you got stuck on "high" or on "low"?
2. Can you identify the symptoms or sensations of being stuck outside of your RZ?
3. Are there places in the therapy sessions presented here that you would navigate in a different way as the therapist?
4. If a person is in touch with his or her body sensations during moments of emotional distress, or just from time to time during the day, how do you think it would impact life's ebbs and flows?

REFERENCES

Citron, S., & Miller-Karas, E. (2013). *Final CRM innovation evaluation report*. Claremont, CA: Trauma Resource Institute.

Felitti, V. J., Anda, R. F., Nordenberg, D., Williamson, D. F., Spitz, A. M., Edwards, V., . . . Koss, M. P. (1998). Relationship of childhood abuse and household dysfunction to many of the leading causes of death in adults: The Adverse Childhood Experiences (ACE) Study. *American Journal of Preventive Medicine, 14*(4), 245–258. Retrieved from https://www.ajpmonline.org/article/S0749-3797(98)00017-8/pdf

Grabbe, L., Higgins, M. K., Baird, M., Craven, P. A., & San Fratello, S. (2020). The Community Resiliency Model® to promote nurse well-being. *Nursing Outlook, 68*(3), 324–336 doi:10.1016/j.outlook.2019.11.002

Grabbe, L., Higgins, M., Jordan, D., Noxsel, L., Gibson, B., & Murphy, J. (2020). The Community Resiliency Model®: A Pilot of an interoception intervention to increase the emotional self-regulation of women in addiction treatment. *International Journal of Mental Health and Addiction*. doi:10.1007/s11469-019-00189-9

Grabbe, L., & Miller-Karas, E. (2018). The Trauma Resiliency Model: A "bottom-up" intervention for trauma psychotherapy. *Journal of the American Psychiatric Nurses Association, 24*(1), 76–84. doi:10.1177/1078390317745133

Gröger, N., Matas, E., Gos, T., Lesse, A., Poeggel, G., Braun, K., & Bock, J. (2016). The transgenerational transmission of childhood adversity: Behavioral, cellular, and epigenetic correlates. *Journal of Neural Transmission, 123*(9), 1037–1052. doi:10.1007/s00702-016-1570-1

Hanson, R. (2013). *Hardwiring happiness: The new brain science of contentment, calm, and confidence.* New York, NY: Harmony Books.

Heller, L., & LaPierre, A. (2012). *Healing developmental trauma: How early trauma affects self-regulation, self-image, and the capacity for relationship.* Berkeley, CA: North Atlantic Books.

Horn, S. R., Charney, D. S., & Feder, A. (2016). Understanding resilience: New approaches for preventing and treating PTSD. *Experimental Neurology, 284*(Pt. B), 119–132. doi:10.1016/j.expneurol.2016.07.002

Jowett, S., Karatzias, T., Shevlin, M., & Albert, I. (2020). Differentiating symptom profiles of ICD-11 PTSD, complex PTSD, and borderline personality disorder: A latent class analysis in a multiply traumatized sample. *Personality Disorders, 11*(1), 36–45. doi:10.1037/per0000346

Leitch, L., & Miller-Karas, E. (2009). A case for using biologically-based mental health intervention in post-earthquake China: Evaluation of training in the Trauma Resiliency Model. *International Journal of Emergency Mental Health, 11*(4), 221–233. Retrieved from https://www.omicsonline.org/open-access-pdfs/a-study-of-stress-affecting-police-officers-in-lithuania.pdf

Leitch, M. L. (2007). Somatic experiencing treatment with tsunami survivors in Thailand: Broadening the scope of early intervention. *Traumatology, 13*(3), 11–20. doi:10.1177/1534765607305439

Leitch, M. L., Vanslyke, J., & Allen, M. (2009). Somatic experiencing treatment with social service workers following Hurricanes Katrina and Rita. *Social Work, 54*(1), 9–18. doi:10.1093/sw/54.1.9

Levine, P. A. (1997). *Waking the tiger: Healing trauma: The innate capacity to transform overwhelming experiences.* Berkeley, CA: North Atlantic Books.

Levine, P. A. (2010). *In an unspoken voice: How the body releases trauma and restores goodness.* Berkeley, CA: North Atlantic Books.

Lowen, A. (1958). *The language of the body.* New York, NY: Collier Books.

Miller-Karas, E. (2015). *Building resilience to trauma: The trauma and community resiliency models.* New York, NY: Routledge, Taylor & Francis Group.

Nummenmaa, L., Glerean, E., Hari, R., & Hietanen, J. K. (2014). Bodily maps of emotions. *Proceedings of the National Academy of Sciences of the United States of America, 111*(2), 646–651. doi:10.1073/pnas.1321664111

Ogden, P., & Fisher, J. (2015). *Sensorimotor psychotherapy: Interventions for trauma and attachment.* New York, NY: W. W. Norton.

Ogden, P., Minton, K., & Pain, C. (2006). *Trauma and the body: A sensorimotor approach to psychotherapy* (1st ed.). New York, NY: W. W. Norton.

Parker, C., Doctor, R. M., & Selvam, R. (2008). Somatic therapy treatment effects with tsunami survivors. *Traumatology, 14*(3), 103–109. doi:10.1177/1534765608319080

Payne, P., Levine, P. A., & Crane-Godreau, M. A. (2015). Somatic experiencing: Using interoception and proprioception as core elements of trauma therapy. *Frontiers in Psychology, 6*, 93. doi:10.3389/fpsyg.2015.00093

Reich, W. (1945/1980). *Character analysis.* New York, NY: Farrar, Straus, and Giroux.

Rothschild, B. (2000). *The body remembers.* New York, NY: W. W. Norton.

Rothschild, B. (2010). *8 keys to safe trauma recovery: Take-charge strategies to empower your healing* (1st ed.). New York, NY: W. W. Norton.

Rothschild, B. (2017). *The body remembers: Volume 2: Revolutionizing trauma treatment.* New York, NY: W. W. Norton.

Steele, K., Boon, S., & Van der Hart, O. (2017). *Treating trauma-related dissociation: A practical, integrative approach.* New York, NY: W. W. Norton.

van der Kolk, B. A. (2015). *The body keeps the score: Brain, mind, and body in the healing of trauma.* New York, NY: Penguin Books.

van der Werff, S. J. A., van den Berg, S. M., Pannekoek, J. N., Elzinga, B. M., & van der Wee, N. J. A. (2013). Neuroimaging resilience to stress: A review. *Frontiers in Behavioral Neuroscience, 7*, 39 doi:10.3389/fnbeh.2013.00039

Yi, C. H., (Gina), Lori, J., & Martyn, K. (2008). Development of prenatal event history calendar for Black women. *Journal of Obstetric, Gynecologic & Neonatal Nursing, 37*(4), 464–473. doi:10.1111/j.1552-6909.2008.00255.x

Index

abstinence-only model of treatment, 241–242
acceptance and commitment therapy (ACT), 141
Ackerman, Nathan, 114
active listening, 46
Adaptive Information Processing (AIP) model, 260–261
Adler, Alfred, 140
Adlerian psychology, 139
Adverse Childhood Experiences (ACEs), 277
affirmations, 46
Ainsworth, Margaret, 75
Albert Ellis Institute, 163
altruism, 97
ambivalence, 225
American Group Psychotherapy Association, 95
American Psychiatric Association, 96, 206
American Psychological Association, 206
annihilation, 3
assertiveness training, 150–151
Association of Medical Educators and Researchers in Substance Abuse (AMERSA), 223
attachment
  ambivalent/anxious, 6
  assessment in psychodynamic psychotherapy, 3
  bonds, 113, 115–118
  disorganized, 75
  infant's style of, 75
  model, 2
  related trauma, 184, 189
  theory, 75, 205
attention deficit hyperactivity disorder (ADHD), 18, 74
authenticity, 21
authentic self, 21
automatic thought record (ATR), 150
Axline, Virginia, 73, 75
  Dibs: In Search of Self, 73

Beck, Aaron T., 140, 162–163
Beck Anxiety Inventory, 141
Beck Depression Inventory, 141
behavioral activation, 163
behavioral rehearsal, 151
Beyond the Hot Seat (Feder and Ronall), 96
bibliotherapy, 152
bilateral stimulation (BLS), 264
Bion, Wilfred, 78
biopsychosocial theory, 205
body image, 18
borderline personality disorder (BPD), 184
Bowen, Murray, 113–115, 223
  Family Therapy in Clinical Practice, 114
Bowlby, John, 75, 205
Bugental, Jim, 56
Bugental's existential approach, 59

case formulation, 209
catharsis, 98
child psychotherapy, 73–74
cliché, layer of personality, 20
client-centered therapy. *see* person-centered therapy (PCT)
cognitive behavioral therapy case study
  client background, 65–167
  commentary, 158, 180–181
  therapeutic sessions, 154–157, 167–180
    coping strategies and healthy ways/ effective communications, 175–179
    Patient Health Questionnaire-9 (PHQ-9), 166–167, 170–171, 173, 176, 179–180
    problem-solving and setting goals, 173–175
    review of COPE program, 179–180
    self-esteem and positive thinking/self-talk, 170–171
    stress and coping, 171–173

cognitive behavioral therapy (CBT), 17, 74, 139–141, 161–163, 206
ABCD model, 140, 162–163
assessment in, 143–144, 164
behavioral techniques
assertiveness training, 150–151
behavioral rehearsal, 151
bibliotherapy, 152
contingency management, 151–152
exposure therapies, 153
guided relaxation, 152
homework, 153
meditation, 152
mindfulness training, 152
psychoeducation, 153
shame-attacking exercises, 152
social skills training, 152
COPE (Creating Opportunities for Personal Empowerment) manual, 165
definition of mental health and psychopathology in, 142, 163
philosophy and key concepts of, 141–142, 163
therapeutic goals in, 142–143, 164
therapeutic interventions in, 144–150
automatic thought record (ATR), 150
distancing technique (analogical comparison), 147
downward arrow, 146–147
idiosyncratic meaning, 147
labeling of distortions, 147
Socratic Dialogue (SD), 144–146
steps for cognitive restructuring, 148–150
therapists' interventions, principles, 164–165
cognitive dissonance theory (Festinger), 224
cognitive distortions (CDs), 141, 147–148
cognitive processing therapy (CPT), 141
cognitive restructuring, 163
Community Resiliency Model (CRM)®, 273
stabilization skills of, 274
compassion, 224
complicated bereavement, 207
congruence, 46
contingency management, 151–152
checklist for, 151–152
Corey, Gerald, 96
Corey, Marianne Schneider, 96
corrective recapitulation, of primary family group, 98
creative arts, 19
creative experiments, 23–24
Cycle of Experience, 19–20

daughter technique, 147
defenses, 3
denial, as defense, 3

despair, 56
Developmental Stage theory, 56
dialectical behavior therapy (DBT), 74, 141, 183–184
assessment in, 187
assumptions in, 185–186
case study
client background, 193–194
commentary, 202
therapeutic sessions, 194–202
definition of mental health and psychopathology in, 186
philosophy and key concepts of, 185–186
skills modules, 188
therapeutic goals in, 186–187
therapeutic interventions in, 187–193
behavioral hierarchy of problematic behavior, 188
chain analysis, 197
commitment strategies, 189
communication techniques, 193
diary card, use of, 190–193
finding freedom, joy, and spirituality, 189
functional behavioral analysis, 193
individual therapy, 188
pretreatment stage, 189
processing of traumatic memories, 189
self-monitoring in, 190–193
solving routine problems of living, 189
stability and behavioral control, 189
validation, 189–190
treatment stages, 188–189
dialectical theory, 185
dialectic behavioral therapy (DBT)
discord, 224
disorganized attachment, 75
dissociation, as defense, 3
Dissociative Experiences Scale (DES), 262
distancing technique (analogical comparison), 147
distress tolerance skills, 188
downward arrow, 146–147
dysfunctional patterns, 119

Eastern philosophy, 19
effective communication, 118
Ego, Hunger and Aggression: A Revision of Freud's Theory and Method (Perls), 18
ego functioning, 3
ego integrity, 56
ego psychology, 2
ego strength, 3
ego (wish), 1
Ellis, Albert, 43, 140, 152, 162–163
How to Live with a Neurotic, 140
Rational Living training institute, 140

EMDR International Association (EMDRIA), 260

Emotionally Focused Therapy for Couples (Greenberg and Johnson), 114–115

emotion-focused family therapy (EFFT), 113–116

emotion-focused therapy, 18, 43

emotion regulation skills, 188

empathic attunement, 118

empathy, 46

enactment experiments, 119

Epictetus, 140

Erikson, Erik, 56, 163

Everett, Geneie, 274

evidence-based psychotherapy, 18

evocation, 224

Existence: A New Dimension in Psychiatry and Psychology (May, Angel, and Ellenberger), 56

Existential–Humanistic Institute in San Francisco, 56–57

existential psychotherapy, 55–57
  assessment in, 57–58
  definition of mental health and psychopathology in, 57
  philosophy and key concepts of, 57
  therapeutic goals in, 57
  therapeutic interventions in, 58–59
    experiential reflection, 59
    I–thou relationship, 58
    presence, 58–59

existential psychotherapy case study
  client background, 59–60
  commentary, 69–70
    behavioral changes, 70
    identification of beliefs and regrets, 69–70
    new awareness and insights, 70
  therapeutic sessions, 60–69

existential therapy, 18

experiential learning, 74

experiential reflection, 59

explosion, layer of personality, 21

exposure and response prevention (ERP), 153

exposure therapies, 153

expressive arts therapy, 18, 43

eye movement desensitization and reprocessing (EMDR), 18, 153, 183, 239, 259–261
  assessment in, 262–263
  case study
    assessment in, 266–268
    body scan, 271
    client background, 264
    closure, 271
    commentary, 271–272
    desensitization, 268–270

floatback memory, 269–270
    history and treatment planning, 264–265
    installation, 270–271
    moment-to-moment dissociation, 266
    preparation, 266
    reevaluation at next session, 270
  definitions of mental health and psychopathology in, 261–262
  eight-phase protocol for, 263
  philosophy and key concepts of, 261
    Adaptive Information Processing (AIP) model, 260–261
  therapeutic goals in, 262
  therapeutic interventions in, 263–264

family psychotherapy, 113
  assessment in, 117–118
  Bowen's approach, 113–115
  definition of mental health and psychopathology in, 116
  Greenberg and Johnson's approach, 113–116
  Minuchin's approach, 113–114, 116
  therapeutic goals in, 117
  therapeutic interventions in
    dysfunctional patterns, 119
    effective communication, 118
    empathic attunement, 118
    enactment experiments, 119
    shaping competence, 119
    unbalancing techniques, 119

family psychotherapy case study
  client background, 119–120
  commentary, 136
  therapeutic sessions, 120–136

family systems theory, 223

family therapy, 18

Feder, Bud, 96

Frankl, Viktor, 56

free will, 55

Freud, Anna, 74

Freud, Sigmund, 1–2, 74
  drive theory, 1–2
  model of psychoanalytic psychotherapy, 1–2

gender identity, 18

Gestalt Center of New Jersey, 18

gestalt psychology, 19

Gestalt therapy, 17–18, 96, 242
  assessment in, 22
    content factors, 22
    process diagnoses and factors, 22
  case study (*see* Donna (Gestalt therapy case study)

Gestalt therapy (*continued*)
  client–therapist relationship
    body awareness, 23
    dreamwork, 23–24
    empty-chair dialogues, 24
    exaggeration, 23
    focusing, 23
    language of responsibility, 24
    metaphor and imagery, 23
    moments of healing, 24
  concepts and methodologies, 18
    figure (foreground) and ground
      (background) formation and
      completion, 19
    layers of personality, 20–21
    notion of awareness and contact, 19–20
    organismic self-regulation, 19–20
  definition of mental health and
    psychopathology in, 21
  moments of healing, 23
  therapeutic goals in, 21–22
  therapeutic interventions in
    creative experiments, 23–24
    I–thou relationship, 22–23
Gestalt Therapy: Excitement and Growth in the
    Human Personality (Perls), 18, 21
Gestalt therapy case study
  client background, 24–25
  commentary
    figure/ground formation and
      completion, 37
    I–thou relationship, 37
    organismic self-regulation, restoration
      of, 37
  psychotherapy sessions, 26–36
gradualism, 248–249
Greenberg, Leslie, 113–116
grief, 207
group cohesion, 98
group psychotherapy, 95–96
  assessment in, 100–101
  definition of mental health and
    psychopathology in, 100
  philosophy and key concepts of, 96–100
    altruism, 97
    catharsis, 98
    corrective recapitulation of primary
      family group, 98
    development of socializing techniques,
      98
    existential factors, 99
    group cohesion, 98
    imitative behavior, 98
    imparting information, 97
    installation of hope, 97
    interpersonal learning, 98
    psychoeducational groups, 99

    psychotherapy groups, 100
    self-help groups, 99–100
    support groups, 99
    universality, 97
  short-term, 95
  therapeutic goals in, 100
  therapeutic interventions in, 101–102
group psychotherapy case study
  adjourning or terminating phase, 109–111
  client background, 102
  commentary, 107, 109–111
  forming or orienting of group, 102
  norming or cohesiveness stage, 105–107
  performing phase of group development,
    107–109
  storming or transition stage, 103–105
  therapeutic sessions, 102–103
group therapy, 43
guided relaxation, 152

harm reduction psychotherapy, 241–243
  abstinence-only model of treatment,
    241–242
  assessment in, 246–247
  definitions of mental health and
    psychopathology in, 245
  "intrinsically unique" starting points, 243
  philosophy and key concepts of, 244–245
    incremental behavioral changes, 244–245
    person-centered principles, 244
    psychological issues, 245
    therapeutic progress, 245
  principles, 243
  therapeutic goals in, 245–246
  therapeutic interventions in, 247–249
    gradualism, 248–249
    identifying motivating factors, 248
    incrementalism, 248–249
    MI techniques, 247–248
    redefining success, 248
    refusal skills and relapse prevention,
      249
    therapeutic relationship, 247
harm reduction psychotherapy case study
  client background, 249–250
  commentary, 256–257
    gradualism, 256
    motivating factors, 256
    pattern of recidivism, 256
  therapeutic sessions, 250–256
healthy people, 21
Herman, Judith, 184
  three-stage sequence of trauma treatment
    and recovery, 184
high contact therapy, 206
homework, 153

Horney, Karen, 140
Human-to-Human Relationship Model of
    Nursing, 55

id (instinctual wish), 1
idiosyncratic meaning, 147
imitative behavior, 98
imparting information, 97
impasse, layer of personality, 20–21, 23
implosion, layer of personality, 21
incrementalism, 248–249
Individual Psychotherapy, 140
installation of hope, 97
Institute for Rational Living, 163
Integrative Therapy for Complex Trauma and
    Structural Dissociation (Steele, Boon, &
    Van der Hart), 274
interpersonal analysis, 2, 19
interpersonal deficits, 207
interpersonal disputes, 207
interpersonal effectiveness skills, 188
interpersonal learning, 98
interpersonal psychoanalysis, 205
interpersonal psychotherapy (IPT), 205–206.
        see also IPT case study
    assessment in, 208–209
        case formulation, 209
        interpersonal inventory, 208–209
    case study
        client background, 211
        commentary, 220
        therapeutic sessions, 211–220
    definition of mental health and
        psychopathology in, 207–208
    linkage between mood disorder and
        problematic interpersonal situation, 207
    philosophy and key concepts of, 205–207
    therapeutic goals in, 208
    therapeutic interventions in, 209–211
        active treatment phase, 209–210
        termination, 210–211
    therapeutic relationship, 208
    types of interpersonal issues
        grief or complicated bereavement, 207
        interpersonal deficits, 207
        interpersonal disputes, 207
        interpersonal role transitions, 207
    view of depression, 206–207
Interpersonal Psychotherapy of Depression, 206
interpersonal role transitions, 207
intersubjectivity, 2
intrapsychic conflict, 3
I–thou relationship, 22–23, 58

Jennings, Hellen H., 96
Johnson, Sue, 113–116

Khantzian, Edward John, 243
    rule of empathy and relationship building,
        247
    Treating Addiction: Beyond the Pain, 243
Kierkegaard, Søren, 55
Kirschenbaum, Howard, 43
Klein, Melanie, 74–75
Klerman, Gerald, 206
Knapp, Dr. Michelle, 242
Kouw, Will, 55
Kozikowski, Adam, 242

labeling of distortions, 147
Lacanian psychoanalysis, 2
Leitch, Laurie, 274
Levine, Peter, 273
life experiences, 139
Linehan, Marsha, 184–185
    Cognitive-Behavioral Treatment of Borderline
        Personality Disorder, 185
    Skills Training Manual for Treating Borderline
        Personality Disorder, 185
logo therapy, 55
logotherapy, 56

major depressive disorder (MDD), 206
Marlatt, Alan, 243
    Harm Reduction: Pragmatic Strategies for
        Managing High-Risk Behaviors, 243
May, Rollo, 56
meaning therapy, 56
meditation, 152
mentally healthy person, 2
Meyer, Adolf, 205
Miller, William (Bill) R., 223–225, 242, 247
Miller-Karas, Elaine, 274
mindfulness, 188
mindfulness training, 152
Minuchin, Sal, 113–114, 116
Moreno, Jacob L., 96
motivational interviewing (MI), 223–225, 242,
        247–248
    assessment in, 226
    case study
        client background, 228–229
        commentary, 239
        therapeutic sessions, 229–238
    definitions of mental health and
        psychopathology in, 225–226
    mnemonic OARS, use of, 228
    philosophy and key concepts of, 225
    principles of, 224
    therapeutic goals in, 226
    therapeutic interventions in, 227–228
Motivational Interviewing Network of
        Trainers (MINT), 223, 225

National Institute for Health and Clinical
Excellence, 206
NeuroAffective Relational Model (Heller and
LaPierre), 274
New York Institute for Gestalt Therapy, 18
nondirectiveness, 45

object relations, 2
older adults, and psychotherapy, 55–56
omnipotent control, as defense, 3
organismic self-regulation, 19, 21–22
organismic theory, 19

Patient Health Questionnaire-9 (PHQ-9), 166–
167, 170–171, 173, 176, 179–180
Paykel, Eugene, 206
Perls, Fritz, 17–18, 43, 96
Perls, Laura, 17–18
personality disorders, 18
personality layers, 20–21
person-centered therapy (PCT), 18, 41, 73, 242,
247. see also PCT case study
assessment in, 45
case study
client background, 46–47
commentary, 52–53
dealing with anticipatory grief, 52
reentry into therapy, 51–52
therapeutic sessions, 47–51
definition of mental health and
psychopathology in, 44
necessary conditions for, 42
philosophy and key concepts, 43–44
practice of framing directives, 42
therapeutic goals in, 44–45
therapeutic interventions in, 45–46
facilitative conditions for, 45–46
women and, 42
Piaget's theory of cognitive development, 163
play therapy, 43, 73–74
approaches in, 74–75
assessment in, 76–77
corrective environment, 73
definition of mental health and
psychopathology in, 75–76
nondirective, 74
philosophy and basic assumptions of, 75
primary caregiver, role of, 75
reenactment of traumatic events, 74
therapeutic goals in, 76
therapeutic interventions in, 77–78
holding environment and containment, 78
use of interpretations, 78
therapeutic play, 74
therapeutic relationship in, 75

play therapy case study
client background, 78–80
commentary
emotional activation of termination, 91
holding environment, 91
therapeutic sessions, 81–91
postmodernism, 57
posttraumatic stress disorder (PTSD), 18,
73–74, 183–184, 260–261
complex, 274
primitive idealization and devaluation, as
defense, 3
projection, as defense, 3
psychic conflict, 1
psychic determinism, 1
psychoanalysis, 18
psychoanalytic program, 1
Psychodrama, 96
psychodynamic psychotherapy, 1–2
assessments in, 3
case study
therapeutic goals in, 2–3
therapeutic interventions in, 3–5
psychodynamic psychotherapy case study
client background, 5
commentary on sessions, 13–14
approach to environment, 14
defensive structure, 14
development of positive feelings, 13–14
improvement of ego strength, 13
persuasion of happiness, 14
regulation of emotions, 14
conceptualization of attachment pattern, 6
denial and projection, 6
history of maternal deprivation, 5–6
idealization of parents, 6
psychodynamic formulation, 6–7
relationship with boyfriend, 6
transcript of treatment, 10–13
treatment and goals, 7–10
psychoeducation, 153
psychoeducational groups, 99
psychological health, 21
psychopathology, 2, 21
psychoses, 18
psychosexual stages of development, 1
psychosocial theory of development, 163
psychotherapy groups, 100

rational emotive behavior therapy (REBT),
139–140, 152, 158, 163
reality, 185
redecision therapy, 18
reflection, 46
refusal skills and relapse prevention, 249
Reichian psychoanalysis, 19

relational and attachment-based
    psychotherapy, 2
Rogers, Carl, 41–43, 73, 75, 242, 244, 247. see
    also person-centered therapy (PCT)
    On Becoming a Person, 42
    Client-Centered Therapy, 42
    Counseling and Psychotherapy, 42
    The Life and Work of Carl Rogers
        (documentary), 43
role, layer of personality, 20
role-plays, 96
Rollnick, Stephen, 224–225, 242, 247
Ronall, Ruth, 96
Rosenthal, Dr. David, 74

schizophrenia, 18
Schneider, Kirk, 55–56
self, 20–21
self-help groups, 99–100
self-medication hypothesis of substance use,
    243
self-perception theory (Bem), 224
self-support, 21
Sensorimotor Psychotherapy (Ogden), 274
sequential reasoning, 146–147
shame-attacking exercises, 152
shaping competence, 119
Shapiro, Francine, 260–261, 263
socializing techniques, 98
social skills training, 152
Socratic Dialogue (SD), 144–146
soft determinism, 140
Somatic Experiencing®, 273
Somatic Trauma Therapy (Rothschild), 274
splitting, as defense, 3
structural family therapy, 113–114, 116
substance use disorder (SUD), 241–242
Sullivan, Harry Stack, 140, 205
superego, 1
support groups, 99
supportive psychodynamic psychotherapy, 2
systems family therapy, 113–115

Taoism, 19
T-group (training group), 96
theory of containment, 78
therapeutic progress, 245
Three Approaches to Psychotherapy, 43
transference neurosis, 2–3

trauma and stressor-related disorders, therapy
    for. see dialectical behavior therapy
    (DBT)
trauma-focused CBT (TF-CBT), 153
Trauma Resiliency Model (TRM)®, 273
    assessment in, 277
    case study
        client background, 281–285
        commentary, 285
    definition of mental health and
        psychopathology in, 275–276
    Event History Calendar, usee of, 277
    origin, 273
    philosophy and key concepts of, 274–275
    self-stabilization and trauma-processing
        techniques, 274
    therapeutic goals in, 277
    therapeutic interventions in
        presence, 278
        reflection, 278–279
        skills for stabilization and reprocessing
            traumatic experiences, 279–281
        therapeutic relationship, 277–278
traumatology, 184
Travelbee, Joyce, 55

unbalancing techniques, 119
unconditional positive regard, 45
universality, 97

Veterans Affairs, United States Department
    of, 206
Victims of Violence Program, 184

Weissman, Myrna, 206
Whitin, Ernest S., 96
Winnicott, D. W., 75
wisdom, 56
withdrawal, as defense, 3

Yalom, Irvin, 55–56, 95
    The Theory and Practice of Group
        Psychotherapy, 56, 96

Zen Buddhism, 19

Printed in the United States
by Baker & Taylor Publisher Services